"In advancing biomedical rese ... the term 'state of the art.'

I have received credit for maintaining the state ... for more than forty years in conceiving and developing mechanical cardiopulmonary critical care ventilators and pulmonary therapy respirators. Of great personal interest has been the clinical management of bronchitis before it becomes chronic and emerges into pulmonary emphysema. Early 'self management' including physical and mental care is a critical aspect of overall therapeutic logic for those with bronchitis before it becomes chronic obstructive lung disease (COPD). It is believed there are currently more than 50 million COPD patients in the United States alone that are now under various therapeutic regimes.

Because of the progressive physical and mental impaction of COPD over time, each patient must rationalize the importance of optimal health through understanding. The application of 'preventive medicine' from both mental and clinical points of patient understanding will continue to play a vital role in our aging populations.

Over time, I have become familiar with the 'existing text books directed toward health maintenance' from both physiological and psychological directions which I have encouraged COPD patients to become familiar with.

In my opinion *Optimal Health Revolution* is the 'state of the art' in terms of self-practice of personal health and preventive medicine, which must be the key to long-term health management in all individuals. Your ability to capture the interest of the reader by making them realize 'how they can influence their own health' is way beyond any other existing health care publication authored by physicians directed toward the quality of life.

Your 'step by step presentations relating to personal health care' will serve to increase the individual's quality of life as well as provide for the reduction of clinical intervention through understanding, the cost of which is breaking the world's economies.

Dr. Johnson, I want to thank you for your dedication in authoring a 'state of the art,' comprehensive, understandable book on how we can care for ourselves by understanding who we are and our unique needs. Your book truly reflects upon your years of personal physician-patient health care experience."

—Dr. Forrest Bird, M.D., Ph.D., Sc.D.,
member of the Inventors Hall of Fame (for the respirator)

"Living well into one's later years involves, primarily, the avoidance of early experiences with a small number of chronic diseases of aging, including cardiovascular disease, dementias, bone and joint diseases, various cancers, and type 2 diabetes. The severity and age of onset of all diseases of aging are determined by environmental and genetic interactions, which are mostly modifiable. Although there are many books that address a specific disease or biological mechanism, Dr. Johnson provides a scientifically-based integrated perspective on how we can all live well for more years. The author's concept of 'optimal health' is appealing. It does not mean trying to remain age thirty forever, but considers how to be happy and active at every stage of the lifecycle.

The science of disease is constantly evolving, but it is clear from this book that there is enough known today for all of us to act differently to increase our likelihood of optimal health as we age."

—KENNETH KORNMAN, Ph.D.,
Chief Scientific Officer at Interleukin Genetics

the

OPTIMAL HEALTH

REVOLUTION

How inflammation is the
root cause of the biggest killers

How the cutting-edge science
of nutrigenomics can transform
your long-term health

DUKE JOHNSON, MD

BENBELLA

BENBELLA BOOKS, INC.
Dallas, Texas

Copyright © 2008 by Duke Johnson, M.D.

BenBella Books, Inc.
6440 N. Central Expressway, Suite 503
Dallas, TX 75206
BENBELLA www.benbellabooks.com
Send feedback to feedback@benbellabooks.com

Printed in the United States of America
10 9 8 7 6 5 4 3 2 1

Library of Congress Cataloging-in-Publication Data is available for this title.
ISBN 978-1933771-82-3

Proofreading by Stacia Seaman
Cover design by Laura Watkins
Text design and composition by Laura Watkins
Indexing by Shoshana Hurwitz
Printed by Bang Printing

Distributed by Perseus Distribution
perseusdistribution.com

To place orders through Perseus Distribution:
Tel: (800) 343-4499
Fax: (800) 351-5073
E-mail: orderentry@perseusbooks.com

Dedication

This book is dedicated to my precious, loving, and supportive wife Tracey. Our marriage is a priceless treasure, and she owns my heart completely and forever. To me, she is the most beautiful woman in the world because she is beautiful both inside and out. Though we've been married for twenty years, it only seems like two. The fruit of our love is manifested in three wonderful daughters: Amber, Katie, and Bethany. These beautiful girls have many God-given talents, but the greatest quality of each is a heart's desire to do what is right.

Secondly, this work is dedicated to my parents, Wayne and Ruthie Johnson. My father is my hero, a genius, oftentimes the wind beneath my wings and the greatest earthly personification of love that I know.

Thirdly, I'd like to acknowledge Dr. Sam Rehnborg, the president of Nutrilite Health Institute. The mentoring I've received from this extremely intelligent and humble man is without equal, and he has significantly shaped my work. His commitment to excellence is demonstrated by the more than one hundred top-notch, full-time scientific researchers at the Nutrilite Health Institute, to whom I'm blessed and privileged to have access.

Fourthly, this book is dedicated to Nutrilite Health Institute, Nutrilite Health Institute Scientific Advisory Board, Amway Corporation, Bill Dombrowski, and all the affiliated corporate staff and thousands of business associates around the world who have entrusted me with their health. It has been a great honor to be the Medical Advisor/Director to Nutrilite Health Institute these last twelve-plus years.

Fifthly, and most importantly, this book is dedicated to my loving God, who's the source of any talent and good within me. (Jeremiah 9: 23, 24). Despite my shortcomings and failures, His love and grace sustain me.

I'm extremely thankful for the outstanding work done by my literary agents, Dr. Uwe Stender, President of TriadaUS Literary Agency, and Lisa Berkowitz at Berkowitz & Associates. Their expertise was obvious immediately. Glenn Yeffeth and his staff at BenBella Books have been wonderful to work with, and I am very blessed to be associated with such a supportive publishing company. I also greatly appreciate the excellent editing support provided by David Bessmer.

I will be forever thankful to Dr. Reggie Edgerton, Ph.D., who was my major professor at the UCLA Graduate School of Kinesiology where I received a Master's of Science degree. This visionary genius was seemingly twenty years ahead of his time and he not only opened the door to my future but also taught me how to scrutinize a scientific study in order to discern the truth.

Finally, this book is dedicated to Rich DeVos, the multibillion-dollar cofounder of Amway Corporation and a heart transplant recipient. After requesting a description of my preventive medicine work with Nutrilite Health Institute, he responded, "In other words, you want to prevent happening to others what has happened to me." When I responded in the affirmative, he stated, "Then keep it up; it's a good work." Thank you, Rich. I think of your kind statement often.

TABLE OF CONTENTS

PREFACE

A Life-Changing Experience

Some major life decisions take years to crystallize. My decision to switch from emergency medicine to preventive medicine took place in one day—almost in a single moment.

I loved practicing emergency medicine. I loved it for the challenge of the continuous stream of important decisions. I loved it for the feeling of accomplishment at the end of each day. I was fortunate to have received an excellent education at the UCLA School of Medicine and felt well prepared to meet the daily challenges of my job.

The day that changed my life started like any other day in the Southern California ER where I worked—a twelve-hour shift with a stream of patients hurt in auto accidents, suffering abdominal pains, chest pains—people suffering from injuries and diseases both acute and chronic.

Chronic diseases are those that progress for a long time—diseases people live with for months or years. This day would be the culmination of many years of treating young people with devastating chronic diseases. What I'm about to describe had happened many times before in our emergency room, and though every patient is important, my experience with one family changed me forever.

Paramedics brought in a thirty-eight-year-old man in full cardiac arrest—that is, his heart had stopped beating. After following the national guidelines for treating cardiac arrest for approximately forty-five minutes, we were getting very little response from the man's heart, and I knew he had little chance of recovery.

I walked out to the waiting room to talk to the man's family—to tell them what we had done and that the picture did not look good. At moments like this I always feel it is best to ease the families into understanding their loved one's situation, rather than shock them later with a sudden announcement of death. I value life tremendously and believe that we should do everything in our power to sustain and protect it. After assuring the man's family that we would continue to do everything we could, I returned to the emergency room and fulfilled that promise. But, despite the best efforts of a great emergency room staff, the patient died. We usually won these battles, but we lost this one.

I looked at the door to the waiting room, and dreaded going through it. The man's young wife and sweet ten-year-old daughter were waiting outside. I had already seen the great love they had for the husband and father who now lay motionless on our cardiac gurney. Sometimes the door from the emergency room to the waiting room is the heaviest door in the world.

As I opened the door, both the wife and the daughter could tell by the look on my face that they would never again see alive the man they deeply loved. They clutched one another as if suddenly alone in a terrifying world. The pain expressed on their faces came from the deepest parts of their souls. It was so abject and genuine that my heart was also broken. I couldn't speak. All I could do was put my hands on their shoulders and cry with them. This must have been a great man; his family was very special.

What makes this story even more tragic is that it didn't have to happen. The man had risk factors for heart disease that were largely preventable, if he had only known what they were and what to do. It was at that moment twenty-two years ago that I decided to pursue preventive medicine. Though I have great respect for emergency medicine and the thousands of lives saved every day by the dedicated doctors and nurses who practice it, I felt a new moral compulsion. I could no longer sit in an emergency room waiting for the next patient to land there on account of years of lifestyle behaviors that insidiously but persistently destroy from within. I wanted to prevent chronic diseases from occurring, rather than trying to treat them after it was too late.

As I reflect on the events of that fateful day I still feel the pain, and it still motivates me. In my preventive medicine work, I've been fortunate to witness dramatic improvements in the health of countless individuals who decided to change their lifestyles in pursuit of longer, healthier lives.

If this book causes just one person to change his or her lifestyle to reduce the risk of chronic disease, then all my effort in research and writing will be worth it. My sincere desire is that that one person is you.

PART I:

The Time for
an Optimal Health
Revolution Is Now!

CHAPTER 1

What Is the Optimal Health Revolution and Why Is It Essential?

You don't have to get type 2 diabetes.

You don't have to die prematurely of cancer, heart disease, Alzheimer's, or any other chronic disease.

You don't have to spend truckloads of money on health care to give yourself a better chance of living longer.

You don't have to feel old at forty, fifty, sixty, or even seventy years old. It's never too late to add energy and years to your life. It doesn't make any difference how old you are today. What makes a difference is how committed you are to the Optimal Health Revolution. Certainly, those who become part of the revolution as children (or even in the womb) will have the greatest benefits, but it's never too late to join.

The Optimal Health Revolution is a process of changing the way you live, so that you can live longer and in better health—so you can live a life filled with energy and vitality.

Yes, I know.

I know, I know, I know. Many quacks, charlatans, and hucksters in the health business have used the word "revolution" to describe their product.

1

A plastic and aluminum gimcrack designed to give you twelve-pack abs in only sixty seconds a day? A fitness revolution!

A little pill that causes pounds to melt away like butter in the summer sun and only causes permanent heart-valve damage in *some* of the people who use it? A weight-loss revolution!

A diet book that tells you to eat nothing but orange vegetables every second Thursday and to eat essentially the same diet as a mountain lion the rest of the time? A nutrition revolution!

But we all know that a *real* revolution isn't a gimmick or a quick fix or a fad.

A revolution starts with a fundamental change in what we think. It starts with a new way of understanding the world. Understanding becomes belief. And belief changes the way we live and behave for the rest of our lives.

The Optimal Health Revolution is real. It started with a breakthrough in our understanding of the fundamental cause of the various chronic diseases that are the biggest killers in modernized nations. That understanding lets us see how to live in a way that gives each of us the best chance for a long, healthy life.

And the best news is that joining this revolution is easy and inexpensive. No matter how busy you are, you have time for this revolution. No matter how stressful your life, you can cope with this revolution—it helps relieve stress rather than adding to it. You can adopt these changes into your life (and your family's) one at a time, rather than changing everything overnight. This is a nonviolent revolution.

For me, getting you to take that first step is the toughest part. Once you decide to revolt from your current lifestyle, the path to your best health—optimal health—gets easier and easier with each step you take. It's a great journey because of all the things you'll gain along the way: good health, energy, increased activity, freedom from disease, freedom to do more things with your family and friends, freedom to pursue hobbies and sports and all the things you love best—while avoiding the sorrows of illness and the pain of premature aging.

That seems like an easy choice to make, doesn't it? Yet I know that many people have become discouraged after following failed fads, or simply because there is so much confusion due to the "experts" constantly contradicting one another. Many people have simply lost hope.

This revolution invites you to rise up from hopelessness, cut through confusion and destroy the fad-based health-and-fitness culture that takes your money and gives you nothing but failure in return.

Revolution? Or Just Another Fad?

At this point, you might be asking yourself this question:

Who is this guy, and how do I know he isn't just the latest fad monger?

At least, I *hope* you're asking that. Being a health revolutionary requires healthy skepticism.

Here is my answer.

I am Duke Johnson, M.D., and I hate fads—*especially* if the fads hurt people.

More to the point, I have been blessed with the opportunity to develop a unique view of world medicine.

I have served as Medical Advisor, then Medical Director, for over twelve years at a prominent medical institute in Southern California. Our institute brings in clients from around the world for an entire week of health evaluations and instruction. (When you see your family doctor for your annual physical, you might get fifteen minutes with him or her, if it's a slow day.) At our facility, clients are provided with physical assessments that include things like state-of-the-art preventive blood panels. Clients receive health-care instruction that focuses primarily on preventing chronic disease. I have evaluated thousands of individuals from many different countries, following their traditional diets, beliefs, and lifestyles. We conduct follow-up exams and evaluations after clients have returned to their home countries and followed our advice for a while. Few physicians have had this kind of opportunity. My daily work involves integrating a great variety of culturally influenced lifestyles into alignment with optimal health. Through this experience, we've gained special insight into the development of chronic disease that the vast majority of health-care providers don't have.

Also, I have traveled around the world extensively, both for speaking engagements and to conduct my work. I have visited and performed health evaluations on people in every inhabited continent. I have studied scores of different medical traditions around the world, and I have found that they *all* have deficiencies. There isn't a perfect system anywhere. However, this experience has provided me with some fascinating and unique insights. The purpose of this book is to share those insights, to help you protect yourself from chronic disease in spite of your busy lifestyle. And the positions taken here are well validated by the nearly nine hundred scientific references in this book.

I have visited the historical locales of other health traditions and interviewed their current practitioners. I have incorporated many of the best global health-care practices, but only those that can withstand scientific scrutiny. Some of this scrutiny has been unwelcome, but I have too many friends and clients suffering from chronic diseases to worry about whether my conclusions are popular or politically correct in every country. We're talking about life and death here. Truth trumps popularity and political correctness.

For more than twenty years I have been deeply involved in a unique method of preventive medicine that is different from what most doctors practice. I practice in an environment that liberates me from the box in which most western doctors are trapped. I call their box "the ICD-9 code mentality" (ICD-9 stands for International Classification of Diseases, 9th Revision). In the United States, insurers pay doctors for treating diseases listed in this classification system. A similar coding system is used by the World Health Organization in classifying and tabulating statistics. ICD-9 is a widely accepted and very useful reporting system. However, the practice of paying doctors for reporting treatment of the diagnosis codes has been a major factor in leading the medical profession to focus on treatment far more than on prevention. When doctors can't get paid much for disease prevention, we can't really blame them for focusing on treatment.

To me, this is like focusing all of a society's fire-safety efforts on funding fire departments, while ignoring the concept of fireproof buildings.

Physicians have limited time for reading and continuing education, so they devote most of it to disease management rather than the massive amount of literature available on prevention. I know. I've been there. During the years I worked in emergency and family practice, my preventive medicine work typically amounted to telling my patients to lose weight, writing Lipitor® prescriptions, and so on. I wasn't providing them with the tools they really needed to keep from getting sick in the first place. This book is my response to all those years of frustration.

Today my work is primarily preventive screening, and it is not dependent on insurance payments. Not only has my focus changed radically; I have had time to study the vast new body of scientific literature on prevention.

To the doctors who read this book: I am in no way trying to impugn your integrity or ethics. I've been mired in the ICD-9 mentality myself. I sympathize with your frustration. One of my goals is to help our profession break out of this box and focus more on prevention.

And of course, doctors aren't the only people who need to break out of the old ways of thinking. This revolution starts with *you*—with taking responsibility for your own health. Not that you haven't wanted to. If you're like most people, you just haven't understood what to do. The result: your thinking, your beliefs, and your lifestyle are leading you down the path to premature death from chronic disease.

This book will take you in the opposite direction. I'll show you the way to optimal health through prevention—and not the token prevention practiced by many today. I'll show you one of the great discoveries of our age: the underlying medical cause of virtually all chronic disease. And I'll show you how we can use knowledge from many disciplines, including the new science of nutrigenomics, to neutralize the enemy.

Optimal Health Defined

Since optimal health is the goal of our revolution, it's probably a good idea to define it at the outset.

Let's start with *your* definition.

What comes into your head when you think of optimal health? Is it an image of a skinny starlet or a fashion model? The ripped muscles of an action hero or professional athlete? If so, the diet and health fad industry has gotten into your head and is running the show, as they are with millions of other people.

But here's the revolutionary question: Is that really what you want to look like? Why? Is it because that movie star is sexy? Is looking hot the ideal, or is living a long, healthy life a better goal?

Think about it. Are professional athletes and movie stars the longest-living people on the planet? No. Absolutely not. Many of those jocks got bulked up and extremely "cut" by taking steroids. And too many actresses and fashion models are literally dying to be waif-thin. A huge percentage of these people have achieved their body shapes in ways that are destructive to their health—steroids, weight-loss pills, appetite suppressants, amphetamines, malnutrition, anorexia, bulimia or myriad other methods that may be legal but are generally unstudied scientifically and can lead to premature death.

Industrial societies, particularly the United States, are deeply confused about what constitutes health and fitness. The idea is to live as long as you can, free of chronic disease. But most of what we do in the pursuit of "fitness" leads us in the opposite direction—toward an unattainable goal of what we should *look* like, by means that sap us of strength and energy, make us more prone to chronic disease, and ultimately shorten our lives.

So why does the media keep pointing to these impossibly skinny or buff people as our ideal? Why do you think? Money. The fitness and weight-loss industries make billions trying to help you attain a goal that is impossible for nearly everyone, and is unhealthy in the first place. If you hear somebody say, "I'm going to look like her or die trying," place your bets on the latter. The idea that we *can* look like that is almost as crazy as the notion that we *should*.

This revolution isn't about how you look. It's about how you *feel*, about staying healthy and living longer. You and I aren't going to look like a twenty-something movie-star when we're seventy, no matter what we do. But when we're seventy I want us to be healthy, vital, and enjoying life.

Yet every day, every hour, we're being sold an idea that's killing us. It's time we all rise up in revolt against the culture that keeps selling it.

Now here's *my* definition of optimal health. Optimal health is the best health you are capable of, given your past and your genetic heritage. You may have made mistakes in your lifestyle up to now. You may not have the best genetics. But the optimal health pathway leads you to the longest, healthiest life possible for *you*, starting today. We won't all live to the same age. But the earlier you start, the longer and better life you can live.

You'll notice I have written an entire book about attaining optimal health. That's because it's a broad subject, and the plan for getting there addresses many aspects of your life. If this were a single-focus plan, I could publish it in a brief article in one of those magazines you pick up in the supermarket checkout line and stuff into your grocery cart along with the corn chips and double-sugared energy cola. The issue of health is so oversimplified in modern culture worldwide, it's a crime. For most people it's nothing more than, "I'm fat. I need to go on a diet." For the few who are naturally scrawny it's, "I'm thin. I can't possibly be at risk."

That kind of simple-minded single focus is making the diet and fitness industries vastly rich while causing the premature death of millions. It's time to revolt against that kind of thinking. The way to optimal health and longevity involves broad lifestyle changes. It's a real revolution, not a phony quick fix. If you join this revolution, you *will* lose weight—assuming you have excessive body fat to start with. But you will lose it as a result of achieving a healthy lifestyle, not the other way around. Losing weight will be a healthy side effect of reducing your risk of chronic disease and early death.

So let's begin. Down with weight-loss diets! Join the Optimal Health Revolution!

A Worldwide Revolution Against a Global Problem

The truth is that the health of essentially everyone in the industrialized world is being impacted negatively, and we all need to join the Optimal Health Revolution. For most of the time that humans have been on this planet, health has been a matter of fate. You got sick or you didn't. You lived a long time or you didn't. However, we live in an age in which there is more and more you can do to maximize your lifespan and the degree of health you will enjoy while you are alive.

With the knowledge and technology now available, achieving optimal health is like a contest between you and the factors that work to shorten your life and damage your health. What are those factors? I'll discuss them in later chapters. But here is a point I want to make first:

The rules of the game have changed.

What made people ill and shortened their lives two hundred, one hundred, or even fifty years ago isn't the same set of health risks as the ones we face today. Knowing your opponent is the first step in devising a successful plan for winning the revolution. How did we get into this health crisis? Let's take a brief look at history.

Despite thousands of years of experience in Eastern and Western medical traditions, and despite breathtaking scientific advances in our lifetimes, there is still a fundamental global problem that isn't being addressed: We're all dying of the same chronic diseases. It's true around the world, and the prevalence of these diseases is getting worse, not better.

The World Health Organization (WHO) states that there is an epidemic of obesity occurring around the world,[1] to the extent that there may now be more obese people in the world than starving people. On balance, that's a good thing. It is a sign of real social, political, and economic progress that more people are dying from excessive junk-food consumption than from starvation. But both extremes are forms of malnutrition, and the nutritional deficiencies of the affluent also take millions of lives prematurely, even if not as rapidly as starvation.

The WHO also states that there's an epidemic of type 2 diabetes (previously referred to as adult-onset diabetes) occurring around the world.[2] Expenditures for treating type 2 diabetes have quadrupled in Japan over the last ten years, and have doubled in most other industrialized nations.

For all its advances, medical science still has much to learn—which means I do, too. However, the Optimal Health Revolution doesn't involve complex schemes or formulas. It is based on the best of scientific literature from the last twenty years, combined with our experience with our institute's clientele—more than 15,000 people from all over the world.

Bookstore walls are lined with the work of authors who offer bits and pieces of the master plan for optimal health, but I haven't seen anyone who has been as fortunate as we have been in having the unique view of world medicine necessary to bring it all together.

My first critical insight into global health occurred ten years ago, in the course of customizing our program for each country whose residents came through our doors. This work required gathering information from the WHO and the ministries of health for many nations in order to customize our program for each country. As we gathered data from around the world, I began to see a disturbing trend. Whether participants of our program were from China, Malaysia, India, Thailand, Japan, Russia, Korea, Hong Kong, Brazil, Argentina, Venezuela, Great Britain, Germany, Austria, Italy, Poland or the U.S., they all had the same risk factors for major chronic diseases and were beginning to show evidence of these diseases. With technological advances, we have begun to adopt very similar lifestyles globally.

Modern Times, Modern Diseases

At the beginning of the twentieth century, heart disease and cancer were not nearly as high on the list of major causes of death as they are today. However, in the last century industrial civilization has seen the greatest changes in diet and lifestyles in the history of the world.

Automation—on the job, at home, and in transportation—has dramatically decreased our daily exercise and the number of calories we burn. We eat a great deal more meat, most of it produced by industrial means. Our other foods are highly processed.

Hollywood loves to depict primitive humans as hunters—people who feasted daily on buffalo, antelope, wooly mammoth, and the occasional anachronistic dinosaur. In truth, though, until recently most humans' diets have primarily been plant-based. This is especially true over the last few thousand years—that is, since the introduction of agriculture.

Throughout history, meat has been very expensive. The wealth of ancient kings was often recorded in terms of the number of animals they owned. If you were among the very few who were rich, you could eat a lot of meat. Everybody else ate mostly foods derived from plants.

And the rich weren't always better off for it. Consider the case of the *Beefeaters* of London. These guys were, and are, officially called the Yeomen Warders of Her Majesty's Royal Palace and Fortress the Tower of London, and they are the ceremonial guards of that establishment. A few centuries ago they were a real, working security outfit. According to legend, they received the sobriquet Beefeaters because their kings believed that a hefty meat ration would result in the strongest and best guards; their payment in meat at least seems well documented. Legend also has it that these fellows became not only beefy, but particularly gout-afflicted. Gout is an inflammatory disease of the joints that results from the

9

formation of uric acid crystals within the joints. Uric acid is a byproduct of purine metabolism. The Beefeaters, and others of their ilk, got most of those purines from beef. So it is no surprise that gout used to be referred to as a "disease of the rich." Nowadays it is a disease cheaply available to almost everyone in a developed nation.

With industrialization came many advances in medicine, public health, agriculture and food processing. Infectious diseases (smallpox, tuberculosis, malaria, and others) and malnutrition receded from being the major causes of death that they were at the turn of the twentieth century. Since then, heart disease and cancer have become the two leading causes of death. This happened partly by default; we all have to die of something, and old age is a risk factor for heart disease and some cancers. However, there are other factors that have elevated the rates of these diseases—risk factors ranging from pollution to diet to changing lifestyles. I'll discuss these factors in detail later.

About one-third of deaths in the U.S. are from cardiovascular disease (heart attacks and strokes.) About 22 percent of Americans die of cancer. This increasing trend in chronic diseases over the last sixty years in the U.S. can be seen in Figure 1.1. Though we have had a decline in heart disease recently, the absolute number of deaths from the six leading causes in the U.S.—heart disease, stroke, cancer, chronic obstructive pulmonary disease, diabetes, and accidents—continues to increase.[3]

As industrialization has spread throughout the world, the chronic dis-

FIGURE 1.1

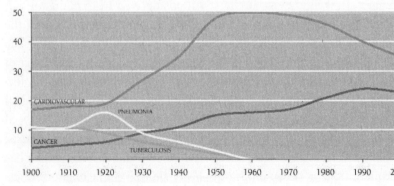

Source: cdc.gov/nchs/about/major/dvs/mortdata.htm

eases associated with our modern lifestyles have become global diseases. Heart disease and cancer are the leading causes of death in almost every industrialized nation on the planet. Some nations' ministries of health list heart disease and cerebrovascular disease (strokes) separately, but they are essentially the same disease process, and when put together they rank first in every industrialized nation.

Japan and the United States are distant and culturally different from each other, yet the history of chronic disease over the last century is similar in both countries. Figure 1.2 shows statistics from the Japanese Ministry of Health. As you can see, their chronic disease pattern changed rapidly—right along with their lifestyle—after World War Two. Heart disease and cancer began to rise almost immediately, and the trend continues. As in the U.S., the rate of heart disease has leveled off, but recent data point to another possible rise in the near future, because of

FIGURE 1.2

ANNUAL MORTALITY TRENDS FOR LEADING CAUSES OF DEATH IN JAPAN (1930–2000)

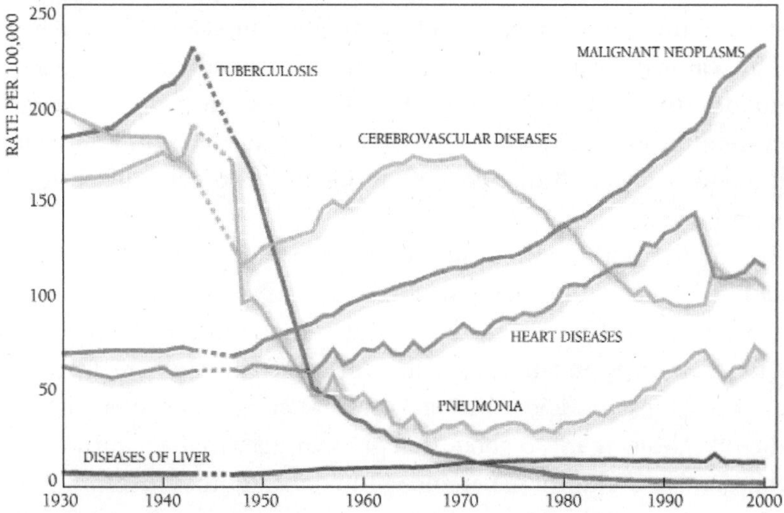

Source: Japan Ministry of Health

the dramatic increase in type 2 diabetes. Cancer has been rising at a phenomenal rate in Japan that still continues today.

I could show you local statistics from talks I've given all over the world, and the pattern would be almost identical to those you see in the

11

U.S. and Japan. The only difference would be the years when the chronic diseases started rising. In South Korea they started in the 1960s, in Brazil and India in the 1980s, and in China in the 1990s. (As of this writing, 43.8 percent of Chinese adults die of vascular diseases and 22.3 percent of cancer.)[4]

There is no doubt that this is a global health trend. The medical traditions of all regions and cultures are fighting to stop these epidemics, and they are all failing.

Doctors, scientists, and ordinary people everywhere have gone to great lengths to reverse these health trends. But we're still sinking deeper into trouble.

Bust That Fad!

The U.S. is the world leader in faddish attempts to combat heart disease, cancer, and every other health condition. If there is a fad anywhere in the world, it was probably tried in the U.S. first. There is no end to the parade of American physicians, scientists, and supplement marketers who offer the latest "scientific breakthrough" in the form of a book, video, treatment or device that will magically turn you into a Greek god or goddess overnight with minimal effort. (There are some supplement manufacturers, though, who act with integrity and support their claims with good science. I'll discuss how to identify these manufacturers in chapter 8.)

Around the world, uninformed, often desperate people spend billions of dollars (or the equivalent in local currency) in futile attempts to improve their health. It pains me to watch the uninformed spend their precious resources on faddish products or books, most of which are swill delivered in pseudoscientific packages. Many of our contemporary snake-oil salesmen are so good, though, that you need a solid scientific background and clinical experience to understand their deception. Fad marketers know this. That's why they are able to make millions—billions collectively—before they are exposed. Recently, while speaking in Munich to a group of physicians from nine Eastern European countries, I was amazed to find out that their patients were more familiar with some of the worst U.S. fads than we are in the United States.

In short, chronic diseases aren't the only opponents you have to beat to win optimal health. Health hucksters are the enemy, too, and avoiding them has to be part of your strategy. So one of my functions as a leader of the Optimum Health Revolution is to be a Fad Buster. Throughout this book, I'm going to use this symbol:

$$\boxed{\mathbb{FB}}$$

to call out unscientific fads that are being sold as magic bullets for achieving better health. This concept won't be popular among the purveyors of the fads in question, but I feel obligated to point out these false directions for your protection.

I am certainly not going to address all the fads that are out there. If I did, you would ruin your health trying to carry this book around. But we will be looking at some of the most popular and deceptive ones.

Getting the Big Picture

A major problem with most health-care programs around the world is that they treat various health problems separately, rather than taking a whole-lifestyle approach.

Some approaches come close but are missing important pieces of information. Practitioners of Eastern medicine who attempt to balance all aspects of their patients' lives generally have the right idea, but they often fail to incorporate the latest Western scientific advancements, and are often overwhelmed by the new problems presented by global industrialization. Also, they are often limited by their traditions or spiritual influences.

The problems with both traditional Eastern medicine and expensive Western medicine will be covered in greater detail in chapter 5. Suffice it to say that we must have the courage and patience to forge a new pathway to optimal health. Our global problems with chronic diseases did not develop overnight, nor will they disappear overnight. We need to confront these worsening health trends globally, with maturity and patience.

But I don't want you to worry about that. Global public-health problems are for people like me to worry about. All you have to worry about is yourself and your family. That's the game you're in, and the prize for winning is a longer, healthier life.

Some of the players on the other side are easy to see and avoid. Others are stealthy and hit you from your blind side. But the good news is that we now have a winning strategy—one that addresses all the aspects of your life that affect your health. The knowledge we've gained from our global experience can help you win your best life.

Thousands of people I've spoken from nearly thirty countries (as of this writing) have let me be their optimal health leader, and I would be honored to be yours, too.

A Lifetime of Prevention Is Worth a World of Cure

Two major problems with most of the world's health-care approaches is that they lack the understanding of what true prevention is and are too exclusively focused on treatment of disease. They fail to fully understand the risk factors for heart disease (chapter 9), cancer (chapter 10), type 2 diabetes (chapter 12), and the causes of obesity (chapter 11), and thus fail to incorporate them into their counsel to patients. Treatments based on incomplete knowledge are sometimes worse than the original ailment.

At my institute, we teach that there are fifteen risk factors for heart disease and sixteen risk factors for cancer. A *risk factor* is any lifestyle component or biological trait that increases the risk of a chronic disease. Most risk factors are preventable, but very few people even know what the risk factors are for the most common chronic diseases. Knowledge of risk factors is so critical for optimal health that almost all of the steps of the Optimal Health Revolution involve risk factor reduction.

A critical strategy in our plan is to help you confront risk factors in a way that is simpler to understand and carry out than you would ever expect. Like a good football coach, I don't want you to have to think about everything you do all day. I want to make executing this game plan instinctive and natural.

Nor do I want you to be afraid of losing the game by making a single mistake. You don't have to be perfect with your execution. Just begin taking the steps you can now, and you will improve your health. Once those steps become second nature, add some more. Once you understand how critical these steps are and begin to make changes, you will be on the way to winning optimal health.

How will you know when you've won the game? I'll answer that question in the last chapter.

Most medical traditions recognize some of the risk factors for chronic diseases. But why go into a game knowing only part of your opponent's playbook? Our defense against chronic disease is weaker when we don't understand all the risk factors we face. In Western medicine, progress is often slowed by the process of approval and acceptance by governments and the vast majority of the medical community. Eastern medicine often fails to take advantage of the newest and best research and appropriate statistical evaluation. Even if the risk factors are understood, many medical traditions don't deal with them completely or appropriately. There are risk factors for all chronic disease, but I will focus on heart disease, cancer, obesity, and diabetes because of their worldwide prevalence and worsening state.

For Those of You Who Thought This Was Just Another Diet Book . . .

Sorry. You need to change your focus. Obesity has become a monstrously fad-ridden industry, in which each new fad addresses only one or two aspects of your lifestyle. Most people who buy these books, products and programs lose little or no weight, and fewer still keep the weight off. Many, perhaps most, damage their health in the process of losing and regaining weight.

FB

THE HIGH-FAT DIET

One popular fad, which has finally lost much of its momentum, teaches that we need to lose weight by eating a high-fat diet. Not only is this diet largely unsuccessful in the long run (see chapter 11), but high-fat diets are associated with increased risk for five different cancers, according to the National Cancer Institute (see chapter 10). It may be true that for a generation we were oversold on the value of cutting all possible fat out of our diets. But the recent high-fat fad treats carbohydrates—which we get from foods that are often also the source of hundreds of excellent natural antioxidants, phytonutrients, and fiber—as the scourge of mankind, while promoting highly oxidized fats that are loaded with carcinogens. This popular diet is like recommending smoking to someone in order to help them lose weight. Certainly there are poor sources of carbohydrates, but that shouldn't make us conclude that all carbohydrates are bad. We cannot, in fact, live without them. They are the fuel for our bodies' engines. This is one example of why faddish programs based on partial scientific knowledge are not only ineffective long-term, but also sometimes dangerous.

It's time to stop the fad-of-the-year approach to weight control.

The Optimal Health Revolution isn't about losing weight. It's about winning a longer life and living in better health. But if you follow this plan for optimal health, you should in fact lose excess weight. Reducing the risk factors of chronic disease will do that for you. You don't lose weight permanently and safely by cutting out all carbs or all fats or taking a pill or squeezing a spring-loaded gizmo between your knees at a cost of three easy installments of $39.95. You do it by living the simple, healthy lifestyle taught here.

And the best part is that instead of sacrificing your health in order to look thinner, you'll lose weight as a side effect of lowering your risk of chronic disease.

How to Use This Book

Most health-care traditions don't fully understand the underlying process that is common to almost all chronic disease (chapter 2), including the worldwide epidemics of type 2 diabetes and obesity. I'm incredibly excited about how the vast majority of medical and scientific literature has begun pointing to a very consistent theme for reducing the risk of all chronic disease. Once we can grasp this concept, and some new advances in science (chapter 4), understanding how we need to live in order to reduce the risk of chronic disease will become increasingly simple.

What is this great new insight? I can hardly wait to share it with you. But I want you to truly understand it. That means we have to talk a little science throughout the book. Please don't let that intimidate you! I'll do my best to make it easy for those of you who don't have a scientific background. Stay with me and the reward will be a thorough understanding of how to live for optimal health.

You *could* cheat and skip to the last chapters, but I don't want you merely to *know* how to change the way you live. I want you to *believe* you should—and that requires understanding *why*.

So think of this book in part as a mystery novel. The end won't mean much to you if you don't follow the whole plot.

For those readers who do have a scientific background, I have provided nearly nine hundred scientific references to support the positions I have taken. I will add this caveat: I take positions that many in the food industry will not like, positions that expose that industry's almost universal tendency to value profit above health. I recommend that any doubtful reader check the references provided. You'll find that my conclusions are consistent and scientifically solid.

A couple centuries ago the world was ignorant about health. Now there is so much information, much of it false and conflicting, that even well-educated people don't know what to think, believe, or do. Information and knowledge are not the same thing.

My purpose—my passion—is to unify, simplify, and present the knowledge I have gained, with the help of my colleagues, in my twenty-two years of practicing preventive medicine and evaluating thousands of people from around the world—so you can put that knowledge to work in your life.

I want to help you sort through the scientific literature, which at times provides conflicting results. I want be your advocate and to open your eyes to the fads and fallacies that are being sold to you daily. I want to break your false, unreachable Hollywood images of optimal health and give you the healthiest one.

If you're looking for a quick fix, you won't find it here.

If you're looking for a path to a lifetime of better health, please read on. Carefully. Take your time. Get it right.

It's time to stop the narrowly focused quick fixes that in fact fix little or nothing. Let's join the Optimal Health Revolution together. The first step in this revolution is to understand the common theme underlying all chronic disease. That's chapter 2.

It's not too late to lower your health risks. It doesn't matter how often you have failed in the past. This is a completely new approach to health, and as you take the right steps you'll begin to feel the difference.

Our institute has thousands of successful clients who have preceded you. Now it's time for you to know the truth.

PART II:

The Consistent Underlying Theme for All Chronic Diseases

CHAPTER 2

The Danger That Lies Beneath It All

THERE WAS A TIME WHEN I WAS NOTED FOR MY GREEN THUMB, BUT THAT WAS AFTER AN EPISODE OF PAINTING. A GARDENER I AM NOT.

I once bought some weed killer with the aim of perfecting my lawn. I sprayed the few weeds, taking the utmost care not to squirt a single droplet of poison on my grass. Nonetheless, my lawn broke out in brown spots like a fifteen-year-old with a bad case of acne. What had happened? I had read the label on the weed killer so carefully! Well, the manufacturers had simply failed to mention that this product was absorbed into the roots of the weed and would travel to the roots of my beautiful lawn.

A well-kept garden is one of the most beautiful sights on earth, but growing vegetables or flowers requires careful planning, strategy, and constant tending. Gardens have many enemies: frost, insects, weeds, neighborhood dogs that use your property as a beautifully landscaped latrine, wild critters that see your garden as an all-you-can-eat smorgasbord, and brainless neighbors who apply weed killers on windy days. Not to mention one's own errors: overwatering, underwatering, overfertilizing, underfertilizing, and all the other secret ways of committing herbicide.

To me, the trickiest enemies are weeds. If you are too aggressive in your efforts to control them, you can kill the plants that you wanted to keep. But if you are not diligent, weeds will overwhelm your garden and choke out the flowers or vegetables you planted.

The most difficult weeds I have battled are those that spread by rhizomes, like Johnsongrass. (Nice name, right? It was probably one of my horticulturally challenged relatives who introduced this species to the Western Hemisphere a couple of centuries ago.) Rhizomes are plant stems that extend horizontally, usually underground. They terminate in new, above-ground plants with new root systems, which in turn produce new rhizomes. Johnsongrass can produce seven tons of rhizomes per acre. To rid an acre of Johnsongrass, you pretty much have to pull up all seven tons of rhizomes.

But people don't realize that. Not knowing what kind of insidious plant-monster they're dealing with, they think that each upstart is a separate little weed, easily killed. They don't realize that an evil underground network is threatening to choke out every garden plant in its path.

The alert reader will have sensed the growth of a creeping metaphor here.

There is a single, insidious, underlying factor in most chronic disease. It attacks our health the way a Johnsongrass rhizome network undermines a garden, sending up new shoots at its ends—in this case chronic diseases such as heart disease and cancer.

This is still news to much of the medical profession. Most doctors continue to focus their work on outlying shoots of the weed, thinking they are separate, single plants. When they make some progress in killing off a few of those shoots, there is great rejoicing, followed by publication in medical journals and celebrations in the popular media. And we continue to ignore the root cause. And people continue to get sick.

What Is the Root Cause of Chronic Disease?

A few years ago, I had an epiphany. I felt as if I had struck buried treasure while rooting around in my garden. Suddenly the jumble of thousands of scientific facts I'd accumulated over the past seventeen years of preventive medicine research began to fall neatly into place.

What I realized was that underneath the cacophony of conflicting expert opinions, **there are common elements in scientific literature that point out the way to reduce the risk of chronic disease.** And that way is a lifestyle that is surprisingly simple and easy to live.

Vast tracts of complicated scientific literature address certain risk factors for chronic disease: inflammatory markers (such as cytokines), nutrigenetics, nutrigenomics, and other complex areas of scientific exploration all point in one direction. I quickly began to see how thousands of studies from many different disciplines all converged and agreed.

You're shortly going to see this concept, too, and you won't need a science degree to grasp it. All you have to do is read this chapter and the next. I hope this new understanding changes your life as it did mine — because it will protect you from going down the blind, often dangerous alleys suggested by pop diets and other health fads in your pursuit of optimal health.

Mine is not a lone voice in the wilderness. Hundreds of scientists throughout the world have contributed to the information that I'm about to share with you. I am certainly not the only person who understands the meaning of this scientific literature — in fact, my knowledge pales in comparison to that of some experts. However, I do have a unique perspective on the scientific literature, through the extensive experience that I have been fortunate to have as medical director of an institute with an international clientele. This perspective includes a twenty-two-year data bank of personal consultations with our 15,000 patients who live in a great variety of cultures around the world, with differing diets, toxic exposures, belief systems, health-care systems, and so on. There are few (if any) doctors who have a similarly vast and varied clientele.

As I mentioned, research and experience have led us at the institute to teach a longer list of risk factors for heart disease than is common in the medical establishment. We do this in no small part because many heart attacks occur in people who have no documented clinical heart disease, and who lack the cardiovascular risk factors commonly accepted by established medicine.[5]

My flash of insight hit me in 2004 while I was reviewing the fifteen risk factors that I teach for heart disease and the sixteen for cancer. We had noted very interesting trends in scientific literature concerning C-reactive protein (CRP), which is a marker of inflammation found in the blood, similar to how a white blood cell count (WBC) is a marker for infections, even though inflammation and infection are not the same thing.

Specifically, I noted that high levels of CRP were associated with increased risk not only of heart disease, but also of diabetes, smoking, and many other cardiac risk factors. So I decided to see if there were research data indicating that CRP is elevated in all thirty-one of the risk factors I recognize for both heart disease and cancer.

To my great surprise, our review of scientific literature showed that **elevated CRP accompanies all of our risk factors for heart disease and cancer,** *as well as* **many other chronic diseases**.

This knowledge does not represent any breakthrough at the level of basic research—many scientists have connected CRP and other inflammation markers with some risk factors and diseases. What our survey accomplished was to dig up research studies that associated inflammation with *almost all* chronic diseases and *almost all* the risk factors for each of them. But, most important, **we could see deeper connections supporting the idea that inflammation is a** *cause* **of these diseases**. This was the real breakthrough, clearing away what had been the darkest cloud of confusion for most researchers.

We had discovered the evil plant-monster that spread, rhizome-like, under the ground to do damage everything in the garden of optimal health. It is chronic, excessive inflammation. The reason for the dramatic rise in chronic inflammation? **Almost every aspect of our "normal" industrialized lifestyles stimulates our immune systems to become chronically overactive.** This overactivity results in a chronic release of the molecules that cause inflammation. Until we focus our effort on this root cause, we will have only marginal success at controlling the individual diseases that pop up from its unseen roots.

For example, medical science has had some real successes in recent years at reducing heart disease deaths in some industrialized nations. Unfortunately, this has caused many doctors to develop a false sense of security; they feel as if the battle against heart disease is actually being won. But soon the worldwide epidemics of obesity and type 2 diabetes will cause death rates from heart disease to rise again. While doctors have been celebrating the apparent drop in the rate of heart disease in some industrialized countries, they have neglected the root disease hidden under the surface. Until the entire underlying root cause of chronic disease is killed off, these diseases will continue to spread.

The epidemics of obesity and type 2 diabetes are growing because we aren't treating the root cause: chronic, excessive inflammation. That's right, chronic inflammation enhances obesity development, too.

Why Is Chronic, Excessive Inflammation the Monster?

Let's begin by defining inflammation.

Inflammation is a nonspecific protective immune system response to cell injury or irritation that is characterized by capillary enlargement, attraction of white blood cells to the area, redness, local swelling, and partial reduction of normal cell function. This immune-system response is the same whether the damaging agent is infection, a foreign body, decreased oxygen, radiation, chemicals, trauma or extremes of temperature. Its purpose is to repair damaged tissue, but the reaction can be harmful, especially if the stimulus of the inflammation is chronic. CRP is simply a generalized marker in the blood that indicates whether or not inflammation is occurring somewhere in the body. (There are markers of inflammation other than CRP as well.)

You know from personal experience what inflammation is. It's the warm, red, swollen tenderness you get around a cut, a scrape, or a burn—especially if the area gets infected. It's part of your body's attempt to heal that injury and fight off infection. If the process is allowed to persist too long, though, the local tissue won't work normally.

What does that have to do with heart disease, diabetes, cancer, or obesity? Stay with me a little longer, please.

Below is the list of risk factors for heart disease that I will explain in greater detail in chapter 9. Each of the end notes cites a study that links that risk factor to elevated CRP levels. By "link" I mean that people who have these risk factors also have elevated CRP levels that indicate chronic inflammation.

1. Genetic factors[6]
2. Diabetes[7]
3. Smoking[8]
4. Hypertension[9] (HTN causes inflammation and inflammation causes HTN)[10, 11]
5. Lack of exercise[12]
6. Depression[13]
7. Hypothyroidism[14]
8. Obesity[15]
9. Stress[16]
10. Elevated lipids[17, 18]
11. Elevated homocysteine[19]
12. Lack of intrinsic faith[20, 21]
13. Inadequate fruit and vegetable consumption[22]
14. Inadequate omega-3 levels[23]
15. Elevated C-reactive protein[24]

As you can see, high levels of inflammation are present with every risk factor for heart disease. We now could see an underlying theme for all fifteen risk factors.

The next question had to do with cause and effect. Was it just coincidence? Did the risk factors all cause inflammation? Or was inflammation the underlying cause of all the risk factors—or at least a factor in making them worse?

Once we had established the remarkably consistent correlation between elevated CRP and cardiovascular risk factors, we moved on to the cancer risk factors (chapter 10) to see if the pattern continued.

1. Genetic factors[25]
2. Smoking[26]
3. Lack of exercise[27]
4. Obesity[28]
5. Stress[29]
6. High lipid diet[30]
7. Inadequate fruits and vegetable consumption[31]
8. Excessive alcohol consumption[32]

9. High salt intake[33, 34, 35]
10. Pollution[36]
11. Smoked or charred foods (this type of cooking increases chemicals called heterocyclic amines or HCA, which increase inflammation)[37, 38, 39]
12. Excessive sunlight[40]
13. Certain infections[41]
14. Vitamin D deficiency[42]
15. Elevated CRP[43]
16. Insulin resistance and type 2 diabetes[44]

Again, the correlation was 100 percent for the sixteen cancer risk factors!

So—there is an inflammatory response noted in the body connected not only with heart disease and cancer, but with all of the risk factors for those diseases. Furthermore, risk factors for other diseases, like type 2 diabetes[45, 46] and obesity[47] (with persistent inflammation interrupting normal metabolism), are also associated with inflammation. In addition to risk factors, chronic inflammation is also associated with the risk of the above mentioned diseases as well—heart disease,[48, 49, 50, 51] diabetes,[52, 53, 54, 55, 56] cancer,[57, 58] and obesity.[59]

And that's not all.

Further investigation revealed that elevated CRP is present with many other chronic diseases: age-related macular degeneration,[60] Alzheimer's,[61] Crohn's disease,[62] Parkinson's disease,[63] asthma,[64] osteoarthritis,[65] stroke,[66] and others. Inflammation is not only associated with certain digestive conditions, but is the link that can lead to cancer development in people with these disorders.[67, 68, 69] In fact, the list of chronic diseases associated with elevated CRP goes on and on, and the prevalence of most of these diseases has been *increasing* over the last few decades. Chronic inflammation underlies essentially every chronic disease that has increased rapidly in the last several decades.

And if this wasn't enough reason for you to want to reduce chronic inflammation, it is also associated with muscle loss,[70] accelerated aging,[71, 72, 73] and reduced longevity![74]

Still, it remains a question to many scientific investigators whether or not inflammation is a *result* of these risk factors and diseases or a *cause*. In the next chapter I'll show why **inflammation is primarily a *cause* of chronic disease**, and in some cases a result as well.

But first, an important disclaimer. Persistent inflammation is not manifested every second in the blood of every person who has chronic disease, nor does a negative CRP test mean that you are disease-free. There are many markers in the blood for inflammation. It's like high blood pressure. Not every person who suffers from hypertension has it elevated constantly, twenty-four hours per day. Similarly, chronic inflammation is statistically a common factor for many chronic diseases and is responsible for a great deal of chronic illness, but its momentary presence is not necessary for diagnosis. We still have to consider the many risk factors for chronic disease. If you have risk factors for chronic disease—trust me, you have or you will soon have chronic inflammation. And yet—a sound understanding of chronic inflammation is critical to your quest for optimal health.

Inflammation is the star player, the big scorer, on our opponent's team. Our game plan for optimal health has to be built around it.

Finally, there is another phenomenon related to inflammation that cannot be ignored. Our institute constantly reviews statistics that issue from the Centers for Disease Control, the World Health Organization, and the ministries of health of many countries. Long ago it became clear that severe upswings in the rates of chronic diseases had begun in the 1950s and 1960s in many countries. We now know this upswing is related to the spread of inflammatory lifestyles, which trigger our immune systems to be constantly active.

INFLAMMATION AND WEIGHT LOSS

Modern society's obsession with weight is another area that can't be addressed sensibly or successfully when treated as an isolated problem. Treating obesity as another isolated "weed" in our garden is doomed to fail, because the problem is related to a deeper root cause.

This is why most weight management programs fail. They

are attempts to pluck the visible part of the weed while leaving the extensive, unseen root system intact. This is not to say that simply reducing inflammation will result in weight loss; that hasn't been studied as of yet. But, until persistent inflammation, which interferes with normal metabolism, is reduced, your weight loss efforts will be much more difficult and perhaps too discouraging. Some weight loss programs have been successful because they unknowingly reduce inflammation with exercise, increased vegetable intake, etc. Other fads don't work well because they increase inflammation with the removal of natural anti-inflammatory oils, such as omega-3, and allow you to eat processed foods or have you cook with and eat foods loaded with omega-6, such as corn oil.

There's a great deal of interaction between the risk factors for obesity and those for all other chronic disease. This is why **it is imperative that we help you change your total lifestyle.** It's the only way to treat the underlying problem, the only way to achieve optimal health.

So what changed in the 1950s and 1960s? What are the factors that have led to this global health problem? In order to understand this thoroughly, we must begin by learning how the body responds to stressors. Then we can look for the global trends that have led to this chronic inflammatory state in so many people.

Ultimately, the key to living an optimally healthy life is to reduce the inflammation that is associated with these chronic diseases. How do you do that? You can begin by reading the next chapter.

CHAPTER 3

Inflammation —
Life Under the Volcano

DID YOU EVER HAVE ONE OF THOSE DAYS, A DAY WHEN ALL YOUR PLANS BREAK DOWN, BECAUSE EVERYTHING THAT CAN GO WRONG DOES?

First the alarm clock doesn't go off. Already running late, you find that a virus has invaded the house and the kids are throwing up all over the floor. The poor dears are so sick, they can't even hit the buckets you placed by their beds, and they're spewing faster than you can clean up. The water heater being overtaxed, you shower in a spray of sleet. Then your mother-in-law calls to say that she needs to live with you for a month because her house just burned down. She's so distraught that you postpone asking if she had kept up the insurance payments—a point of particular importance, since you cosigned on her mortgage.

Finally, you decide to deal with the chaos in the manner of responsible heads of households everywhere—by leaving for work—but you can't find the car keys. Your frenzied search is distracted by the only child in the house who isn't sick, your three-year-old, demanding to know where his favorite toy is, nonstop like a looped recording.

Your eventual discovery of the car keys is followed by another: The car has a flat tire. You change it and leave the premises like a person fleeing a major volcanic eruption, only to find that every slow driver in the county has chosen the same route as you and that a conspiracy of traffic engineers has programmed every light to turn red at the sight of your car.

By the end of the day, you yourself are in eruption. You've been spouting smoke and steam and setting off seismic tremors all day. As soon as you walk in your front door, you stub your toe on the lost toy. This is all it takes for the pressure to reach its critical level. The top blows off the mountain. You try to vent your rage elsewhere than at your family. The dog is an easy target, but she exits as if fleeing the pyroclastic flow at Pompeii. Your spouse and children smile nervously, in feigned sympathy, while furtively noting escape routes. In the next room, your mother-in-law picks up the telephone to call 911.

In the coming week, as the lava cools and hardens, you will apologize repeatedly at work and at home for the verbal abuse you spewed at innocent people that day. You are so ashamed of your behavior that several years later you will write of the incident in the second person, as though it happened to someone else.

And yet, who hasn't had a day like this? Sometimes problems pile up faster than we can deal with them, and we are overwhelmed—and the result is that we become emotionally inflamed.

Have you sensed in this long description another metaphor? It's true: The same thing can happen with our immune systems, except that the inflammation isn't figurative. When the immune system is continuously turned on or over-stimulated, its response can damage innocent tissue, just as out-of-control emotions can damage relationships with colleagues and family.

In order to protect our health, we need to control the causes of excess inflammation.

The previous chapter explained that inflammation is a consistent theme with virtually all chronic-disease risk factors. We have seen how chronic, excessive inflammation—as signaled by elevated C-reactive protein (CRP) and other blood factors—corresponds with all the risk factors for heart disease and cancer. Elevated CRP is also associated with many other chronic diseases, including Alzheimer's and Parkinson's. There are many other blood markers for inflammation, but CRP is the one that has been studied the most.

So the next question is: What is the *source* of chronic inflammation?

Many scientists are conducting research in order to answer this question. We're gaining new insight almost daily. The research done so far points consistently to one conclusion: Dramatic changes in our lifestyles over the last several decades have caused the steep rise in chronic inflammation. These lifestyle changes will have different effects on the bodies of different people because of our genetic differences, but we have all been affected to some degree.

I hope that all the Fad Buster items I put in this book will teach you at least this: To maintain your health you need to maintain a healthy skepticism. To that end, I don't want you to take what I am saying about inflammation on faith. I want you to understand the science. Unfortunately, reading the scientific support for my conclusions about inflammation can be tough going for people without scientific educations, and for most folks it is about is exciting as watching your fingernails grow.

So I am caught between a rock and a hard place. I want to convince you with facts, but I don't want to bore or intimidate you, for fear that you will put the book down and not reopen it. So here is what I will ask you to do (that is, those of you who don't have much scientific background): Just stay with me for a few minutes. I'll do my best to explain the science by analogy. I'll keep it brief. If it is still tough going, just think of it as being like your first attempt to read Shakespeare. The language seemed impenetrable at first, but in the end you were surprised at how well you understood the text. And unlike a Shakespeare play, this stuff only goes on for three or four pages.

The truth will set you free — in this case, free from chronic diseases that stand between you and a lifetime of optimal health.

I will begin with a very basic explanation of how your immune system works, and I'll conclude by giving you the appropriate steps to take to reduce the chronic inflammation that causes chronic disease. As new research is published, you can refer back to this chapter to help you understand what effects certain lifestyle habits have upon your health.

Immune System 101 (A Very Short Course)

The immune system protects us from attacks on our health and well-being. You probably know that it protects us from bacteria, viruses, and parasites. It also protects us from many substances that it recognizes as foreign or damaging to our bodies.

There are two categories of immune-system function: *innate* and *acquired* immunity. The difference between them is a bit like the difference between a police force and a militia or national military force.

The *innate* immune system is like a police force, which is on duty all the time, enforcing laws ranging from jaywalking to felonies, and chasing down lawbreakers. It provides the first response to any emergency presented by an infection or foreign substance, but only responds generally and in the same way to each.

Acquired immunity is more like a militia. Rather than being on active duty all the time, a militia is only called upon at times of special need, like natural disasters or civil insurrections or attacks by a foreign enemy, and it can be trained to deal with very specific threats.

Acquired immunity is also referred to as *adaptive immune response*, in which cells called *lymphocytes* produce antibodies specifically adapted to certain diseases. Adaptive immunity has a memory. It's why most people only get certain diseases once—like measles, mumps, or chicken pox. Once your adaptive immune system makes antibodies to fight off such diseases, it recognizes them the next time around and kills them off before they get started.

Acquired immunity is like a state or national military force in that it takes it a bit longer than the on-duty police force to respond to an emergency, but it is more specialized and better trained in certain emergency functions. Once the acquired immunity kicks in and identifies the specific organisms or substances to attack, it takes command over parts of the innate immune system to help fight off the threat.

Both the innate and acquired immune systems use white blood cells as troopers and soldiers. One of the ways your doctor can tell if you have an infection is to count your white blood cells. When your immune system is very active, it makes more white blood cells and sends them into the blood stream to carry out their duty.

The Acquired (Adaptive) Immune System

The acquired or adaptive immune system doesn't have much to do with our discussion of inflammation. All you need to know is that the source

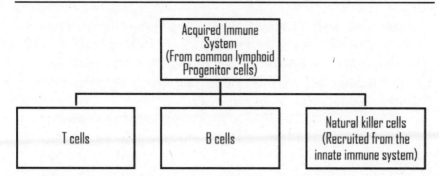

of its white blood cells is the bone marrow. The acquired immune system employs three kinds of white blood cells: T cells, B cells, and natural killer cells. Natural killer cells lack specific receptors, so while they act with the acquired immune system, they are really part of the innate immune system. Among other functions, natural killer cells attack abnormal cells that can develop into tumors. That is, they help keep cancer and other tumors from forming and growing.

The Innate Immune System

The innate immune system is of special interest in regard to chronic inflammation.

Like the acquired system, it derives its cells from the bone marrow, which gives rise to many different cells, including neutrophils, eosinophils, basophils, mast cells, and monocytes. Monocytes become macrophages (Greek for "big eaters"). Neutrophils, eosinophils, basophils, and monocytes circulate mainly in the blood. Mast cells and macrophages are distributed throughout the body.

FB

THE ANTIOXIDANT CRAZE

Neutrophils and macrophages have the ability to gobble up and destroy stuff. This is called *phagocytosis* (Greek for "eats cells"), a process that uses very powerful chemicals such as oxygen radicals and peroxides, which are *oxidants*.

No doubt you've heard a lot about how *antioxidants* are good for you. They are, in moderation. But some health food stores, supplement manufacturers, and faddish health programs try to convince you that the more antioxidants a product contains, the better it is. **The truth is, if you take *too many* antioxidants, you may neutralize your body's ability to kill foreign substances or abnormal cells.**

Naturally, there are loonies on the other side who say you don't ever need any supplements. I'll straighten this out in chapter 8.

For now, let's say it's better to base your antioxidant intake on solid science rather than the "advice" of someone whose primary motivation is profit.

Neutrophils are the most numerous and important cells used by the innate immune system. These cells eat foreign particles and secrete chemicals that affect our bodies. Monocytes and other cells secrete a group of chemicals called *cytokines* (Greek for "cell movers"); these are proteins that affect the behavior of cells. Cytokines also cause inflammation. (You can read more about how cytokines work in Appendix A.9.)

Time out for a quick review. Inflammation has four main characteristics—redness, heat, pain, and swelling—but if allowed to persist long enough, the surrounding tissue won't work well (dysfunction). You can easily see inflammation (not to mention feel it) when it occurs on or near your skin—as when you've been cut or pick up a splinter. You might feel it when it's internal, too—for example, if you have appendicitis. *But* most internal inflammation isn't noticeable at all—for example in the linings of your blood vessels. Such inflammation can only be detected using blood tests such as the CPR test.

Okay, back to cytokines.

During inflammation, blood vessels become larger and increasingly permeable, which is the medical term for leaky. This happens because cytokines make the inner lining of blood vessels (the endothelium) become slightly "sticky," so that white blood cells can attach to these linings and then transfer through the blood vessel wall. These white blood cells then travel wherever they are needed, propelled by other cytokines. This movement of white blood cells through the walls of blood vessels is critical to fighting infection. It is one of nature's ingenious and beautiful designs. But, this process can cause reactions in the walls of blood vessels that lead to the formation of plaque deposits on those walls.

And those plaque deposits are what we mean when we talk about *atherosclerosis*, or coronary heart disease. They are the deposits that can shut down coronary arteries, starving heart muscles for oxygen.

That's what we call a heart attack.

So far I've only scratched the surface of how the immune system works. It involves entire classes of chemicals I haven't mentioned. But I hope you are beginning to see how complex and powerful the immune system is—how intricate its system of controls, how various the substances and functions that spur it into action.

The point I've been leading up to is this: Once the immune system is stimulated into action, certain functions are triggered that can be harmful or damaging. This is why chronic over-stimulation of the immune system is not a good thing.

The immune system was designed to act quickly and powerfully to protect us from infections. Normal immune system function is a thing of power and beauty. Yes, sometimes it malfunctions or is temporarily overpowered, and we become ill before the immune system finally wins the day. But we are exposed to trillions of bacteria and viruses, and the immune system vanquishes nearly all of them without our becoming sick.

The immune system was designed to fight infection and foreign invaders. It was designed to act quickly, raising our body temperature and recruiting many cells into action, thus rapidly repelling each assault. But in peacetime, as it were, the immune system is supposed to be at peace, its function minimal. It is not supposed to be turned on continuously. If this happens, we get unwanted damage, just as if a militia force continued to shoot up the place in the absence of any enemy invaders.

This phenomenon is probably best seen in the effects of CRP.

CRP: The Symptom or the Cause?

We've touched on this before. We know that elevated levels of C-reactive protein always indicate inflammation. But is elevated CRP merely the result of an inflammation, or is it the cause?

The quick, easy answer is that it's both, but that doesn't tell us much. What's important to understand is that if we constantly over-stimulate our immune systems, thereby causing chronic inflammation, **we are damaging our bodies**. As you will soon see, many normal behaviors associated with our modern lifestyle over-stimulate our immune systems. We have to stop living this way if we want to slow down the epidemics of chronic disease.

How do we do that? Please keep reading. I'll tell you soon.

When the immune system is functioning normally, CRP has many benefits. Among other things, it binds to the walls of bacteria and fungi, stimulating the complement system. This triggers many functions of the immune system, including phagocyte activity, that kill off the invaders.

However, CRP is destructive to our health when it is abnormally produced—that is, at low levels but constantly. Here are some examples of the harm it does:

- Decreases the release of nitric oxide, which is needed to help the inner lining of the blood vessels to relax.[75]
- Stimulates interleukin-6 release and increases the transfer of destructive white cells to blood vessel walls.[76]
- Increases the rate of blood clotting and of damage to blood vessels.[77]

All of the above contribute to the formation of the blood vessel disease atherosclerosis, which is the cause of heart attacks and strokes. So it's easy to see that CRP is not just a marker of inflammation, but a cause of chronic cardiovascular disease.[78]

Moreover, we now see how CRP and other inflammatory chemicals contribute to abnormal cell development when the immune system is abnormally and chronically stimulated. This is most likely why CRP and other markers are elevated in every risk factor that we have discussed for cancer.

More Evidence That Inflammation Causes Chronic Disease

Many leading researchers still do not suspect a single root cause for insulin resistance, metabolic syndrome, the epidemic of type 2 diabetes, the obesity epidemic, dramatically rising cancer rates, and increases in other disease such as Alzheimer's. They lack a few key facts, or haven't put those facts together to solve the puzzle. Many have known that inflammation is associated with chronic diseases, but fewer are convinced that it is a cause rather than an associated factor.

And yet, a review of those puzzle pieces is compelling. Here is a list of facts that support the idea that inflammation is a cause of chronic disease.

1. Inflammatory markers, when stimulated chronically, are destructive to normal tissue.
2. Non-disease entities, such as consumption of foods that contain bad fat and exposure to pollution, stimulate both inflammatory marker production and diseases. In other words, common behavior in healthy people stimulates the immune system even when no disease process has started.
3. Chronic inflammatory diseases unrelated to the cardiovascular system—for example, chronic periodontal disease (inflamed gum tissue)—are associated with increased cardiovascular disease.[79]
4. Genetic variations that cause over-expression of interleukin-1 are associated with a more than three-fold increased risk of heart disease.*
5. Many people already have advanced atherosclerosis by the time insulin resistance, metabolic syndrome, or elevated cholesterol is first diagnosed. In other words, the chronic disease was progressing

---

*Sir Gordon Duff, M.D., Ph.D., at the University of Sheffield in the U.K., along with a group of scientists at Interleukin Genetics in the U.S., have done extensive research into the genetics of interleukin-1. Some people have been found to have a genetic predisposition for increased interleukin-1 inflammatory response, resulting in increased CRP and subsequent development of three- to four-fold increase in the risk of heart disease. The specific locations on the DNA have been identified and now can be specifically tested for commercially. I routinely test for this genetic predisposition at the institute where I consult.

Also, the researchers have found that there are some specific location abnormalities on the interleukin-1 gene that further increase the risk of heart disease, but do not increase CRP levels. Therefore, it becomes even more important to understand the "big picture" of inflammation—and to test for it—in order to estimate your genetic risk of developing heart disease and other chronic diseases. Now that this test is available, it is important for you to have it.

Fortunately, clinical trials involving specific supplements have already been done to show what we can do to reduce the expression of these genes. There are now natural products that have been clinically shown to reduce not only interleukin-1 production, but interleukin-1 gene expression as well.

rapidly long before the more acute disease was noted.

6. Some researchers are convinced that the rapid release of fatty acids from the visceral fat cells of obese people leads to insulin resistance, yet are unaware that the immune system, when chronically activated, may stimulate such energy release even in patients who are not obese or overweight.

7. Statin drugs, which are prescribed to reduce cholesterol levels, also reduce inflammation *and* seem to reduce the risk of other diseases, like colon cancer.[80] A huge study called the Jupiter Trial,[81] involving 17,802 people in twenty-five countries, gave a statin drug called Crestor® to people with low LDL cholesterol but elevated CRP, and reduced heart attacks, stroke, and cancer deaths in just two years. A different study which gave this same class of drugs to people with low LDL cholesterol and low CRP had no benefit.[82] The difference between these two studies shows obviously that lowering elevated CRP provided the benefit seen for both heart disease risk and cancer deaths!

8. Aspirin, an anti-inflammatory, not only reduces the risk of heart attacks,[83] but also prostate[84] and colon cancer,[85] among others.

9. The rates of most chronic diseases have risen sharply in countries that have become economically developed or Westernized—as in Japan following World War Two. This trend continues today as more countries become industrialized.

10. Some researchers have presented a very convincing case that the Mediterranean diet promotes good health primarily because it is rich in omega-3 fats,[86] healthy oils, and vegetables, all of which are anti-inflammatory.

11. Rheumatic and other inflammatory diseases, such as lupus, increase the risk of apparently unrelated diseases, like diabetes.[87]

12. Osteoporosis has been found to be caused by chronic inflammation. Osteoporosis, or thinning of the bones, occurs naturally with age but especially in post-menopausal women. Initially, osteoporosis was thought to be due to the withdrawal of estrogen in women. But when pre-menopausal women had their ovaries removed, thus creating a surgical menopause, it was noted that inflammatory cells increased immediately and were associated with bone thinning.[88] In

the same study, when inflammatory chemicals were blocked after surgery, almost no bone thinning occurred. Therefore, estrogen withdrawal during menopause is associated with increased inflammation. In further support of this, many studies have shown that inflammatory chemicals stimulate bone absorption.[89, 90, 91] Perhaps we will be able to protect more women from the risks of post-menopausal estrogen exposure in the future.

The list increases almost daily as new research unfolds.

There is a growing number of scientists who agree that inflammation is at the root of many chronic diseases.[92] Among them is Dr. Peter Libby, M.D., Professor of Medicine at Harvard Medical School and Chief of Cardiovascular Medicine at Brigham and Women's Hospital in Boston, who states in a review article, "While diseases such as atherosclerosis, rheumatoid arthritis, cirrhosis or interstitial lung disease may manifest in different ways, the same fundamental mechanisms and mediators drive the same process."[93]

FB

A MATCH IN A WINDSTORM

The immune system is incredibly complex, with many checks and balances and thousands of components. This book only mentions a few.

The immune system can generate thousands to millions of specialized white blood cells very rapidly—cells that are armed with toxic chemicals to kill invading viruses, bacteria, parasites, and abnormal cells, and which are smart enough not to attack the body's own normal, healthy cells.

And yet...fad hawkers want you to believe that the doorway to optimal health can be opened by a simple, single key—like reducing carbs or fat in your diet or taking a certain mystery supplement or doing ab crunches.

Even faddish things that *are* generally good for us, like the jogging craze or antioxidant supplements, are narrow in focus.

But most fad products don't even rise to that level. They're like trying to keep warm in a howling blizzard by lighting a match.

We need a comprehensive approach—a broad change in lifestyle—to achieve optimal health, because the opponent we face isn't a single player but a team with thousands of players that come at us from different directions with different skills and tactics.

The good news: The tactics we need to defeat chronic disease are, in fact, simple and easy—even if they are many. Any positive change in lifestyle is likely to improve our chances, but achieving *optimal* health means that we need to keep adding positive changes to our lives until we have countered the many, many ways in which our diets, our industrial environment and our modern lifestyles have compromised our immune systems by keeping them constantly turned on. Only a plan that involves a complete understanding of the whole picture and utilizes all the best resources, including nutrigenomics, will work for the rest of your life. That's what we have provided to you here in this optimal health manual.

What Keeps Our Immune Systems in Overdrive?

By now we know a better way to ask that question: What are the behaviors unique to industrial societies that over-stimulate the immune system, leading to chronic inflammation and resulting disease?

And we do know the main problem is behavioral—that it has to do with some combination of our own personal choices and environmental change brought about by human activity. It can't be due to genetic changes alone. Human genetic makeup doesn't change that fast or for no good reason.

So what are the significant lifestyle changes that have taken place in the last fifty years—the changes that have caused epidemic rises in chronic disease? Here are some examples of new factors in our lives that increase chronic inflammation:

- **High consumption of simple sugars**, like fructose (which we get in the ubiquitous processed-food component corn syrup),[94] increases CRP levels. See Appendix B.1 for more information about high fructose intake.

- **Trans fatty acids**, another too-common component of the modern diet,[95] are associated with elevated CRP levels.

- **High cholesterol intake.** When high levels of cholesterol were fed, in the form of mass-produced eggs, to otherwise healthy, lean, insulin-sensitive people, it caused their CRP levels to increase, as well as the bad cholesterols in their blood.[96]

- **Pollution**, as noted in the last chapter, is also associated with elevated CRP. We can't personally control some kinds of pollution, especially those which are airborne. But a good deal of chemical pollution comes to us in what we eat and drink. For example, diets high in animal fats are harmful not only because of the fats, but because mass-produced meat contains harmful chemicals such as herbicides, pesticides,[97] hormones, and antibiotics.

Solid research has shown that reducing those risk factors we've been talking about also reduces CRP levels in the blood. *So lifestyle modification is absolutely necessary in order to reduce the production of CRP.*

To sum up, our industrialized lifestyles are chronically inflammatory. To reduce the risk of chronic diseases such as heart disease, cancer, type 2 diabetes, and others, we need to reduce the inflammatory stimuli to which we are chronically exposed.

To that end, let me introduce to you . . .

DR. DUKE'S GAME PLAN

Seventeen Steps for Reducing Chronic Inflammation
You can reduce chronic inflammation in your body by taking these simple steps. The documentation for why these steps work is presented throughout this book.

1. **Reduce the risk factors for chronic disease.** This is the most impor-

tant, effective step you can take. These risk factors are listed and explained in chapters 9 through 12. Since virtually all of these risk factors are associated with inflammation, it follows that you can reduce inflammation by eliminating them from your life. In fact, research has shown this to be the case. Moreover, you don't have to achieve risk-factor perfection to improve your health. Reducing just one risk factor can make a very big difference for you.

2. **Consume natural anti-inflammatories like omega-3**. Modern diets have turned away from healthy oils like omega-3, which is a natural anti-inflammatory, in favor of cheap, inflammatory oils like corn oil. Increasing your intake of healthy polyunsaturated fatty acids (by eating cold-water fish and using olive and canola oils) has been shown to reduce inflammation.

3. **Exercise**. Research has shown that exercise is also associated with reduction of inflammation. I know lack of exercise is one of the risk factors included in item #1 on this list, but I can't emphasize it enough. Modern technology has left us increasingly motionless, on the mistaken theory that banishing all physical labor is a good thing. Technology has eliminated motion from almost every aspect of our lives, from the automobile to the escalator to the remote control to the personal computer. This "progress" is taking years off our lives. Human beings need to move to be healthy. (Disclaimer: Get your doctor's clearance before beginning any new exercise program.) Even simple walks near your residence, playing with your children in a park, etc. is exercise and will be beneficial. You don't have to join a club to participate in exercise which will reduce your risk of chronic disease. Even leisure-time walking has been shown to reduce inflammation,[98, 99] and adding dietary supplementation provides greater anti-inflammatory benefits.[100]

4. **Take a good multivitamin/multimineral** as described in chapter 8.[101]

5. **Reduce saturated, trans and omega-6 fatty acids in your diet.** These are the fats associated with inflammation. To avoid them, you will commonly also have to avoid processed foods, unless they are specifically labeled as containing no trans or saturated fats. Dark meats and partially hydrogenated oils contain omega-6. Oils that are higher in omega-6 are corn, safflower, cottonseed, sunflower,

peanut, sesame, grapeseed, primrose, and soybean oils (although soybean oil also has some omega-3). The *only* oils we recommend are canola and virgin olive oils.

6. **Take reasonable levels of antioxidant/anti-inflammatory supplements**, especially those that are rich in phytonutrients (like resveratrol), from concentrated food sources. Antioxidants have been shown to reduce inflammation (see chapter 8, where I'll also deal with the people who say supplementation is bad or dangerous). Among the nutrients or components that have been shown to reduce inflammation are: Coenzyme Q10,[102] lycopene,[103] magnesium,[104] glucosamine,[105] and quercetin.[106]

7. **Eat seven to nine servings of fruits and vegetables per day.** There is no substitute for eating vegetables and fruits. They are loaded with natural antioxidants and phytonutrients that reduce inflammation.[107] For example, one group of plant chemicals or phytonutrients has both antioxidant and anti-inflammatory qualities.[108] Examples in this group and food sources are quercetin (onions, kale, blueberries, broccoli and tea), flavenols (green tea and cocoa), hesperatin (tomatoes and oranges), flavones (parsley, celery), isoflavones (soy), and anthocyanins (grapes, beans, onions, and berries). Hopefully, you can see why there is no substitute for seven to nine daily servings of fruits and vegetables of different colors.

8. **Avoid processed foods.** I mean foods laden with high-fructose corn syrup, partially hydrogenated oils and other chemicals. The more chemicals added to your food via processing, the greater your chance of chronic inflammation. Yes, I know that heat-and-serve processed foods make your life easier. They can also make it shorter. So give it a try. Shop for helpful cookbooks, surf the Internet. You can find plenty of ways to make fast, easy meals using healthy, unprocessed foods. I will list the food additives to avoid in Appendix B.1. Some food additives, like high-fructose corn syrup, increase inflammation.[109]

9. **Avoid fast food.** Studies have shown that eating fast food increases the inflammatory response in the body.[110] This is most likely related to the quality of fast food due to its cheap ingredients which are inflammatory and mentioned elsewhere.

10. **Eat organically grown and raised fruits, vegetables, meats, and dairy products.** The herbicides, pesticides, hormones, and antibiotics used in industrial farming and food production are still present when you serve meats, fruits, grains, vegetables, and dairy products to your family. Usually these chemicals are absorbed and stored in the fatty portions of the plant or animal. Stuff that is sprayed on plants is still there when it is fed to the animals you're going to eat—and when it's fed to you. Antibiotics and hormones are given to animals to make them grow faster in the weeks before they are slaughtered. When *you* eat these products, they are then transferred to the fat deposits in *your* body and stored there. These chemicals can build up and cause chronic inflammation. The different classifications of organic foods are explained in Appendix A.10. Some manufacturers try to imply that their products are more organic than they really are. The more a product is truly organic, the better it is for you. Don't forget to always wash the organic produce, though, because it can still have bacteria on the outside.

11. **Eat carbohydrates with a low glycemic load.** That means they are low in simple sugars. The higher the sugar load in your diet, the greater your risk of elevated CRP.[111, 112] One study reports a 28 percent reduction in CRP when patients were given a whole-food vegan diet rich in soluble fiber.[113] Note that I only recommend that you use the low glycemic carbohydrates, not the low glycemic meal plans or diets. The reasoning for this is explained in Appendix C.

12. **Follow the nutrigenomics guidelines in chapter 4.** All recommendations in this book—including Appendix B, which includes a one-week sample 2,000-calorie menu and a section on food contents to avoid—are all based upon the best nutrigenomic scientific information. The menu I created in Appendix B.4 is compared with the USDA "My Pyramid" diet to show you how I would significantly improve upon that menu by using nutrigenomic information. The "My Pyramid" diet is widely considered in the scientific community to be a rather sound program and menu, but I think we can make it better.

13. **Take low-dose aspirin or another anti-inflammatory.** (Of course, do this only with the clearance of your doctor.) Established medicine

has recommended aspirin to patients for years to reduce the risk of having heart attacks because of its tendency to reduce clotting in the arteries. However, we found to our surprise a few years ago that people who have taken aspirin for many years also have a reduced risk of colon cancer. The aspirin helped reduce the inflammation that can lead to chronic diseases in addition to heart disease.

I'm hesitant to suggest this, though, because blocking inflammation with medicines is associated with frequent complications, such as increased infections,[114] poor heart or circulatory effects,[115, 116] lung complications,[117] ulcers,[118] and other possible complications.[119] Despite these significant negative side effects, there are more than 80 million prescriptions written annually just in the U.S. to treat inflammatory diseases. This number doesn't even include over-the-counter use. Nevertheless, anti-inflammatory medicines have a definite role and have been extremely beneficial. The message here is that you should talk with your doctor so that you use them as little as possible, knowing that there are side effects and problems associated with their use. Overall, the ideal scenario is to reduce all inflammatory sources in our life through lifestyle change and natural anti-inflammatory food components as much as possible. This book is dedicated to teaching you to accomplish this goal in the best way possible.

14. **Take adequate amounts of vitamin D.** Vitamin D supplementation has been shown to be associated with reduced inflammation.[120, 121] Vitamin D and calcium together have been shown to also reduce inflammation.[122] Additional information concerning vitamin D will be presented in chapter 8.

15. **Get adequate sleep.** Inadequate sleep increases inflammation.[123, 124, 125, 126] (See chapter 6.)

16. **Reduce salt intake.** High salt intake increases inflammation.[127]

17. **Talk to your doctor.** If you rigorously follow the first sixteen steps, you often won't need medication. But if you can't reduce your chronic inflammation to a healthy level, then talk to your doctor and he or she may recommend taking prescription medicines, such as statins, which have been shown to reduce CRP. From the results of the Jupiter study discussed earlier, the greatest benefit of statins

seem to be in their ability to reduce inflammation. ❖

This list hits the big things, the high-reward lifestyle changes. Making these changes is certain to reduce inflammation in your body dramatically. I know it's a longish list, and some of the changes I suggest may seem difficult now. But please, please don't let that intimidate you. You don't have to go whole-hog on every item on the list to significantly improve your health. Even one or two sincere, consistent changes can make a dramatic difference in your chances of developing disease.

Do what you can now. Try to do more later.

Chapter 13 will list Twenty-Five Easy Steps to Optimal Health. Taking those steps will help you reduce inflammation and your risk of chronic disease. I've taken a lot of science and broken it down into easy steps for you. Please be patient, though, and don't skip ahead. There's more you need to learn.

An Important Note About CRP and Judging Inflammation Status

There are many inflammatory molecules in the body, and just because CRP is not elevated, that doesn't mean that one of the others aren't elevated. Generally, I don't recommend that we base our interpretation as to whether we have chronic inflammation on blood values, like CRP, alone. (Occasionally it is useful, but I don't recommend it as the gold standard by any means.) Please remember that CRP can be elevated with recent colds, infections, skin wounds, significant arthritis, chronic gum disease, and the like. In these cases, your immune system is functioning appropriately to protect you. When I refer to chronically elevated CRP, I mean those situations where you don't have one of these conditions and yet your CRP is still elevated. (More than one measure of CRP would help you understand what your baseline level is.) This concept is why many researchers have been confused by CRP levels and their prediction of chronic inflammatory status. The vast majority of studies haven't controlled for these temporary or confounding conditions/situations. We have discussed CRP extensively only because a great deal of research has been done on this molecule. There is increasing evidence, though, that CRP *is* a good marker to determine heart disease risk.[128, 129] Obtaining a CRP as a baseline and a generalized monitor of inflammatory status probably is reasonable but many questions still remain.

This is the reason why I don't recommend that everyone race out and get inflammatory panels at this point or base everything you believe about your health on the CRP alone. We are working with such panels now, but it is too early to make any recommendations. I can assure you based on a vast body of scientific research that if you have risk factors for chronic disease (as will be explained in chapters 9 through 12), you have chronic inflammation. If you aren't doing essentially all the seventeen steps above to reduce inflammation, you have chronic inflammation to some degree. Determining the number of risk factors for chronic disease is probably the best way for most of us to determine our inflammatory status. This is why it takes a revolution in thought about lifestyle and health.

Hopefully you can clearly see that a fad diet that helps you lose a few pounds is bound to fail eventually because true success in achieving optimal health should be defined as longevity and reduction in chronic disease rather than looking like your favorite movie star. What good is it to get thin from a method that will cause you to die prematurely?

Now that we have helped you build an understanding of inflammation's role in chronic disease, let's move on to a discussion of two exciting new fields of science — nutrigenetics and nutrigenomics.

Don't let the scientific jargon stress you out. You're about to learn a great deal about how to eat and live in order to achieve optimal health.

The recommendations in this book are largely based on these fields of study. They are new areas of science that most "experts," including most physicians, know almost nothing about. Once you grasp these concepts — and they're not difficult — you will be in the vanguard of preventive medicine.

CHAPTER 4

Nutrigenetics and Nutrigenomics: The New Health Sciences

By now I hope you understand that attaining optimal health has to do with the complex relationships between the food that we eat, our behaviors, and our genetic makeup. You've seen that inflammation is now understood to be a common, underlying cause of chronic disease.

Now it's time to learn about two relatively new areas of scientific study that are revealing the fundamental ways in which nutrients and genes interact. You already have some understanding of nutrigenetics (even if you haven't heard the word before now) but the concept of nutrigenomics is probably new to most readers.

Long scientific dissertations have already been written on these two new sciences. You will be relieved to know that I'll only spend a few pages on them here, and I'll discuss them in simple terms. But the information you're about to absorb is critical to an understanding of eating for optimal health. It will also help you understand why single-issue fads are wrong-headed and generally bad for you.

Also, these next few pages will further confirm why the recommendations in this book, though based in part on very recent research, will stand the test of time—specifically, because they are in agreement with human genetics.

In fact, all aspects of this book are in agreement with the best and most advanced science.

Nutrigenetics

The term *nutrigenetics* was first used in a book by Dr. R.O. Brennan in 1975. It is the study of how genetic differences cause people to respond differently to the same nutrients. This happens with regard to both macronutrients (proteins, carbohydrates, and fat) and micronutrients (vitamins, minerals, and phytonutrients). Let me give you some examples.

DNA molecules in the nuclei of our cells are the memory banks containing all the genetic information we need in order to grow from a single cell and live. Each cell in body contains the same DNA. DNA is like an ingenious computer program, directing all our body's specialized cells to function in different ways and to make different chemicals as needed.

Each person is born with a genetic program that is absolutely unique, except in the case of identical twins, who have identical programming. Variation in certain DNA segments is the reason no two people look exactly alike, except identical twins. (Their environments are not exactly the same, though, so even identical twins begin to look different over time.) We have the same kind of differences in the parts of our genetic programming that affect our health. *Polymorphism* is the term applied to variations in a particular DNA segment between individuals. When you walk down the street and see people with black, brown, red, and blond hair, you're looking at an example of polymorphism.

Researchers have discovered DNA segment variations, or polymorphisms, that will cause some people who are given a moderate-fat diet to respond with high triglycerides and low LDL levels in their blood.[130] If you had this variation in your genes, you could sit at the dinner table with your spouse, enjoying the identical meal, but your bodies would respond to that meal in very different ways. Your family doctor might be haranguing you to change your diet, get more exercise, and take a medication, while telling your spouse he or she was doing fine, even though you were eating the same diet.

This is why *there is no single diet plan that is ideal for every individual in the world.*

Another example of nutritional polymorphism is the different ways people respond to salt. Salt causes some people's blood pressure to rise, but not others'.[121, 132] This helps explain why there has been confusion about salt intake and hypertension over the years. In most people, salt intake does not cause blood pressure to rise, but for some it's a real problem. So the news media broadcast confusing, conflicting reports about salt, while the food marketing industry tells us all to fear sodium and buy low-sodium products (less salt, higher price), even though moderate salt intake is only a problem for some of us.

The confusion created by the daily barrage of health reporting in popular media can be very discouraging. One day a certain food is a panacea for our health problems, and the next week we're told that same food portends certain untimely death. Sometimes these conflicts of information arise from poor research or poor interpretation, including shoddy use of statistics. Sometimes it's because different studies were performed on groups of people with different characteristics, or from different cultures with different sets of genetic tendencies. The most reliable research usually comes from the most respected journals, where the authors' professional peers have reviewed the research.

As the science of nutrigenetics expands and develops, we will soon be so well informed about our genetics that each of us will know which foods or substances to avoid and which ones to favor. You will base your decisions not on popular opinion, but on what is best for *you*, given your specific genetic makeup. It's hard to say how soon custom diet recommendations based on each individual's nutrigenetics will become commonplace, but this field of research is already beginning to have an impact.

Nutrigenomics

Nutrigenomics is probably a very new concept for you, but it has even greater impact on your health than nutrigenetics. Nutrigenomics is the study of how the nutrients we eat interact with our DNA. Both macronutrients and micronutrients can affect how our DNA is expressed. They are not merely sources of calories or isolated molecules that perform specific jobs. The quality of the diet that we eat is absolutely critical to our health, because it literally affects our genes.

I will provide several dramatic examples of discoveries in the area of nutrigenomics. You'll notice a direct correlation between risk factors we'll be discussing all through this book and the new nutrigenomic research.

Omega-3 fatty acids in the diet reduce the ability of the DNA to make the enzymes needed to produce the inflammatory molecule interleukin-1.[133, 134] All the nagging you'll be getting from me about taking your omega-3? Now you know why. Omega-3 literally suppresses the body's ability to make this inflammatory molecule. It is a natural anti-inflammatory—medicine in the form of salmon fat and olive oil. Obtaining omega-3 from natural sources is generally very safe, but some of you may find supplementation more convenient. (Warning: Before you begin taking an omega-3 supplement, you should consult with your doctor, especially if you are on blood thinners such as warfarin.)

Nutrigenomics research has provided a new perspective on the incredible influence omega-3 has in our lives. In light of our new understanding of inflammation's role in chronic disease, you can see why cultures like Greece and Italy, whose traditional diets included large amounts of omega-3, had lower incidence of chronic disease. We've known for quite a while that the so-called Mediterranean diet has great health benefits. Now, thanks to nutrigenomic research, we know why. Today you can rest assured that there will be little media panic over conflicting findings regarding omega-3, because its effect has been observed and proven at the level of DNA function.

You may have heard about the scientific research which has shown that severe calorie restriction results in increased longevity. If you're like me, you'd find that this type of lifestyle is very difficult to follow, though. You should be greatly relieved to learn that the main factor most likely involved in the benefit of severe caloric restriction[135] was also found—through the study of nutrigenomics—to be controlled by omega-3! In other words, instead of starving yourself with extremely severe caloric restriction in order to live longer, you can most likely achieve the same benefit from omega-3.[136, 137]

Another example: Vitamin D affects the immune system in several ways. It seems to slow down inflammation and boost antibody production, and it may promote T-cell activity, too.[138] It functions as a hormone and has many other effects on the body. Vitamin D is regenerated by exposure of the skin to sunlight; you can get more of it through supplementation or dairy products that are vitamin D fortified. Recent research has found that in extreme northern and southern latitudes, many Caucasians have low vitamin D levels toward the end of winter. This problem is exacerbated by our replacing milk consumption with sweetened drinks. In light of its effect on our immune system, it's easy to see how low levels of vitamin D are associated with increased cancer risk.

One researcher has concluded that approximately *fifty human genetic diseases* can be treated or reduced with multivitamins, based on the action of vitamins at the DNA level.[139] Given the high amounts of processed food and fast food in the typical diets of industrialized nations, a multivitamin has long been considered a good idea. Our modern diets leave some huge nutritional gaps that need to be filled. Nutrigenomics only lends further support to this recommendation. Unfortunately, there are thousands of physicians around the world—typically doctors who were last exposed to nutritional training thirty years ago in medical school—who discourage their patients from taking supplements, because they are unaware of current research.

Yet another example: Zinc has been shown to reduce inflammation by suppressing interleukin-6 production at the DNA level.[140] This helps explain how zinc has been associated with reduction of certain chronic diseases. Vitamin E has also been shown to have anti-inflammatory effects because of its ability to suppress the production of interleukin-1 and tumor necrosis factor.[141]

In addition to diet, our behavior can influence gene expression. Exercise has been shown to do this.[142] In fact, exercise triggers the expression of many genes in a progressive order, depending on the duration and intensity of the workout.[143]

These findings show that many of the activities and risk factors that we participate in affect our body at the most basic level. This is why all of the risk factors that I will teach you in chapters 9 through 12 are important to your health.

Nutrition scientists have found that that cruciferous vegetables (like broccoli, Brussels sprouts, cauliflower, kale, mustard greens, rutabagas, and turnips) affect the genes of enzymes that can reduce cancer risk.[144] A component in green tea helps keep cells from becoming cancerous.[145] Resveratrol, a chemical found in grapes and other foods, has shown anti-inflammatory and anticancer effects by reducing interleukin-8 production.[146] (Much of the cardiovascular benefit ascribed to red wine is probably from this phytonutrients, which are also found in grape juice.) Components of garlic have been shown to stimulate production of enzymes that help destroy dangerous chemicals.[147] A compound in black tea has been shown to reduce inflammation through its effect on the DNA.[148]

Foods can also stimulate DNA in harmful ways. For example, high dietary fructose increases inflammation.[149] Dietary intake of inflammatory omega-6 fatty acids (found in cheap oils, dark meat, and fast foods) has been shown to cause our DNA to effect the production or release of the worst forms of cholesterol.[150]

These are only a few examples from the growing body of knowledge that is nutrigenomic research. Prospective studies on food intake that are currently ongoing will soon provide more information about how food influences our DNA.[151, 152] I hope this information has helped you see how important what we eat and drink is to our health. Too often we think of food as nothing more than filler to reduce our hunger pangs. We feel we're too busy to read food labels, which sometimes tell us that what we are about to eat can be very dangerous to our health. When you pick out fresh produce or meat, you at least glance at it to see if it is moldy or spoiled. You need to do this with packaged foods, too, by reading the labels. Taking this kind of precaution now is especially important, since many of the effects of poor nutrition and harmful ingredients don't show up for months or years.

That's true for fast foods, too, not just packaged ones. If you rely on fast food to streamline your busy life, then chapter 11 will provide a lot of insight into how that can increase your risk of disease. The fast-food industry does *not* have your optimal health at the top of its list of priorities.

Someday perhaps everyone will have his or her DNA sequenced at birth, so that we can design an optimal nutritional plan for each person's life. I'm not recommending that now—the cost would probably be so high that it would give you a heart attack, which would more or less offset any benefit. However, specific genetic testing is already coming into use, and it will soon be common for patients with family histories of certain diseases or those who have significant health problems themselves. Some genetic tests available today will likely prove to be excellent screening tests, especially in the area of inflammation tendencies, such as interleukin-1.

The main idea I want you to take from this chapter is that **what we eat and drink has a powerful effect on our health**, now and for the rest of our lives. Your diet affects every level of organ and cell function. I also want you to understand that the risk factors I've listed and the recommendations I make are based on both solid, traditional research and newly unfolding areas of study that involve gene expression. When you grasp these simple concepts, you won't be chasing every new fad the promises you better health. You will understand that optimal health is a total-lifestyle thing.

And here's the best news: As complex as the science is—involving thousands of chemicals, billions of cells, and terribly complex codes written in microscopic DNA strands—the game plan for optimal health is pretty simple and very easy to follow.

Because it involves general and gradual lifestyle change, this game plan is easier to follow than almost all the fads. (That's why they're fads: People pay their money, follow the fad for a while, and then drop it because it turned out to be a big pain with little or no gain.)

In order to win your best life, you *will* need to change your lifestyle. But you can do so confident that the recommendations this book makes are based on powerful scientific research.

The sciences of nutrigenetics and nutrigenomics will soon make big, exciting changes in our lives. When broad genetic testing becomes commonplace, it will be possible to determine in detail which foods and drinks are best for you, and which ones to avoid. Diet and supplementation will be personalized, custom-designed exactly for your own genetic makeup. This science will take much of the guesswork out of interpreting new research and applying it to your personal health. Many of the conflicts in scientific information will be resolved. These new frontiers hold great hope for improving your health.

If you would like to learn more about nutrigenetics and nutrigenomics, I would suggest an outstanding book by Artemis Simopoulos, M.D., of the Center for Genetics, Nutrition and Health in Washington, D.C., entitled *Nutrigenetics and Nutrigenomics*.[153] However, this book is definitely written for people with strong scientific backgrounds.

I could write an entire book just on nutrigenomics, but I will limit the topic at this point. So you can relax! But know that all the recommendations in this book are based upon this newest science of nutrigenomics and are very consistent. My teaching doesn't involve contradictory guidelines that will sometimes increase inflammation and other times decrease it, as most other authors who aren't knowledgeable about nutrigenomics have done. At the institute where I consult, we work with many of the leading researchers in this field.

In the next chapter we'll tackle an issue that has been a source of frustration and misinformation for millions of people around the world for decades—the difference between Western and Eastern medicine.

Many proponents of fads and popular health programs have told you that Eastern medicine, with its focus on balance, has all the answers for achieving optimal health. Others preach that Western medicine, based on science and technology, is the only "real" medical discipline. In reality, both traditions have weaknesses. *People all over the world are dying of the same diseases*, no matter what medical tradition holds sway in their countries.

Since I treat thousands of people from all around the world—people who live with many different medical traditions—I have a unique perspective. I have documented how these traditions affect the health of our patients. It isn't theory at our institute.

So whether your preferred path to a healthy life inclines more to the mystical or the scientific, the next chapter should make the truth clear.

PART III:

Pathway to Optimal Health

CHAPTER 5

Eastern vs. Western Medicine:
Where the Twain Shall Meet

had just finished speaking to a convention of five thousand people in Utah when a well-dressed, white-haired businessman approached me. His expression betrayed anxiety, even fear. I do my best at these occasions to fill people with hope and encouragement, so I wondered what I might have said wrong.

I wish the problem *had* been some blunder on my part. Instead, I quickly learned that the man was worried about a serious heart ailment. He had been experiencing palpitations for some time because of an abnormal heart rhythm, for which his physician had prescribed a strong anti-arrhythmic medication. I knew this medication is not routinely given unless the abnormal rhythm is fairly dangerous, so I asked if he was taking it as prescribed. He said that he wasn't, in a tone that bordered on defiance.

The man didn't want to talk to me about his prescription, but to find out what herbal remedy he might take in its place. I was momentarily dumbfounded by this, and his wife must have noticed the shocked look on my face. She explained, reluctantly and with a hint of despair in her voice, that her husband refused to take the medication because he didn't trust Western medicine. She was a registered nurse, but neither her professional training nor her love for her husband had been enough to break down the stone wall he had built around the idea that the Western approach to medicine was somehow fraudulent. The emotion I saw in his face was the fear that his decision could be fatal.

I told him that yes, herbs are the basis of some cardiac medications used today, but it wouldn't be wise to depend on herbs to treat this arrhythmia. We spoke for several minutes. I encouraged him to get back on his medication. Unmoved, he solemnly walked away.

I wish I had had time to find out why he felt so strongly. Perhaps he or a loved one had some horrible experience with a doctor or hospital. Unfortunately, the guy isn't alone in his distrust. Many people reject Western medicine altogether. If you are one of those, I beg you to read this chapter, leaving your mind open just a crack. There is a solution. I want to help you see it.

Paranoid or disillusioned individuals aren't the only people perpetuating an unreasonable bias against Western medicine. Sadly, our mail, newspapers, magazines, and airwaves are rife with solicitations to buy products, services, and literature promoted as "alternative medicine." And sadder yet, many of these sales pitches come from physicians, scientists, and other people claiming expertise—all bashing Western medicine and its practitioners.

Some of these people claim that physicians make decisions about your health in order to earn kickback payments from pharmaceutical companies or hospitals. Or they use phrases like, "We'll tell you what your doctor is hiding from you . . ." or "Our revolutionary product cures . . ." Of course they present themselves as having pristine integrity, but the truth is that they just have a product to sell—generally a product of unproven value.

Of course, when it comes to health claims and marketing, everybody is bound by professional codes and the law, at least in most countries. In the U.S., a doctor caught taking kickbacks can lose his license and go to jail. And such a doctor is very likely to get caught. Both the government and insurance companies monitor not only physicians' referrals and prescriptions to make sure they are appropriate, but their investments as well.

The law requires pharmaceutical companies go through long, expensive research and testing processes to get new drugs to market. On the other hand, supplements, including herbals, aren't subject to mandatory testing to prove claims prior to marketing. As a trade-off, their makers aren't allowed to promise health benefits or cures without proving those claims through research, but there are plenty of ways to let people know that a certain herb is supposed to "support the normal function" of your heart, prostate, or whatever.

Unfortunately, too many advertisers push beyond the limits of the laws governing health claims, and sell a lot of questionable products before the Food and Drug Administration reins them in.

And yet, the noisy lunatic fringe wants you to believe there is a conspiracy among doctors and drug companies, in which doctors profit from writing prescriptions. This claim is mind-boggling to me. I don't get paid for writing prescriptions, and I don't know of anyone who does. It is both unethical and, to my understanding, illegal. I've heard that there are doctors in very influential university or governmental positions who receive significant amounts of money from pharmaceutical companies to influence their opinions and practices, but if these relationships do exist, they are outside of my radar screen. Nevertheless, I have read a lot of biased research and suspect that there probably are physicians who have "sold their soul" to pharmaceutical companies. (I'll discuss these misleading people in chapter 8.) That said, though, the average physician I know has high integrity concerning such matters. No physician of any quality would choose to prescribe a drug simply because he or she was invited to a continuing-education dinner.

And then there are the crazy claims that the medical profession is withholding cures for cancer—sort of like the old stories about oil companies buying up the patent on the mythical one-thousand-mile-per-gallon carburetor. Aside from the obvious—that doctors devote their lives, including many years of grueling, expensive education, to healing people—there is a fundamental flaw in virtually any similar medical conspiracy theory. For a conspiracy to be successful, there have to be a lot of like-minded people "in on it." There is no such thing as a conspiracy involving hundreds of thousands of medical professionals, scientists, and drug-company employees. Do you believe that not one person out of that many would come forward? Such a whistle-blower would become the most famous doctor in the world.

And whoever brought that cure to market would become the richest doctor in the world. It would be worth the trouble just to be rid of the billing and management problems!

Another of my favorite phony claims is that physicians typically die young, proving that they don't know what they're talking about. Though the newsletters and ads that contain such startling discoveries sound convincing, they're unfounded.

According to a 2003 study, the average physician's lifespan is seventy-six years, which is not significantly different from the general population's.[154] My family doctor, who passed away at ninety-four, would hardly agree with the foolish claims concerning physicians dying young. In a study of the thirty-four scientists in the world known to be over one hundred years old, six were physicians.[155]

The urban legend that physicians live to only fifty-two years of age, propagated by self-proclaimed scientific "experts," seems to have arisen from a scientific study of the lifespan of doctors who graduated from a medical school in Japan between 1926 and 1974. This time period conveniently includes World War Two. The authors of this study state: "This [physicians' average lifespan] was not different from the future life expectancy...of the general population."[156] Sadly, a great many people died too soon in Japan and elsewhere during that time.

Not only did those Japanese physicians have the same lifespan as the general public, but theirs is obviously not representative of the lifespan of physicians all over the world today, as these "experts" have implied. Anyone who has spread this information is either uninformed, didn't check the sources of their facts, or purposely passed on misleading information. If a company has tried to mislead you in the past, they will mislead you in the future.

Talk about one's own integrity is cheap when you aren't required to back it up. Buyer beware!

I know well over a thousand physicians, and the vast majority live very healthy lives. As knowledgeable doctors, most choose lifestyles that correspond closely the reduced risk factors I describe in chapters 9 through 12. The most common risk factor I see in physicians is stress.

There's a surprise! Medicine is a high-stress profession. Doctors frequently make life-and-death decisions. They work long hours. But they knew that going in. It's the extraneous problems of rising liability insurance premiums, the endless red tape of insurance billing, changes in government insurance and regulations, and rising overhead costs that are most responsible for driving physicians out of the medical practice. Those physicians who leave the profession still love the art of medicine and patient care, but are unable to tolerate the rest.

The Problems with Western Medicine

Thanks for bearing with me through the preceding screed. Those things need to be said. I feel better now.

On the other hand, there *are* significant problems with Western medicine. Medicine is a business, the livelihood of millions of people. In the West, health care is paid for by private, group or government insurance. With the rapid rise of health-care costs, medicine has become very political. For example, few people realize that when a plaintiff in a malpractice case is awarded millions of dollars by a jury, the cost is paid by the malpractice insurance company, not the doctor who was sued. That means the cost of the judgment is shared by all physicians, who in turn to pass their increased costs on to all patients—or rather, to the insurance companies, to which patients pay premiums. Even truly frivolous lawsuits are expensive—it costs thousands in legal fees to get them dismissed.

A more fundamental problem has to do with the way Western companies buy health care. The problem is pretty much the same whether a given nation has a private or government health insurance system, or a mixture of both as in the United States.

The problem is this: Physicians are paid for diagnosing and treating disease, but not, generally speaking, for preventing it. I don't mean to say that doctors are cynical about this—the profession is conscientious about counseling people to lead healthier lives. But the economics of Western medicine make it impossible for doctors to spend any serious amount of time on preventive medicine.

Because physicians are paid for treating sickness or injury, that is where their primary focus has to be. Disease diagnosis becomes their main emphasis by default. Certainly, much of doctors' work involves prevention; a common example would be treating elevated cholesterol with medication in order to reduce the risk of heart disease. But that is still based on a diagnosis (hypercholesterolemia), and involves a treatment that is quick and easy for the doctor—he or she just writes a prescription.

Ideally, that doctor would have spent hours with that patient years prior, counseling him on how to avoid high cholesterol in the first place. Even once the problem arose, there should have been extensive education on diet, exercise, lifestyle, and the use of natural products to significantly lower the patient's cholesterol. Unfortunately, though, no insurance company will pay a physician the money he or she needs to stay in practice for seeing only two to four patients per day. Time is money. In fact, many of the medical groups that employ physicians carefully monitor the average time each doctor spends with patients. If the doc moves too slowly, or if he doesn't see enough patients per day, he's encouraged to speed up or move on to another practice. In some respects, Western medicine is woefully far behind Eastern medicine when it comes to prevention and seeing patients as complete individuals.

However, based in science and grown in wealthy societies, Western medicine has provided the greatest health-care advances in the history of the world. Antibiotics and vaccines save millions of people from lethal diseases that only a few decades ago spread fear and misery throughout the world. Technological and surgical advancements now prolong and save lives with procedures that until recently seemed like the stuff of science fiction.

And yet, physicians are human. Sometimes they make mistakes that result in harm or death to their patients. None of us is perfect, but in modern societies we tend to set a very high standard for physicians. It's understandable that a person like the man I met at that Utah convention—or someone who has lost a loved one through a doctor's error—might distrust Western medicine.

If that is the case, where does one go?

The Problems with Eastern Medicine

A few years ago, young woman called our office for help because she was unable to sleep. The cause of her insomnia was heartbreaking: her thirty-year-old husband had recently died. He came back from a morning run one day, opened the kitchen door, and dropped dead in front of his wife and their small children.

We were stunned because he was a patient of ours, and we knew he did not have a problem with his heart. His only risk factors had been mild hypertension and being slightly overweight. Upon careful questioning, his wife told us that he had recently started taking an herbal product to lose weight. It contained ma huang, also known as ephedra, a substance that can cause abnormal heart rhythms. An autopsy revealed that the young man did not die of a heart attack, but of an abnormal heart rhythm. He had significant amounts of ephedra in his blood.

His wife successfully sued the supplement manufacturer, but whatever judgment she received obviously could never have compensated for the loss of her husband.

FB

SAFE, ALL-NATURAL, USED IN CHINA FOR 5,000 YEARS!

"Natural" is another of those advertising buzzwords that we mistakenly equate with "good, safe, and pure."

You want some enlightening examples of "all-natural"? Poison mushrooms. Toxic berries. Cocaine. Heroin. Snake venom. And that ma huang stuff you just read about.

Health food stores offer many genuinely natural products that are not safe. Ma huang continued to be sold for about eight years *after* our patient died, until it was finally outlawed in the U.S. Shortly before it was banned, ma huang was a billion-dollar industry, even though its health risks were well known.

Another common advertising claim is that a product must be safe if it has been used for centuries or millennia. Ma huang has been used in China for 5,000 years, and it isn't safe. Many traditional herbs contain heavy metals (which are widely used in the Ayurvedic medicine of India) that are toxic to the liver. Just because people have used them since the dawn of civilization doesn't mean they are safe. (You'll note that most of the people born since the dawn of civilization are now dead, and most of them lived short, sickly lives compared to humans today.)

Many Eastern medicine practices haven't undergone the types of rigorous, double-blind, randomly selected research that most components of Western medicine do. Without scientific scrutiny, it is almost impossible to tell if any appearance of benefit was merely due to placebo effect or coincidence.

Last year, a man in his twenties sought medical attention because of a sudden loss of speech. He had had similar episodes since he started taking herbal weight-loss products six months prior, but this was the worst.

A CAT scan revealed that he had bleeding inside his skull. Ephedra again? Nope. The label on his weight-loss product proudly announced that it was ephedra-free. But it did contain bitter orange, which is suspected of being just as dangerous. It's true that this patient had a preexisting health problem, but that's all the more reason he shouldn't have been taking this supplement. Bitter orange and similar natural products can be purchased from health food stores today, but that does not mean they are safe for you.

Some argue that we tend to use herbs differently in the U.S. today compared to traditional herbalism. I agree. But people also died from toxic stuff they got from traditional herbalists.[157, 158, 159] Carefully controlled, high-tech analysis has *not* been done on traditional herbs until recently, and the research is grossly incomplete. What we do know is that people have died from toxic herbal exposure for thousands of years, and their herbal practitioners didn't know why. I have visited the offices of traditional herbal practitioners in the Far East. I find that these practitioners are uniformly unable to list the active biochemical ingredients in the bat wings and turtle ashes they have on display.

I mean no disrespect. But like Western medicine, the Eastern tradition has its problems.

In addition to its technological deficiencies, many aspects of traditional medicine practices are heavily influenced by religious belief. Many ancient civilizations saw disease and its treatment in light of their religions. I don't want to challenge anyone's religion, but religious tradition doesn't guarantee positive medical outcome. Many of today's successful treatments have evolved through centuries of trial and error.

Eastern medicine is influenced by Eastern religion. Principles of yin and yang, Chi, meridians, yoga, meditation, and acupuncture all have religious connections. Many of these treatments have been studied scientifically to determine their health effects and found not to be any more beneficial than a placebo.[160] Studies that do report positive findings frequently were not double-blind (where neither researcher nor subject knows who is getting the treatment) or lacked adequate controls.

Some Eastern treatments, especially herbal remedies, have been beneficial to millions for millennia. But this doesn't mean that a Westerner has to go East in order to become healthy. Some well-known mind-body authors write as if the only path to good health is through their particular religious practices. That's silly. I've evaluated the health of thousands who currently live in Eastern countries and are practicing believers in Eastern religions. As a group, they are just as sick as Westerners, with the same chronic diseases and death rates. Nearly one in five type 2 diabetics in the world lives in India. (It's estimated that it will be one in four by 2030.[161]) The World Health Organization estimates that over 60 million people will die of chronic disease in India in the next ten years.[162] In China, a leading child-health researcher commenting on the increase of obesity among Chinese children in the last decade states, "The speed of growth is shocking."[163] The crisis that is the growth of chronic disease isn't a Western phenomenon. It is global.

Again, I do not disparage any Eastern religion. My position is just the opposite. Some in the West have broken important Eastern religious practices into "fun exercises" for profit, which I think is quite demeaning. I respect the world's major religions too much to agree with important doctrinal practices being converted by hotel spas, health clubs, and gyms into a degrading form so that they can make money.

What I want to clarify is that certain "expert" authors are extremely biased and have misled people. I have many clients and friends who hold their Eastern religious beliefs deeply, and I respect their beliefs. In fact, for reasons I'll discuss in chapter 9, I encourage all people to pursue their beliefs sincerely. My point is simply that there is not necessarily any health benefit in changing your religion from Buddhism to Judaism, from Christianity to Hinduism or the like. Your religious decisions should be based on faith or beliefs, not health reasons, as some promote.

If you're paying attention, you're probably now a step ahead of me. You're probably saying to yourself, "The Eastern and Western traditions both have their strengths and weaknesses. Isn't there a way to combine the best of both worlds?"

Voilà!

Preventive Medicine: The Best of Both Worlds

Oh, East is East, and West is West, and never the twain
shall meet . . .

So wrote Rudyard Kipling. But what did *he* know?

Preventive medicine, as practiced at our institute, is a fusion of the best of the two medical traditions. We have sought to bridge the gap, and have made considerable progress in doing so.

Specifically, we employ the best of Eastern preventive practice, including scientifically justified use of herbal supplements, while applying the rigorous scientific standards of Western diagnostics, medications, treatments, and procedures only when necessary.

This isn't "alternative" medicine. It is a synthesis of the best of East and West, supported by sound scientific research.

Here's what happens when a client comes to us for a health assessment.

We survey our patient's nutritional and health habits and obtain accurate determinations of his or her basic metabolic rate. Given that information, we provide education on balanced nutrition and guidance on caloric intake, all based on the best research, including nutrigenomics. After examining our client's exercise habits, medical history, and health assessment, we provide customized exercise and lifestyle programs to fit his or her daily life.

Our cutting-edge health assessments include specialized blood profiles that measure levels of antioxidants, fatty acid profiles including omega-3 fat, and hs-C-reactive protein, among other factors. We run sub-maximal cardiac stress tests and check for the development of atherosclerosis with a test that measures carotid intima media thickness (CIMT). We screen for osteoporosis, and for those with risk factors or evidence of bone thinning we provide DEXA scans for accurate assessment.

We obtain risk factor histories and run genetic tests and other studies, all designed to identify any tendencies or risks for chronic disease and inflammation. All of these tests are necessary to make the best lifestyle recommendations—accurately and in detail. They all fit together beautifully.

We conclude with personalized physician consultations focused on reducing risk factors and chronic inflammation, so that we can best assist the patient's personal physician.

Ideally, true preventive medicine of the highest degree would begin before conception. A baby's future health is dependant upon the chronic inflammatory status and health of the mother during pregnancy.[164, 165] Our industrialized diets have even affected breast milk contents. As our diets have increased in the intake of inflammatory omega-6 fats found in cheap oils (like corn oil) and dark meats, it has also increased in human breast milk, thus increasing children's chronic inflammation at birth. Human breast milk in the U.S. today has a two-fold higher omega-6 content than in the 1950s.[166,167] This would be true for essentially every developed or industrialized nation as well. Regretfully, modern infant formula manufacturers are duplicating the doubling of calories from omega-6 to make current formulas reflect our current lifestyle and not that of the 1950s.[168] Hopefully, research will be done soon to verify that lowering omega-6 in formulas is the safe direction to take. We certainly have a lot of work ahead of us in order to continue to clarify the most scientific and best pathway to optimal health through true preventive medicine. The exciting part is that we have come a long way and are very confident about our current direction and have great hope for the future.

We have embarked on a new journey in preventive medicine, in which I'm honored to have played a part these last twenty-two years. We have helped thousands of people pull out of metabolic syndrome, beat obesity, and otherwise reduce their risk of chronic disease. We don't merely offer theories. We have numerous documented cases of people moving toward and attaining optimal health. With regard to our ability to prevent or slow down the development of chronic disease, the future looks very bright. The disease trends I discussed in the introduction to this book have worsened because of lifestyle changes. They can be reversed by changing to a healthy lifestyle.

The key component of our plan for achieving optimal health is reducing inflammation. You'll read more about how to reduce chronic inflammation in upcoming chapters, but we needed to deal directly here with biases that many previous authors have presented to you as "truth." Many books and teachers have convinced lots of people that their unscientific way was the only pathway to better health. Their bias has become your unfortunate, unstable platform—which will most likely fail you. You need to let go of a great deal of the unscientific information that individuals with an agenda have taught you. Be a strong member of the Optimal Health Revolution by breaking away from any health teaching that can't be scientifically proven. I'm upfront about my science and have provided hundreds of references so that you can check them out yourself. I'll help you stand on a scientific platform which won't be easily shaken.

To this point, we have discussed the root cause of all chronic disease and how to begin to reduce it. But now we will start to get serious about specific lifestyle changes that will dramatically reduce your risk of chronic disease and lead to potentially huge savings in health-care costs globally.

The next step is to understand the ultimate goal of optimal health as well as the foundational principles to take you there. That's chapter 6.

CHAPTER 6

The Eight Pillars
of Optimal Health

Any successful revolution needs to be based on the right foundational principles, and that foundation for the Optimal Health Revolution consists of eight pillars.

It is critical that you understand this, because one of the problems with living a healthy life today is that there is so much bad advice out there, and people are too quick to heed the advice of anyone who sounds as if he knows what he's talking about.

Here's an example from my own life of the trouble that tendency can cause.

My family and I were moving across the country to a new home. The collection of useless junk we can't live without filled three rental trucks, and we proceeded in convoy, like Columbus coming to the New World with his three ships, only at greater expense and slightly faster.

Our route took us through a major city in the northwestern U.S., where we planned to drop anchor for the night. A street map of this city looks a lot like a plate of spaghetti. I trembled at the thought of driving through it, just as Columbus's crew must have at the thought of sailing into the storm-tossed unknown. So I called ahead to our hotel to get exact, local-expert directions, hoping to eliminate all possibility of getting lost. The sweet, perky young woman on the phone sounded so confident that as I wrote down the directions I felt assured of our successful arrival.

Unfortunately, my young navigator failed to ask if I was traveling from the north or south—an important omission since the freeway exit she gave only exists on the southbound side. We were headed north. Several miles beyond our supposed turnoff, I led the flotilla off the freeway to reconstruct the directions I had received from the hotel's director of guest confusion.

Another problem with Spaghetti City's streets is that most of them are one-way. After a total circumnavigation of a large supermarket I was boiling like a pasta pot, and my kids began to ask, "Are we lost, Daddy?" My wife, sensing that their safety was in jeopardy, assured them that I knew what I was doing and we'd be at the hotel soon.

Several turns later, I found my way into a one-lane street that quickly became too narrow for our trucks. We were run aground in a narrow inlet with no room to turn around. I got out of the truck looking for a tree to kick and encountered the coup de grâce: a sign that read NO TRUCKS. They *could* have posted that sign on the corner, but then I wouldn't have had the fun of having to back our three trucks out of that narrow strait.

Getting out of that mess and on to the hotel was a nightmare. And I made one final mistake: I told all our friends about it, which means I will never be allowed to forget it.

The point is, ask anyone for directions and he or she instantly becomes an expert, regardless of qualification. That applies both to navigation and to advice about your health. We live in an age of astounding scientific advances, but the advice people give us is often on the level of superstition and folklore. In fact, folklore can be slightly more valuable, since science and centuries of experience have proven some folk medicine valid. That's more than one can say for the latest fads you see trumpeted on magazine covers while standing in line at the supermarket.

Everybody has an opinion. Your brother-in-law saw an infomercial at 3 a.m. the other night and now has the secret for adding ten years to your life. The media hit you with a double-barreled barrage of unfounded fear and magic-bullet remedies. First fat is bad, then it's good. Last year carbohydrates caused all our ills, this year they're not so bad. Eat low fat, high fat, low protein, high protein, starve yourself, eat anything you want. Every time I see the latest hot new health product advertised, I think of my Lost in Spaghetti City episode. There is a multibillion-dollar industry selling maps to optimal health, and all they do is get people lost, confused, and frustrated. At best, we get nowhere, winding up back where we started. At worst, that bogus map leads us right off a cliff.

The institute where I consult has developed something better. Over the years, I have led thousands of people to optimal health. I like to think of what we give patients at the institute not as a map but as a plan for winning your best life. If you want to win optimal health in your life, you need to have a plan. And the first thing you need to know is the definition of optimal health so you can truly understand what you're trying to achieve.

Optimal health means having the best health possible given your genetic heritage, personal history, and environment. Ideally, the foundation for optimal health should be started before we are conceived. Many studies have shown that the health of the mother at conception and during pregnancy affects the health of her child both in his early years as well as his adulthood. However, even if your foundation wasn't laid perfectly, it's not too late to make a significant change for the better. We can't change our past, but we can often reverse some of the physical damage we have incurred. We can't change our DNA (yet), but we can certainly modify how our DNA is expressed. We may be powerless to change our city's or nation's environment, but we certainly can change the microenvironments in which we live.

Our genetic heritage is a major factor in our health, but it is not absolute fate. The key words to know are *genotype* and *phenotype*. Genotype is your genetic makeup, which you inherited from your parents. Phenotype is the expression of your genes as influenced by many environmental factors and life experience. Though your grandmother might have lived for a hundred years, you may be less fortunate, as a result of living in a different world and pursuing a lifestyle different from hers. Conversely, just because several members of your family succumbed to a chronic disease does not necessarily mean that you will, too. There may be things you can do to offset the increased risk indicated by your family history.

We have distilled our decades of experience in leading thousands of people from all over the world to optimal health into a few simple principles. There is no magic bullet here, no shortcut to the Promised Land. Rather, I'm offering a realistic plan for achieving an optimally healthy lifestyle, and that plan rests on eight pillars.

Pillar #1: Reduce Your Risk Factors for Chronic Disease

A risk factor is any lifestyle or biological quality or characteristic that can increase your likelihood of developing a disease. For example, smoking is a risk factor for lung cancer. The risk factors for heart disease, cancer, obesity, and diabetes will be explained in chapters 9 through 12.

There are many risk factors for chronic disease, but too often you'll hear that health problems can be corrected by changing only one or two aspects of your life. For example, you often hear that the keys to good health are proper diet and regular exercise. Diet and exercise *are* crucial to optimal health, but they are only two of the risk factors for chronic disease. We need to know and address them all.

The University of Pittsburgh keeps a database of thousands of people who have been able to lose a significant amount of weight and keep it off for over five years—contrary to popular perception, such people are less rare than unicorns. According to a former Acting Undersecretary of the U.S. Department of Agriculture,[169] 90 percent of these people have been able to maintain their reduced weight by both controlling the calories they consume and exercising. However, only 9 percent were able to control their weight by diet alone, and only 1 percent were able to control it by exercise alone.

Jim Fixx, the marathoner whose books and articles spawned a running craze in North America in the late 1970s, died from a sudden, unexpected heart attack at the age of fifty-two. Fixx was a guy who got more aerobic exercise in a month than most diligently healthy people get in a year, but he had other cardiac risk factors. Heart disease ran in his family; his father had died of it in his forties. Also, before Fixx started running, at age thirty-five, he had reportedly been a heavy smoker. Fixx, in changing his lifestyle, probably extended his lifespan significantly, but he was fighting other risk factors that, sadly, ended his life at an early age.

Pillar #2: Exercise

This word strikes fear and revulsion into the hearts of confirmed couch potatoes, but it shouldn't. Even true experts, like Jim Fixx, tend to define exercise in terms of their preferred sport, activity, or school of thought. Hucksters and fad promoters define it in terms of whatever they're trying to sell you, from workout videos to exercise machines that defy parody to expensive memberships at health clubs that, based on the TV commercials, are attended only by people with perfectly chiseled physiques and designer workout clothes.

We are offered the fantasy that we can lose stomach fat by exercising our stomach muscles and thigh fat by working our thigh muscles—along with gimcrack machines to help us do it.

Step aerobics. Low-impact aerobics. Dance aerobics. Kick-boxing. Exercise balls. What's next: pogo-stick parties? Exercise fads frustrate me, because people think that in order to get fit, they have to be chasing every new time-consuming, usually expensive trend, and so they wind up doing nothing at all. Most sedentary folk argue that they don't have time to exercise. This is partly because the "experts" often define exercise too narrowly in terms of organized, costly activities. People can't see how exercise can possibly fit into their lives or their budgets.

FB

YOGA-CISE!

Yoga is both an ancient religious practice and a contemporary fad. Traditionally, it is the practice of assuming various postures to assist in meditation, and it is common to Hinduism and other Eastern religions. In American and much of Western culture, yoga is presented merely as a form of an exercise, something for health clubs to add to their menu of extra-cost activities. My Hindu friends think that trying to separate yoga from its religious heritage is hilarious. To them it is roughly analogous to Rosary-bead aerobics. (I am sorry I wrote that down. Now it's only a matter of time before health clubs have people chanting: "Hail Mary, full of grace; bless me while I run in place.") Doesn't this blending of religious practices and exercise seem a little demeaning and wrong? As I've said before, I respect the world's major religions too much to agree with important doctrinal practices being converted by hotel spas, health clubs, and gyms into a degrading form so they can make money.

Moreover, the majority of people who rely on yoga classes don't develop an adequate level of cardiovascular conditioning. This should be obvious, considering that health-club yoga classes consist mainly of standing, sitting, lying, and stretching, three of which are the chief activities of committed couch potatoes.

Yoga may be beneficial for increasing flexibility and improving strength. However, it lacks cardiovascular benefit—it won't significantly reduce your risk of heart attack or stroke.

Here's the happy reality: *exercise doesn't have to suck up a lot of time.* There is substantial evidence that the "exercise of daily living" is highly beneficial for reducing risk of chronic disease.[170] Here are some examples of the "exercise of daily living":

- Take stairs instead of escalators or elevators. If you work on the fiftieth floor, take the elevator to the forty-eighth.
- Park on the outer edges of parking lots and walk the rest of the way. (You'll also get fewer dings on your car doors.)
- Carry your luggage instead of using rollers.
- Buy a walk-behind lawn mower instead of a riding one—and don't pay some kid to push it.
- If you take a train or bus to work, get off a few blocks early and walk the rest of the way.
- Take a walk with your spouse or play outdoors with your kids.

- Take dancing lessons. I know of people who have lost 20+ pounds (10+ kg) after they joined a dance class and are having a great time maintaining that weight loss.

Activities like these benefit cardiovascular health and burn calories throughout the day, which helps you maintain or lose weight. Of course, an organized, fad-free program of regular exercise is best—whether you pursue it at a health club or at home—but if you do nothing else, add the "exercise of daily living" to your life. It takes very little time and can dramatically reduce your risk of chronic disease.

Science has shown that cardiovascular exercise reduces the risk of many diseases and adverse health conditions, including diabetes,[171] colon cancer,[172] dementia,[173] heart disease (even with walking),[174] stroke,[175, 176] osteoporosis,[177] and others. It has also been shown to reduce mortality rates[178] for older people and even slow the whole aging process (perhaps by as much as twelve years, according to some researchers).[179]

Perhaps one of the most significant contributions that exercise provides to our health is the reduction of inflammation. Leisure-time physical activity reduces chronic inflammation,[180] and it has even been discovered that just six minutes of fast walking will reduce inflammation in the elderly as well.[181] Adding dietary supplementation with antioxidants to exercise provides even greater anti-inflammatory effects.[182]

In short, the benefits of exercise in attaining optimal health are proven and profound. This second pillar of optimal health includes both kinds of exercise: *resistance*, such as weight lifting or push-ups, and *cardiovascular* exercise, which involves raising the heart rate through activities like walking, running, swimming, and bicycling. If you're interested, the U.S. government just updated its guidelines for exercise, and have them online at www.health.gov/PAguidelines. The exercise guidelines from the World Health Organization can be found online at www.who.int/dietphysicalactivity/factsheet_recommendations/en.

Pillar #3: Good Macronutrition

Macronutrition describes the nutrients that make up most of our nutritional intake by weight—carbohydrates, fats, and proteins.

Good macronutrition consists of eating the right types and percentages of these nutrients.

Foods rich in carbohydrates, fats, or proteins have each had their turn to be demonized by diet-fad authors, to the point that if we followed all their advice we would be reduced to a diet of water and sawdust. The truth is that none of the big three macronutrients is inherently bad for you, as long as your intake is balanced, moderate, and from healthy sources.

There are good and bad sources of proteins and carbohydrates. There are good and bad fats. I'll show you the differences later on. For now, let's just say that we need appropriate amounts and sources of macronutrients to achieve optimal health. The Institute of Medicine recommends that the ranges of macronutrients in adults' daily diets should be:

- 45–65 percent carbohydrates
- 20–35 percent fats
- 10–35 percent proteins

A balanced diet must also include good daily sources of fiber.

These ranges differ widely from the recommendations in popular fad diets, because many of these diets have been based on poor or old science or have been no more than educated guesses by the authors.

FB

EATING WELL ISN'T ROCKET SCIENCE

Many fad diets make eating so complex that to follow them you'd need to hire a nutritionist-chef to plan and cook your meals and a security guard to keep your spouse and kids from sneaking out of the house to eat "off-diet" behind your back. Most of us don't have the budget for hired help.

So once again it's Fad Buster to the rescue. An optimal health diet is neither complex nor punitive to your loved ones. Think for a moment about a traditional Asian diet, which is based primarily on carbohydrate-laden rice with a wide variety of fruits and vegetables. Obesity was never a widespread problem in China, Japan, Korea, and the rest of eastern Asia until the last thirty to fifty years, with the advent of worldwide industrialization and food processing. For centuries, chronic diseases and obesity were never widespread in these countries, despite the fact that the people had no idea what carbohydrates, proteins, and fats were. They didn't have any diet-fad authors telling them to binge on fats or to avoid carbs as they would a bubonic rat.

So why are we now led to believe that eating the proper diet is as complex and baffling as quantum physics? Beats me.

As you read this book, you will come to understand how to eat for optimal health. The guidelines are general, not strict. Tastes and cuisines vary between cultures, as do financial resources, local food availability, time for preparing food, education, and personal commitment. It isn't possible to recommend a single diet that will function well for people of all cultures and lifestyles.

In Appendix B.4, I have provided an example of a healthy diet for one week, as well as some sources that I trust for more information and advice. If my sample diet is somehow at odds with your culture, just adapt it as best you can and follow the rest of the guidelines presented in this book.

To be optimally healthy, consuming as much food as possible from organic sources is best (and may also be more nutritious[183]), especially free-range organic sources of protein. The U.S. Government standards for allowing the use of the word "organic" on a food label are defined in Appendix A.10. Commercially grown and processed foods commonly contain many chemicals that are harmful to your health. Mass-produced cattle and chicken meat contains hormones, herbicides, pesticides, and antibiotics. Non-organic dairy can contain similar chemicals. Non-organically grown fruits and vegetables contain herbicides and pesticides. Certainly those in the commercial food industry will scream that there has been no solid evidence that these contents are dangerous, but the studies done to compare the risks have to date been very short in duration, and many worrisome effects don't show up for years or decades. And there's no doubt that chemicals can increase inflammation and thus contribute to chronic disease development.[184]

In light of this warning, I'm very commonly asked if the risks of pesticide residue on fruits and vegetables outweigh the benefits if organically grown food is not available. My answer to that is, "Not at this point." In other words, keep eating your seven to nine (or more) servings of fruits and vegetables daily because their massive phytonutrient load seems to be of greater benefit than the risk of the chemicals they may contain. Fruits and vegetables are themselves anti-inflammatory.[185]

Moreover, pre-packaged and processed foods should be minimized as much as possible. They are almost always made with the cheapest oils, which are inflammatory and contain massive amounts of chemicals and manufactured contents, all of which your body commonly sees as foreign substances. The easiest way to think of this generally is that you should purchase most of your foods from the periphery of a store and the smallest amount from the center aisles, where most of the highly processed items are kept.

More detailed information about macronutrition is presented in Appendix A.8, but here is one final point: size matters. I want you to have a lot of choices for *what* to eat, because the stresses and time constraints of modern life make it hard to stick to rigid diets. However, I want you to be able to control the *amount* of food you eat, without feeling deprived or constantly hungry. Guidelines for making it easier to eat in moderation are given in chapters 11 and 13, as well as in Appendix A.7.

Pillar #4: Good Micronutrition

If macronutrion relates to the bulk of your diet, micronutrition is the stuff that comes in tiny but critical amounts in our food. This includes not only vitamins and minerals, but also phytonutrients. The prefix "phyto" derives from the Greek word for plant. Phytonutrients are active nutrients found in plants that are not defined as vitamins or minerals—for example, lycopene. As with vitamins and minerals, we can also get phytonutrients from food supplements, though it is best to get as many micronutrients as possible from food; that's a big part of the definition of a healthy diet. However, there is a vast body of research literature that clearly points to the need for supplementation for virtually everyone living in the developed world.

In short, yes, most of us need supplements to win optimal health. A lot of doctors will tell you otherwise. They are inadequately informed.

Here's a test. The next time a doctor says that you can get all the vitamins and minerals you need through food alone, ask this question: "How many micrograms of folic acid did you eat yesterday?"

If the doctor makes up an answer just to be smart, ask about international units of vitamin A. Then try C, D, E, and all the Bs. Don't worry about memorizing the essential minerals and the phytonutrients; your doctor will give up while you're still on the alphabet stuff.

My point is that not even medical professionals keep track of their micronutrional intake. It's too hard and too time-consuming. "Excuse me, waitress, before I pay the bill I need an hour or so to calculate the amounts of the twenty-eight essential vitamins and minerals in this meal. Can you ask the chef to send out the recipes? Phytonutrients? Oh, don't bother. I'll just guess at lycopene and lutein and stuff."

Guess what. Even doctors have nutritional deficiencies, because even they can't keep track of what they're getting in their diets.

Another problem is confusion over the official government nutritional guidelines for vitamins and minerals. These guidelines are expressed as Dietary Reference Intake (DRI). You see them printed on the nutrition labels of foods and supplements. They are useful, but you have to understand that they are based on the amounts of nutrients necessary to prevent deficiency diseases, like rickets, scurvy, and beriberi. How many people on your block suffer from these ailments? None? The reason is that in modern society almost everyone gets enough calcium, vitamin C, and vitamin B1 to avoid these deficiency diseases. But that just means we are getting enough micronutrients for *minimal* health. *Optimal* health is another matter. I'm talking about preventing not just deficiency diseases but *chronic* diseases—the ones that kill most people today.

For example, only 30 mg of vitamin C are necessary daily to reduce the risk of scurvy, but higher amounts have been shown to help reduce the risk of strokes and heart attacks.[186] I don't know about you, but most people don't have nightmares about contracting scurvy. That disease does exist in modern society, especially among the institutionalized elderly, but scurvy is to heart disease as the horse-drawn carriage is to the automobile. The latter is considerably more common and a result of industrialization.

And that's why dietary supplements are a critical part of the game plan for winning optimal health. In many cases the micronutrient levels that have been shown to reduce chronic disease can only be obtained by supplementation. There is no way to get optimal levels of them from food alone.

This is especially true of fat-soluble antioxidants such as coenzyme Q10. If you did try to obtain the optimal amounts through diet alone, your food intake would have to contain so much fat that it would become a risk factor.

Chapter 8 will go into more detail about supplementing your diet.

Pillar #5: Mind, Spirit, and Positive Attitude

We have known for years that happy and hopeful people are generally healthier and longer-lived than the perennially depressed, angry, fearful, and pessimistic. Ebenezer Scrooge's nocturnal transformation not only made him a better person, but probably extended his life. Dickens doesn't say, but I think it did.

This phenomenon is not miraculous. Recent scientific research has finally been able to pinpoint the physiological cause and effect: Depression triggers two hormonal pathways that worsen our overall health. I'll discuss this in detail in chapter 9, with regard to cardiac risk factors.

There are now over 1,200 studies that reveal that people with sound, committed faith live longer and better. This might be partially related to the two hormones just cited. It is a fascinating area of research currently being pursued at such institutions as Duke University, the National Institutes of Health and Harvard Medical School, with Duke arguably being the leader in the field.

There is now little doubt that our mental and spiritual health affects our physiological health. Some scientists don't discuss this topic because they can't relate to spirituality, and that bias leads them to consider the research soft science. But the truth is that they haven't examined the evidence objectively, even though it is much more credible than many medical practices that became conventional wisdom prior to being proven invalid. (Example: for decades, postmenopausal women were prescribed hormones to reduce their risk of heart disease; later research found that that doesn't work.)

So just do it. Give it a try. Exercise your faith as you would your body, and apply it to your health. If faith isn't your thing, then accentuate the positive in your life in every way you can. Whether you practice spirituality or not, if you are chronically depressed, fearful, anxious, angry or pessimistic, please accept that your state of mind will damage your physical health and probably shorten your life. There are treatments for these mental and emotional illnesses. Seek them out. In doing so you may be saving your life as well as beginning to live it better.

FB

"THE ONE TRUE FAITH"

In recent years, several authors have suggested that in order to be healthy you must follow their particular religion particular spiritual beliefs. I won't debate their theology, but from a medical standpoint that just isn't true. You don't need to change your religion in order to become healthier. Many authors writing about the mind-spirit-body connection have combined some scientific truth with a biased agendas—much like those we discussed in the last chapter.

Pillar #6: Adequate Rest

Of our eight pillars, this one may need the most shoring up. People in modern civilization don't get enough sleep.

It is believed that in the mid-nineteenth century people averaged around nine and a half hours of sleep per night. Yes, I know. Hard to believe. But you have to understand how radically different life was then, even in the most technologically advanced societies. Most people did hard physical labor all day, so at night they were dog-tired. At a certain hour it got dark. There was no television, no radio. Lamp oil was expensive. So was heating fuel. People doused the lights, banked the fire, and went to bed.

Today, most individuals living in industrialized societies average six hours of sleep per night or less. There was some concern in the 1950s that technology would make life so easy that by the twenty-first century there would be little for the average person to do. We would live in a leisure society. Boy, were they wrong! Technology now enables us to do work that required three people a decade or two ago. And we don't leave our work at the factory or in the fields. Our work—and the stress that goes with it—follows us, via cell phones and the Internet, everywhere in the civilized world and points beyond, including home.

Keeping up with work, driving our kids to all their activities, staying connected with family and friends—the demands on our time are huge. And the one bank from which we can always steal a little time is our sleep.

We don't need all of the nine and a half hours of nightly sleep our ancestors got, but we do need more than six. There are many biochemical reactions that occur during rest that are necessary for both physical and mental health. For example, the hormones leptin and ghrelin are affected by the amount of sleep we get: Sleep deprivation is associated with decreased leptin levels and elevated ghrelin levels, both of which result in increased appetite.[187] So a little more sleep may result in a little less compulsive eating.

There has been a great deal of excellent research lately concerning the importance of adequate sleep. Let me share some of it with you now (and frankly, if this information puts you to sleep, you'll find that's good). Its been shown that chronic sleep deprivation can lead to a shorter lifespan.[188] Sleep also influences many aspects of our lives, including how well we think,[189, 190] sugar metabolism,[191] and immune function,[192] among others. Moreover, sleep deprivation has cumulative effects so that mild, chronic, daily sleep deficiency can add up to important health issues. Chronic sleep deprivation has even been shown to be associated with chronic increased inflammation.[193, 194, 195, 196] Sleep apnea is known to increase heart disease risk, partially by increasing inflammation.[197] Inadequate sleep also increases the risk of obesity.[198]

What is the optimal amount of sleep to get? Between seven and eight hours of sleep a night appears to be the best for the vast majority of adults.[199]

Perhaps there is more to the ancient Biblical recommendation of resting one day a week than we realize. And a little more rest each night helps, too.

Pillar #7: Good Medical Care

"I run twenty-five miles a week and eat handfuls of vitamins, and I'm so healthy I haven't seen a doctor in twenty years."

I wince when I hear people say things like that.

I mean…if you haven't seen a doctor in twenty years, how can you know whether you're healthy?

This is another example of people thinking that there are only a couple of risk factors that stand in the way of optimal health.

In fact, there are several risk factors for heart disease and cancer that can only be assessed by a physician through the use of blood tests—not to mention the value of early detection of those diseases.

I am a doctor, but the last thing I want to do as the author of this book is to replace your relationship with a well-trained physician who values preventive medicine. I want to strengthen your relationship with your doctor by helping you become a more resolute and informed participant in your own health care. And I want you to have regular checkups (see Appendix A.1).

FB

DOCTORPHOBIA

I've received countless newsletters and advertisements from people who want to scare folks away from doctors.

Some of these make wild, paranoid claims about pharmaceutical companies conspiring to bribe doctors in ways that dictate your medical care. I've heard tapes of people purporting to be Nobel Prize nominees making ridiculous claims about physician lifestyles and death rates. I could make a full-time job of responding to such untruths, if only it paid enough.

And of course I am always *shocked,* shocked to find that the authors of these newsletters and books, after asserting their integrity and purity of motive, are happy to offer me the one true product that will guarantee me a long, healthy life, for only pennies a day (or, more often, dollars).

The great majority of these salesmen, even those with professional training, are ill-informed, narrow-minded, greedy, or all the above. Unfortunately, they have scared many people away from obtaining the real health care they need. This leaves anyone who believes these conspiracy claims adrift in uncertainty. Mistrust of professional medicine generally leads people into the hands of untrained quacks with unproven cures and preventatives.

The relationships between governments, pharmaceutical companies, the medical profession, and medical consumers may not be perfect. But in developed nations, governments require the medical profession and drug manufacturers to prove—through extensive testing—that their products and therapies are effective and not dangerous.

The guy on the television selling you the magical cure-all isn't held to those standards.

I wish the medical community would speak out more against the snake-oil marketers who want to scare you away from doctors, but too many of us don't take those guys seriously enough.

If commercial propaganda has led you to develop an unreasonable fear of doctors, please reread chapter 5 very carefully. Doctors can save and prolong your life in thousands of ways that snake-oil salesmen can't.

MORE WEIRD SCIENCE

Here is another example of questionable science based on a doubtful analysis of cause and effect.

Many anti-aging health practitioners have reasoned that since hormones wane with age, taking hormone pills or injections must be a good anti-aging therapy.

By that logic, inducing the teenage afflictions of acne and sweaty feet to elderly people ought to have the effect of a fountain of youth! Yet physicians have administered hormones such as melatonin and human growth hormone with the idea that doing so would promote extended youth. The problem is that hormones have very complex interactions and can be dangerous. Human growth hormone, for example, has been shown to increase insulin resistance (see chapter 12), decrease good cholesterol, and increase the risk of death, none of which I would classify as anti-aging outcomes.

Pillar #8: Healthy Environment and Good Hygiene

Air pollution is associated with many upper respiratory diseases and cancers. It has even been associated with an increased risk of heart disease.[200]

One solution to this problem is to move to Antarctica or an island in the South Pacific. Unfortunately, few of us can afford to do that. In fact, that's why those places aren't very polluted: few people and less industry.

So the idea is to think globally and act locally, as they say.

In fact, pollution can be very local, even originating in your own home or workplace, and there are equally local solutions.

New houses can be loaded with chemical fumes, for example. Radon gas, which is found in the ground and can seep into your basement, is a major cause of lung cancer, especially among smokers, and needs to be detected and controlled.

If you can't avoid pollution in your residence or workplace, you may want to consider a good air treatment system for your home. You can also lobby for one at work.

There have been many horror stories of contamination in water supplies that was discovered long after people had suffered significant exposure. Some of the most dramatic cases have occurred in China.[201] China's economy has boomed in the last twenty years, and along with the economic benefits have come increased water and air pollution. Due to delays in government regulation and antipollution technology, industrial poisons have leached into groundwater and contaminated drinking water supplies in some regions, drastically increasing cancer rates among the residents. *USA Today* reports that residents near the Feng Chan River have a cancer rate that is eighteen times the national average, while the city of Liukuaizhuang has a rate that's thirty times the national average.

These are tragic statistics. China is working very hard to correct these problems, but it takes time. The numbers are lower in most other industrialized nations, but the existence of carcinogens in the air, water, and food in all developed countries is still far higher than a century ago, and people are paying the price with increased cancer rates.

China is not alone in its water problems. Discarded drugs are showing up in drinking water all over the world. One article estimates that 250 million pounds of drugs are dumped into the U.S. water system yearly, and 46 million Americans are exposed to the drugs because water treatment systems don't remove them. Thirty-one of thirty-eight wastewater samples in France showed evidence of drugs that had the ability to mutate genes. Contaminants have been found in Asia, Australia, Europe, and in oceans globally.[202]

Though there are some good sources of municipal water, the only water that I generally trust is water filtered at home. You need to be very careful of bottled water, because it may not be any safer than your own tap water. There are some good bottled water companies, but a lot of it *is* just tap water, bought from municipal water companies, marked up about 10,000 percent and labeled with a picture of a pristine, bubbling spring. Another problem with bottled water is the plastic container it comes in. Some are made with a chemical called BPA (bisphenol A), which has been shown to increase the risk of breast and prostate cancer in rats.[203] (See Appendix B.2 for more.)

Unless you know that bottled water is filtered, save your money. Better yet, buy your own purifier. The best ones are usually a little more expensive, or you should replace your filters often.

Another important component of this pillar is hygiene. In some countries, neither basic sanitation guidelines nor modern fresh water and sewer infrastructure are universally in use. In addition, monogamy is a great defense against a variety of diseases. This may seem like common sense, but optimal health is very difficult to maintain if you frequently expose yourself to the possibly infected body fluids of others.

Are You Running on All Eight Pillars?

These eight pillars are the fundamentals upon which the Optimal Health Revolution is built. They are absolutely critical for achieving optimal health. That said, I sincerely hope you aren't feeling intimidated or overwhelmed right now. If you are, take a deep breath and relax.

Perfectionism is your enemy. Our popular health culture has infected many people with the idea that unless they follow their health plans perfectly, their efforts will be in vain. This notion is wrong. It has discouraged millions from trying at all, leaving them apathetic about their health. Do not fall into this trap! Any step you take toward optimal health will benefit you to some degree.

Few people will be able to do everything that I recommend perfectly, but if you do your reasonable best you will significantly increase your chances of living longer and in better health.

I will cover all the risk factors for chronic disease carefully beginning in chapter 9, but there is one source of inflammation and chronic disease I have to address in detail first. The reason for this special emphasis is because there has been so much misinformation in the media concerning how to deal with it. This source of inflammation even deserves its own chapter.

Chapter 7 is my game plan for managing stress.

CHAPTER 7

Living Your Best Life
in a World of Stress

S tress is like what we physicians scientifically refer to as bowel gas. Everybody has it, no one wants to admit it, and we try to cover it up in polite company. But sooner or later the pressure builds to the point that we feel an urgent need to "vent"—which makes *us* feel better, but doesn't exactly enhance quality of life for people who are close to us.

Almost everyone lives with stress, regardless of nationality, ethnicity, heritage, economic status, spirituality, profession, lifestyle, age, or sex. Anyone who claims to be stress-free either doesn't live in the real world, has a delusional mental disorder, or is a liar. Combinations of the three also occur.

I am fortunate to have traveled the globe and met clients who come from all over the world. Here is what my global experience has taught me about stress: Stress is global. It makes no difference if you are from France, China, Germany, Argentina, India, South Korea, America, Ukraine, Japan, Venezuela, Italy, Australia, or anywhere else in the developed world. Normal people in all these societies and cultures experience so much stress that I realized years ago that we had to help our clients manage and reduce it if they were to achieve optimal health.

I have in fact met people who claim to have found a stress-free way of life: Yeah, right! If I lived sequestered away, had no external goals, only needed to eat, sleep, or spend time in religious devotion, performed a few chores for my room and board, and only communicated with a few like-minded people, then I'd be pretty calm, too. (Well, no, *I* wouldn't, but a lot of people would.)

Anyhow, I'd love to see some of these cloistered people six months after they were expelled back into the wide world and had begun to experience all the chaos most of us deal with daily. How calm and collected would such people be if their lives included a pack of screaming and fighting kids, in-laws, rush-hour traffic, an ill-tempered, power-craving, alcoholic boss, teenage neighbors whose "music" rattles china in cupboards three houses away, last-minute homework, last-minute everything else, running on four hours of sleep a night, recurrent diarrhea, an obese mortgage, and a pocketful of maxed-out credit cards? Come on. Let's get honest about modern life. It's busy, and stress is part of the deal.

As a former emergency physician, I've had more than a little experience with job stress. Before switching to preventive medicine, I worked for years in a busy trauma center in Southern California where I was the only physician on call during my shifts. It was not unusual to have to manage two heart attacks at once. A normal day at the office: The ER is overrun with abdominal pains, chest pains, kidney stones, sprains and cuts and so on when the paramedics call to say they're dropping by with several victims of an auto accident or a shootout.

People react to stress in different ways. I am one of those who thrive on that stuff. That may sounds weird to you, but the truth is I enjoyed my ER work. The busier things were, the more I enjoyed the challenge. I didn't leave emergency medicine because of stress.

The most stressful period of my life was during the years when I had a family practice. I was one of two doctors in a practice that served over eight thousand patients. That ought to be enough for a sane physician, but it wasn't for me. I was also involved in three other businesses. I co-founded a wellness company, had a very successful commercial agricultural business, and participated in a third enterprise. I'm sure it is obvious to you that this is the lifestyle of a crazy person, but the insane are often the last to notice their own insanity.

Our oldest daughter had always been sweet and obedient (except, like every other kid, when she was two). Then, when she was five, she suddenly developed a defiant streak. One day my wife and I were discussing this on the phone when I mentioned that our middle daughter (then eighteen months old) was beginning to copy the defiance she saw in her big sister. My wife was completely puzzled by this. She said I had a serious misperception of our second child. I held my ground. She ended our talk by saying, "Honey, I'm with her all day, every day, and she's not like that."

It was like getting hit in the forehead with a two-by-four. I had a child whom I didn't know. I had to change something, but I had no idea what. Should I quit some or all of my jobs? How much more time did I need to spend with my family? How should I spend it? Is spending "quality time" with your children a legitimate concept or a cheap rationalization? How do I make these decisions, and where do I go for help? Isn't everyone else doing what I'm doing?

Since I had no idea what to do next, and being who I am, I decided to do an extensive review of the literature, both scientific and general, to find answers. I collected and read over 400 articles. To my amazement, nearly all of them argued that the way to manage stress was to get away from it in one form or another. That didn't seem right. I continued to pursue the issue until I arrived at the conclusions I'm about to share with you. We teach these principles at our institute. Thousands of our clients have reported wonderful results. I hope they will help you, too.

The conclusions I reached engendered some pretty big changes in my life. I sold my medical practice and moved my family to a rural area. I had come to see that I had only one shot at raising my children, and I wasn't going to blow it. That's the biggest responsibility most people have, and you don't get do-overs. I immediately shut down two of my "side" businesses, even though one was just starting to become quite lucrative, and dramatically reduced my participation in the third. I began to take every Wednesday off to spend the whole day with our eighteen-month-old. I think we visited every playground and slide park in Southern California. This freed up my wife to spend Wednesdays volunteering at our oldest daughter's school. What we found out was that our oldest daughter needed a daddy, and as soon as I started spending more time with her she returned to being the sweet young lady she is today.

Now we are an incredibly close family. We do just about everything together, because we all genuinely enjoy being around each other. Did these changes impact me financially? You bet. Time with my family was the best purchase I ever made. There's no way I'd trade the relationship that I have with my family today for all the income I've lost over the years. No way at all.

Changing our lives in this way wasn't a snap decision. It took time and deliberation. But we came up with a process that took us from living crazy to actually managing stress.

That process is what I want to offer now for your consideration. It begins with a simple but mandatory writing exercise.

What Is Stress?

Stress is any factor (emotional, physical, social, economic, and so on) that requires a mental or physical adaptive response. These factors can be real or imagined. They can come at us from all directions or spring from within ourselves. Stress is any pressure placed upon you that demands a response.

As if we don't have enough problems with the real, empirical world, much of the stress we feel comes from our fear of things that *might* go wrong but rarely do. What we fear may be imaginary, but the stress is real.

Sources of stress can be work, family, finances, time (or the lack of it), friends, colleagues and acquaintances, national and world affairs, technology, and anything else that causes us to deal with the unexpected or the uncertain. I could devote long chapters to any of these sources, but I want to focus on the one that has changed our lives the most in recent decades—the one that coincides with the rise of chronic diseases. I mean technology.

As I noted in the last chapter, people in the 1950s wondered about how people in the future would spend all the free time they would have on their hands. They believed that technology would soon do most of our work for us—that by the year 2000 we would have a leisure society, in which idleness and boredom would be serious problems.

Readers under fifty may now take a five-minute break to roll around on the floor laughing hysterically.

In the future we actually got, technology hasn't made us lazier; it has enabled us to perform work that took three or more people to do twenty years ago. And because we can, we do. Information and communication technology have made it possible to radically shorten lead times and deadlines, to compress the calendar time necessary to complete work. And because we can, we do. Worst of all, we can't get away from work. We receive text messages in the bathroom, take cell phone calls and answer e-mails on vacation. We can work anywhere, at any time of the day or night. And because we can, we do.

Our time used to be scheduled for us, according the hours kept by our workplaces, schools, retail stores, professionals' offices, and so forth. Today our time isn't managed for us, but it isn't our own, either. We need self-discipline. But discipline is a tactic. First we have to know our goals, our priorities. Those are the things that have gotten lost amid the chaos.

I have a writing exercise for you that is priceless. Please write down the seven greatest sources of stress in your life. Don't read another word until you fill in these blanks. You'll get so much more out of this chapter if you do so.

1. _____

2. _____

3. _____

4. _____

5. _____

6. _____

7. _____

There are very high costs associated with stress. Some studies report that in many industrialized areas, 75 percent of workers report being over-stressed. Some people believe that stress accounts for the majority of visits to physicians' offices, either directly or indirectly. An article in a national newspaper in the U.S. estimated that as many as 400 million workdays in the U.S. are lost because of stress.

I'll demonstrate in chapters 9 and 10 that stress is a risk factor for heart disease and cancer. You've already seen in chapter 2 that stress increases inflammation. It has an eroding affect on three of our pillars of optimal health—reducing risk factors, rest, and mental and spiritual health. Stress has been shown in many studies to decrease immune system function, increase blood pressure, increase depression, and lead to temper control issues. Stress may be normal, but it is not our friend.

Not only does stress harm our health, but so do many of the ways people choose to cope with it. Some of us respond to stress with isolation or anger or impulsive behaviors. Appetite changes are common: some people lose their appetites during stress while others cope by compulsively stuffing or starving themselves: "I may not have control of my life but I do have control of this piece of food." Some of us turn to mood-altering drugs (both legal and illegal), smoking, or excessive alcohol use—quick escapes that damage our health more than the stress we're escaping, while often adding to the stress in other people's lives.

The Seven Most Important Things in Your Life

Now for writing exercise #2. Please list the seven most important things in your life, **in order**. (Ranking them may take more reflection than naming them.) Again, please take a few minutes to actually write down your seven items here.

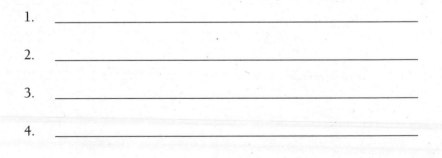

1. _____

2. _____

3. _____

4. _____

5. _____

6. _____

7. _____

Now, please compare the two lists that you have made. Notice anything interesting?

For most people, the two lists are very similar. (If yours are not similar, your path is easy. It means that you have a lot of unimportant things
bothering you. Just get rid of them.) When the two lists are similar, it
means that the most important things in your life are also causing you
the most stress. Therefore, when people tell you that the way to handle
stress is to run away from it, they are really telling you to run away from
the most important things in your life. As if ignoring your job, your family, and your finances is gonna get rid of a whole lot of stress.

I'm not talking about a weekend getaway with your spouse or a golf
game with your friends. Nothing wrong with that. But your problems are
always there when you come home, and they are usually connected with
the most important things in your life.

And there's the rub. Isn't there something *else* wrong if the most
important aspects of your life are also the most troublesome?

One Important Question

Even if you have never made a written list like this before, you have carried one inside you. All I did was to ask you to put it on paper. And that's
important. Looking at that list gives you perspective and objectivity.

Now for the most important question. Let's say you had a friend who
had no idea what was on your list. Say it was me. If I could watch you
live your life for a week—like in one of those reality shows where the
camera is on you all the time—could I figure out what's on your list?
Would observing your behavior for seven days tell me what the seven
most important things in your life are? In order?

**If not, then you are living in conflict with your own goals and val-
ues.** When you do not live according to your internal priority list, you

99

will experience internal conflict and stress. And stress is bad for your health.

This is what happened to me and my family. We thought of ourselves as having well-defined priorities, but you would never have guessed what was important to us by watching the way we lived our lives. We had good intentions, but life kept dragging us off the path. We didn't have a plan for overcoming stress.

Having a list of your life priorities that is well-conceived, refined, and tested is **the basis for your revolutionary plan for overcoming stress.** I don't mean we can eliminate stress. But we can *beat* stress. We can stop letting it spoil our lives. And we can knock it out as a risk factor for chronic disease.

There are other methods that can help you reduce stress, but unless you have this basic game plan in your life, you're just kidding yourself about managing chronic stress.

What do we learn from our own priority list, the seven things that are most important to us? Let's say, as an example, your list looks like this:

1. Me
2. My job
3. My investment portfolio
4. My family
5. My friends
6. Leisure time
7. Home maintenance

Now let's say you have a particular day reserved for your family (#4) and a friend (#5) calls to see if you want to play golf. You'd say no, because you already had something more important planned for that day. Then, a few minutes later, your boss (#2) calls to "request" that you transport your derrière into the office right away for special duty. You say, "Yes, sir!" and drive to work. Your job trumps a day spent with your family. Not that it always *should*. But in your life it usually has to. It's #2 on your list.

This system really makes life easier, because it removes stress from your decisions and your daily conflicts of interest. All the questions were answered *before* the phone calls came. This works well when your family is aware of your priority list and has had an opportunity to provide feedback and work out exceptions to the rules with you.

Here's another example of a priority list. It happens to be mine. That doesn't mean it should be *your* list. But I'd like you to know how I arrived at this one. It took me a few years to get to the final version, and to fulfill it. But it has been invaluable for our family and has reduced my stress dramatically. I have been following this method for about twelve years.

Dr. Duke's own priority list:

1. My faith
2. My wife
3. My children
4. My health
5. My occupation
6. Extended family and friends
7. Hobbies and home maintenance

Anyone looking at my life twelve years ago would have figured that my occupation, medicine, was #1 on my list. I was at the office all day every day. I struggled with how to get my life in line with my priorities. Finally, I realized that I had to change my approach to my work.

I had to make many other changes, too. I moved to a rural area in order to reduce my cost of living, so that I could cut back on my work. (This relocation had some nice benefits for my wife and children, aside from having me hanging around the house more.) I sold my portion of the medical practice to a larger corporation, which freed up a lot of time to spend with my family and friends. It had been my habit to start playing with my kids the minute I got home from work; I changed this to focusing on my wife first. This gave the children a better sense of her rightful importance in the family. Initially, I'd placed my health last on the list. Then I realized that it needed to be moved higher if I wanted the strength and energy to take care of everything else. Getting my life in line with all seven priorities took years to accomplish, but the process has worked amazingly well.

My wife made her own list. The time we spent comparing our lists has been a huge help in reducing conflict and stress in our lives. Though the top three entries are the same on her list and mine, the lower entries don't match, because we have different responsibilities in life. Now when she does things differently from the way I would, her actions make sense to me, because I know her priority list.

I really don't believe that men and women are from different planets. Poor communication just makes it seem that way. And poor communication can be improved.

Maybe you don't like my priority list. No problem! You're supposed to make your own. Sometimes people get upset at me or my family because of the way we have set our priorities. But far too many people are overstressed because they spend too much time and energy trying to please everybody. I know I can't make everyone happy, so I have to focus on living according to what I believe is right.

Spending your time and energy to truly *help* other people is a noble thing. Spending it trying to *please* people usually turns out badly for everyone. It can't really be done.

It takes work to create your list and put it into action. It can be disruptive to others in your life until they get used to the changes you've made. Don't let that stop you.

This process is like pushing a car over a hill. Laborious at first, but once you crest the top, you're coasting.

DR. DUKE'S GAME PLAN

The core of my plan for reducing stress as a risk factor to your health is to follow the process we just discussed. Make that list of the seven most important things in your life, and get your day-to-day existence in line with those priorities.

There are many other ways of reducing stress, but I think they pale in comparison to living faithfully according to your values and beliefs. Most of the methods I'm about to list are the ones to which people turn first. Some of them are escapist and therefore temporary responses to chronic problems. But all these things have benefits, as long as you have your major priorities in place.

1. **Proper nutrition.** People who are stressed have a tendency to eat less. Too often we rely on caffeine for energy or alcohol for relaxation. These chemicals disturb our sleep and leave us more tired and stressed out than before. When we are under unusual stress, it's more important than ever to eat well, because these are times when our bodies typically use up more vitamins, minerals, and vital plant nutrients. If you eat well during stressful episodes, you will function and think better, making it easier to solve your problems.

2. **Day planners and time-management systems.** These can be very helpful in organizing your daily errands and tasks, and in keeping you focused on how much you have to shovel today, rather than fretting about the mammoth size of the pile, which causes many of us to give up before we've even started. These organizers are a great investment.

3. **Enough sleep.** Sleep can raise serotonin levels, which helps us to think more clearly. Sleep is often the first thing we sacrifice when we have too much to do, but getting all the sleep you need can actually help you keep up with life by enabling you to think more clearly and act efficiently. (There's more about the importance of adequate sleep in chapter 6.)

4. **Exercise.** Moderate exercise has been shown to both reduce stress and increase immune system function.

5. **Music.** Among the most misquoted lines in English literature are these, written by William Congreve and correctly rendered here:

Musick has Charms to sooth a savage Breast,
To soften Rocks, or bend a knotted Oak.

This is especially—and clinically—true of certain kinds of music. Music can stimulate the brain to release hormones that cause us to relax and feel at ease. However, research has shown that the brain has certain tastes, as it were, only releasing those hormones in response to certain *types* of music. Generally, for stress reduction the brain prefers a strong melodic theme; it doesn't respond well to lots of percussion or excessive repetition. Research has shown that classical music, for example, regulates stress hormones, boosts immune function, and increases levels of endorphins, the pleasure chemicals in the brain. At the institute, we've found that Johann Sebastian Bach is effective for reducing stress.

6. **Meditation.** This method is greatly misunderstood. People tend to think of only one particular form of meditation, but there are many different types, just as there are many different types of exercise. Not all exercise is good for you (for example, high-impact aerobics' effect on joints), and not all meditation is beneficial, either.

The dictionary defines meditation as an act of spiritual contemplation. Throughout recorded history, it has always been used in a religious context. Once you thoroughly study the subject, you find it naïve to think that one can separate a religious practice from a religion. My point is that if you want to meditate, you should do so in accordance with your spiritual beliefs, rather than paying someone to teach you a "non-religious" way. Not all forms of meditation are equal.

Three major forms of meditation are practiced around the world. Certainly there are variations, but they usually stem from one of these three methods:

- Focusing on an object or a process, as opposed to free thought.
- Repeating reinforcing suggestions to manipulate oneself or one's environment for a desired outcome.
- Reflecting on good thoughts, teachings, or things that have happened in one's life. This form allows a free progression of ideas and thoughts.

If you meditate using a method that doesn't complement your spiritual belief system, it can increase anxiety and stress. Patients have come to my office with extreme stress and anxiety after going to meditation centers that don't correspond to their spiritual beliefs. Studies report that as many as 63 percent of people experience such negative side effects.[204]

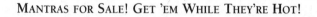

MANTRAS FOR SALE! GET 'EM WHILE THEY'RE HOT!

I'm all for meditation as a stress-relief process, with the qualifications noted above.

However, certain methods of meditation were introduced to the West a few decades ago as a heavily marketed fad. As is usually the case, not all the claims are true. The vast majority of research concerning the health benefits of meditation has been of very poor quality, according to a 450-page scholarly report prepared for the U.S. Department of Health Services[205] and reported by the National Institutes of Health's National Center for Complementary and Alternative Medicine. The report asserts: "Firm conclusions on the effects of meditation practices in healthcare cannot be drawn based on available evidence." Mediation as a health fad is still with us, but I'd rather stand on the best science when it comes to protecting your health.

---

7. **Escape.** My wife and I try to go on an overnight or weekend trip several times a year. Getaway weekends, vacations, retreats, and long walks on the beach have their place—as long as they support your life priorities and aren't the mainstay of your anti-stress game plan. ❖

This life-priorities approach has benefited thousands of people. It will help you, too. It takes a bit of work up front, but the results are eminently worth it. Stress produces inflammation and you need to control it. This approach works beautifully if implemented sensitively, with your whole family in mind.

A final word of advice: Don't measure your stress level by comparing it to those of your coworkers, friends, and relatives. People use this as a rationalization. "I don't have any problems . . . everyone I work with is as stressed out as I am." Yes, you're right. All those other people are as stressed out as you are, and it's damaging *their* health, too.

If stress is affecting your health, work, family or friendships in any negative way, it needs to be seriously addressed.

In the last chapter, I promised to discuss two issues in greater detail before summing up the Twenty-Five Easy and Manageable Steps to Optimal Health. Before I thoroughly explain the risk factors for the major chronic diseases in chapters 9 through 12 (which are fundamental to your understanding of optimal health), I will discuss the other topic—the role that dietary supplements play in optimal health. There are some brilliant scientists who lack fundamental understanding of the role of supplementation and disparage their use. I can relate to those misperceptions because I once had them, too.

The next chapter is devoted to the why and how of dietary supplementation. You will soon have a deeper understanding of why supplements are an important component of our strategy for reducing inflammation and the risk of chronic disease. Supplementation is truly a pillar of optimal health.

CHAPTER 8

Dietary Supplementation's Role in the Reduction of Inflammation

In most team sports, you can't be successful in the long run if you rely only on your starters and your star players. You need skilled players on the bench, ready to fill the gap when a starter has to come out of the game. Star players get injured, they get tired, and sometimes they just have bad days. To win and keep winning, you need backup, and in most sports you need to play your backups often.

Nutrition is a bit like that. You've seen from reading this far that I want you to eat the healthiest diet you can, because good nutrition from healthy food is critical to winning optimal health. You can't get there without it.

But this is the twenty-first century, and most of us find it difficult to eat as well as we should all the time. Actually, that statement is a huge oversimplification of why we need to augment our diet by taking supplements. I'll explain in greater detail presently why dietary supplements are vital to our game plan for winning optimal health.

For now, let's just say that our opponent never lets up. The risk factors for chronic disease are always ready to take over the game. They don't get tired or take a day off. Dietary supplements help us keep our nutrition levels where they should be, even when we can't always eat as we should.

Nutritional Deficiency: Not Just a Third-World Problem

While visiting Cochin, India, my associate Bill met a family that included a beautiful ten-year-old girl. As he spoke with the little girl's parents, he began to notice an unusual hesitancy in her manner—something beyond the normal shyness of children. The child's parents told Bill that she was blind. And as a guy who lives in an affluent Western country, he was stunned to learn that her blindness was the result of a vitamin A deficiency.[206]

Vitamin A is an essential nutrient that is inexpensive and easy to get, either through diet or a supplement. If this child had had access to it, she wouldn't be blind. That encounter still troubles Bill today. And the saddest part is that that little girl's case is tragically common. There are about 2.8 million children under five years of age in more than sixty countries who suffer blindness caused by vitamin A deficiency. Basic nutrients profoundly affect our health.

What's more, this problem isn't confined to poor people or poor countries. Nutrient deficiencies are prevalent around the world, in both developed and developing nations. The World Health Organization reported in 2000 that vitamin and mineral deficiencies afflict one-third of the world's people.[207] Another World Health Organization report states that micronutrient deficiencies are an underlying cause of death and disease worldwide.[208] As will be discussed further in chapter 10, vitamin D deficiency is associated with many cancers and is much more common than most health-care workers realize. A study that assessed a population of normal and apparently healthy volunteers at the European Urban Center found that 34 percent of them exhibited vitamin D deficiency. The study revealed that the deficiency is much more common than previously thought and is not restricted to high-risk groups.[209]

A study in Beijing indicated that vitamin D deficiency occurred in more than 40 percent of adolescent girls in winter.[210] A U.S. study by the Centers for Disease Control found that 42 percent of African American women and 4 percent of Caucasian women of reproductive age were deficient in vitamin D.[211] These were women in the prime of their lives, living in the wealthiest nation on earth. And it's actually much worse than that. These studies were all done *before* current recommendations of increasing the vitamin D deficiency level.

There are many common nutrient deficiencies. An estimated 2 billion people have iron deficiency anemia,[212] and over 2 billion people are at risk for iodine deficiency disorders.[213] That is about *one third of the people in the world*, at the time of the studies. The people of China struggle with deficiencies of zinc, selenium, thiamine, calcium, retinol, and riboflavin, among other nutrients.[214] Globally, over two billion people are at risk for deficiencies in vitamin A, iodine, iron, zinc, folate, and the B vitamins—again, one in three.[215]

There is a great deal more research demonstrating that nutrient deficiencies exist in both developing and developed nations. One study reported significantly below-normal intakes of vitamin E, carotene, and alpha-carotene in U.S. women. More than 60 percent of the women in this study reported dietary copper, zinc, and selenium intakes well below recommended levels.[216] Some 75 percent of elderly men and 87 percent of elderly women in the U.S. have inadequate dietary intake of calcium, an especially serious problem for that age group.[217]

A national nutrition survey in Japan discovered an increasing trend of excessive calorie intake coupled with deficiency in micronutrients.[218] A study of the elderly in Great Britain revealed that vitamin D, magnesium, copper, vitamin C, iron, and folate deficiencies are common.[219] Since vitamin and mineral deficiencies are so common in the U.S. and can lead to DNA damage, one researcher concluded that this deficiency is most likely a significant cause of cancer.[220]

I could cite hundreds of scholarly articles on this topic, but instead I want to note a surprising and encouraging trend. *Average people all around the world are taking nutritional supplements.* And they are doing so without any broad-based push from the medical profession.

Hundreds of scholarly authors have concluded that supplementation will help solve deficiency problems.[221] But the majority of professionals in established medicine around the world act as if they are unaware of these statistics. They seem stuck in the paradigm established by outdated research that says sufficient amounts of all nutrients can be gotten through diet alone.

A scientific review published in the *Journal of the American Medical Association (JAMA)* in 2002[222] stated, "it appears prudent for all adults to take vitamin supplements." Yet many physicians, nutritionists, and dietitians dig in their heels when it comes to recommending supplementation. Globally, the idea of supplementation seems somehow wrong to the medical community. It amazes me that even though everyone knows the industrialized lifestyle has people gobbling vitamin-deficient fast and processed foods, the medical community act as if they would rather leave these people vitamin-deficient than recommend a supplement.

Perhaps some doctors are afraid their patients will over-supplement. Some people do this, and there *are dangers* associated with excess. But a happy medium has to be found, because millions of people around the world are supplementing, despite the feelings of so many in the medical community. Most physicians feel uninformed or uncomfortable with the subject, so it's easier for them to just discourage supplement use across the board. Patients sense this uneasiness and will deny that they are taking a supplement even when asked. (The Mayo Clinic has studied this phenomenon—more on it below.) This is an area in which established medicine is lagging behind the patients it serves.

Data from the National Health and Nutrition Examination Survey in 2002 showed that 52 percent of adults in the U.S. report taking a dietary supplement.[223] The same survey reported only 40 percent in 1994.[224] Moreover, these numbers are likely to be underestimates, given a study done at the Mayo Clinic[225] in which some two hundred subjects were requested to report their supplementation on a written questionnaire and then were interviewed. Dietary supplement use was noted on 30.5 percent of the subjects' written reports, but when interviewed, 61 percent of people said that they were taking supplements.

People are popping vitamins, minerals, and other supplements all over the world. Forty-three percent of Germans report using supplements.[226] Fifty-four percent of Korean senior high school students use supplements.[227] In Denmark, 59 percent of people report the use of some kind of dietary supplement.[228] In Canada, 46 percent of women and 33 percent of men report taking at least one supplement.[229] In Australia, 48 percent of men and 61 percent of women report some supplement use.[230] A World Health Organization survey concluded that 75 percent of the world's population use non-conventional medicinal practices, and most of those involve herbals.[231]

Even though doctors downplay the value of supplementation, many of their smartest, most health-conscious patients supplement their diets. A study by the Fred Hutchinson Cancer Research Center in Seattle obtained supplement information from 61,587 people ages fifty to seventy-six to study their demographics. Use of herbal and specialty supplements was significantly higher among respondents who were older, female, educated, had normal body mass index, were nonsmokers, engaged in exercise, and ate a diet lower in fat and higher in fruits and vegetables.

Meanwhile, as a group, physicians, nutritionists, and dietitians remain undereducated about dietary supplements, and certain recent, biased research hasn't improved matters.

A poorly reasoned review article in the British medical journal *The Lancet* in 2004,[232] along with other research that suffers from bias and poor methodology,[233] only widened the gap between established medicine and the average patient. Too many doctors buy in to research like this. I blame the lack of training in preventive medicine provided by medical schools for physicians' inability to recognize the fundamental flaws in this kind of research. This isn't an attack on the schools; I received an outstanding education, and yet held a similar bias. The problem relates to one I discussed in chapter 5—our profession's focus on diagnosis and treatment of disease, at the expensive of prevention.

For example, researchers tend to study supplements as if they were medicines. One such study found that folic acid didn't reduce incidence of heart attacks *among people with advanced heart disease and multiple health problems*. The study concluded that "such treatment should therefore not be recommended."[234]

Yikes! You missed the point, guys. I'm not talking about *curing* advanced heart disease—I'm talking about *preventing* heart disease through a lifetime of good nutrition.

Unfortunately, many scientists and physicians who read this research decided that since folic acid wasn't beneficial to people who already had advanced heart disease, it had no value in prevention. From there, they leaped to the position that homocysteine must not be a risk factor for heart disease—see chapter 9. (Homocysteine is an inflammatory chemical that can be controlled by adequate folic acid intake.) This is shoddy reasoning. Again, we're talking about *preventing* the disease, not reversing or curing it once the patient is close to death.

Elevated homocysteine is associated with increased inflammation, oxidation, clotting, and other conditions associated with heart disease.[235] It has been shown to be an independent risk factor for heart disease in India where there is less access to folic acid (their foods are typically not fortified with folate as they are in the West.)[236]

Until we have seen long-term, prospective, double-blind intervention studies on healthy people, homocysteine should not be eliminated as a risk factor.

I wish I could fully detail the inadequacies of the research that has been done on supplements, but that would double the length of this book. I'll just say that the worldwide medical community desperately needs to educate itself on this subject. Prevention is a much more sensible approach to disease. It is far easier to prevent a disease than to treat and cure it once it is established—and it goes without saying that prevention is in the patient's best interest.

Look at it this way. I've seen doctors do brilliant, heroic work to save the life of a child who had been struck by an automobile. But if those doctors had been present at the scene of the accident, they would certainly have done everything they could to keep that child from running out into the street.

In the case of chronic disease, we doctors *are* present at the scene. We *can* teach our patients how to avoid being hit by the runaway bus that is chronic disease—or at least how to significantly improve their chances of dodging it.

"I'M NOT A DOCTOR, BUT I PLAY ONE ON TV."

Americans of certain age will remember a TV commercial that began with that line. It's a silly way to add credibility to a sales pitch, and yet, if your doctor isn't giving you sound advice on nutritional supplements, to whom should you turn?

Unfortunately, there is no shortage of pseudoscientists filling air time with infomercials and our mailboxes with sales pitches and "newsletters." It's time for established medicine to embrace the role of nutrition and supplementation in disease prevention, for the protection of their patients. There are too many hucksters out there who are eager to fill in the gaps with misinformation.

Why Do We Need Supplements Now?

As far as we know, early civilizations did not use vitamin and mineral supplements. So why has supplementation become necessary now? The reason lies in the dramatic changes in our lifestyles and technology, especially over the last few decades. Essentially, we have polluted not only our air and water, but our food as well, while taking a great deal of the nutrition out of it.

Before I explain this further, I want to address a question that may have just formed in your mind.

"Dr. Duke," you are thinking, "I know from my extensive reading of history that the average human lifespan in the year 1800 was about thirty years, and by the year 2000 it had risen to sixty-seven years globally and more than seventy-five years in developed countries. So why are you telling me that our diets are worse today than before the industrial revolution?"

I'm giving you an A+ just for asking that question.

Prior to this century, infectious diseases killed off people in huge numbers, including an extremely high number of infants. The average lifespan included those infants in the average. The number is a little misleading, though, because if you look at the ages of famous people, they commonly lived to be in their sixties and seventies. Today we've wiped out most of those infectious diseases, even in poor countries. People now live much longer on the average, but many die far sooner than they should from chronic diseases like heart disease, diabetes, and cancer. As I have demonstrated, the rates of these diseases have risen sharply in the last fifty years. It is possible, maybe even probable, that the average human lifespan could soon begin shrinking if we don't stem these epidemics.

We make food much differently today from the way it was produced two hundred years ago. Then, even in the most advanced countries, most people lived in the countryside and worked in agriculture. They didn't use herbicides, pesticides, or chemical fertilizers, because those things hadn't been invented yet. Crops were rotated to keep the soil rich in nutrients, and they were irrigated, if at all, with uncontaminated water. There was little if any air pollution, so crops weren't contaminated as they are today with chemical particulates that settle out of the air. Food was harvested at its prime and eaten or naturally preserved; it wasn't sprayed with chemicals to make it look pretty longer in the marketplace. Everyone ate organically.

Fresh vegetables were a prominent part of the diet, and only the wealthy ate lots of red meat. Medieval peasants had yet to be introduced to the pleasures of processed corn chips, plastic-wrapped, preservative-laden snack cakes, and artificially flavored beverages.

People got lots and lots of exercise. They had to if they wanted to eat and stay warm, not to mention travel anywhere. Their normal activities of daily living would seem like brutal labor to most of us today, but exercise has extreme health benefits. One of those is that the high caloric demands associated with exercise increase the likelihood that people will consume the appropriate micronutrients (vitamins, minerals, and phytonutrients) as well.

Meals were prepared in the home using natural ingredients. People ate healthy, nutritionally complex whole-grain breads, instead of the white stuff most of us eat today. Take a look at the label of a loaf of white bread—check out the additives, over and above the high-glycemic refined white flour.

Processed foods were rare and none of them contained the cheap partially hydrogenated corn oils, high-fructose corn syrup, or the smorgasbord of chemicals that our food contains today. They also were not exposed to the thousands of chemicals that are a normal part of industrialized life. (For example, just read the fine print on the labels of your personal care items and count the chemicals.)

Of course, we have some significant health advantages today. Western medicine has eliminated most of the acute diseases that used to take so many lives. And our technology allows us to produce, store, and distribute enough food to prevent the famines that used to result from droughts and other natural disasters. (Famine today is generally caused by political disasters, not environmental ones.)

And yet, it doesn't take much imagination to realize that in between disasters, our ancestors' eating and living habits were generally much healthier than ours today.

To attain optimal health we need to replace the good nutrients we have lost and counteract the bad stuff that has been added to our food.

FB

ADAPTOGENS—ADAPTING TO ANYTHING IN THE UNIVERSE

One rather recent concept is that there is a group of plant nutrients that can adapt to many different stresses in your life, becoming everything you need when you need it. Regretfully, the science behind these claims has not been of high enough quality to verify these claims as of yet. A great deal more research by independent groups needs to be performed to verify this concept before recommendations can be made. Until then, be careful of this notion. If the concept is real, good science will prove it

"If You Eat a Balanced Diet, You Don't Need a Multivitamin."

Have you ever heard this statement before? Is it valid? At the least, it's rather confusing because we hear people say that we should take supplements, but then there are doctors who say, "All you're doing is paying for expensive urine because your body doesn't need that much." (I know because I used to foolishly make this statement to patients. I was simply uninformed. I now have thousands of blood reports proving that as people take in more nutrients, we find higher levels of those nutrients in the blood. Obviously, the body does desire more than absolute minimums.) There are even researchers who are apparently trying to hide benefits of supplements in their research, then making statements in their conclusions that supplementation is dangerous. Granted, there are risks, so I will present guidelines here. But the fear tactic used by some simply comes from bias.

The logical question to ask is, "How good is the science of those people who say you don't need a supplement?" Or, "On what basis do they make such statements?" I have already presented some very important statistics, but now it's time to look deeper.

Let's do an analysis here of some of the science upon which these "experts" base their negative statements. You'll soon see that they have serious weaknesses, and that huge misunderstandings need to be cleared up to help reduce the risk of chronic disease.

Governmental Dietary Guidelines

Governmental dietary guidelines are where most health professionals base their statements concerning the need for supplementation, and a misunderstanding of these recommendations is the source of the negative comments presented above. Sadly, most health professionals don't understand the origin or the original intention of such standards. The World Health Organization has dietary guidelines and has written manuals accordingly. Most governments have instituted similar recommendations. In the U.S. they are currently called DRIs (Dietary Reference Intake), and they used to be called RDA (Recommended Dietary Allowance).

These guidelines originated during World War Two. They were written by a committee established by the U.S. National Academy of Sciences because there were severe nutrient deficiencies internationally during the war. The standards were used as nutritional guides to prevent deficiencies for soldiers, civilians, and overseas individuals who were in need of food relief. They have been modified about every ten years or so, but their intention has always been to prevent deficiency diseases like scurvy, beriberi, and others. They were never intended to become what they are today—maximums. Inappropriately, for brilliant scientists and health-care workers all over the world, the minimum nutrient recommendation has also become the maximum, to the point that some professionals will state that any nutrient level above that which keeps you from a deficiency disease is a waste. Is that rational?

Let's take this same reasoning and apply it to money. How many of us will hold to the notion that any amount of money above that which keeps us from starving to death is a waste? Do you really believe that? Of course not. Then why is this same reasoning applied to nutrient levels? Lack of understanding. As noted, I have thousands of blood reports proving that our bodies will absorb—and apparently desire—more than absolute starvation minimums.

As noted in chapter 6, there is a plethora of scientific research that reveals that there are elevated levels of vitamins, minerals, and phytonutrients which can reduce the risk of chronic diseases. I have thousands of articles and would love to write an entire book on this topic. To attempt to get many of these nutrients from food alone, especially fat-soluble nutrients, would require a caloric intake that would result in obesity or create other health problems.

Let's take a quick look at the science used by those who say we don't need supplements. We'll start with an August 2008 study discussing the complexity of gene interaction, nutrients, and disease risk reduction. The authors concluded with a quote:

"There are *analytical challenges* in analyzing the high-dimensional datasets relating genes, nutrients, and other variables *to their influence on health and disease processes*. An even *greater challenge* may be in *implementing population level changes in diet* and behavior to fully exploit the potential of this field." (Emphasis mine.)[237]

What are they saying here? In short, that the interaction of nutrients, genes, and the digestive tract is so complex that we really have no idea what nutrients to recommend at this point.

But wait, there's more!

In a study that looked at our ability to assess the amounts of nutrients people are really getting in their diet by using surveys, the researchers concluded:

> ...*assessing only nutrient intake is inadequate*, since other food components affect its bioavailability. Non-nutrient food constituents, such as phytate and polyphenols, interfere with the bioavailability of iron and zinc.

Bioconversion and bioefficiency of precursor nutrients, such as carotenoids, also affect the estimated intake of vitamin A in its active form. *Different strategies are required to deal with these challenges in assessing dietary intakes of micronutrients* in order to establish the prevalence of inadequate intake, as well as the association between intake and nutritional status." (Emphasis mine.)[238]

Let me tell you what this means in simple language. It says that the interaction of food in the digestive tract is so complex, with chemicals binding nutrients and nutrients changing form, that surveys we have used for years to try to calculate intake are inadequate. We really don't know what's happening in there because it's so complex.

Is there value in taking a multivitamin/multimineral/multiphytonutrient? Deficiencies in certain nutrients—folic acid, B12, vitamin B6, niacin, vitamin C, vitamin E, iron, and zinc—result in our DNA looking as if it had been damaged by X-ray radiation, which, according to one study, increases the risk of cancer.[239] Remedying these deficiencies caused the DNA to look normal because all of these components are necessary for the enzymes which repair DNA to work efficiently. Do you know how much zinc you've had today? Exactly? What about the rest of the nutrients? Wouldn't you rather make sure?

Is there value in a multivitamin that also contains multiphyotnutrients like lycopene? Fifty-seven studies have reported an inverse relationship between the intake of tomatoes or the blood level of lycopenes and the risk of cancer.[240] In other words, as tomato intake and the blood level of a phytonutrient found in tomatoes called lycopene increased, the risk of cancer went down. The benefit was strongest for cancers of the prostate, lung, and stomach, but benefit was also seen for cancers of the pancreas, colon, rectum, esophagus, oral cavity, breast, and cervix. In addition, we have checked lycopene levels on thousands of people and have noted increases in blood levels with lycopene supplementation. Am I saying that supplementation absolutely assures these benefits? No, not until further studies come out that specifically address it. But, with extremely small risk, is it worth waiting ten to twenty years to find out?

Another phytonutrient, quercetin, has been shown to slow and even stop abnormal cells of the prostate.[241] I could go on and on, but the point is that the benefits are there.

The revolution from the antiquated thinking of only focusing on micronutrient deficiencies is long overdue. Using minimum nutrient levels as maximums is silly. Nutrient intake science is far more complex than we realized years ago, so we shouldn't short-change ourselves. I'm not advising that you should ignore maximums, because there are toxic levels of most nutrients (see below), but the blanket "no" reaction to supplementation by health professionals is uneducated at best and increases the risk of disease and mortality at worst.

Are Supplements Safe?

There are risks associated with supplementation just like there are risks associated with any activity we participate in. The risks primarily come from over-supplementation, drug interactions, poor/contaminated supplement sources, or a simple lack of knowledge. This book devotes a great deal of time to providing guidelines to reduce the risks associated with supplementation (see the next section), but what I find particularly irritating is when uninformed physicians or scientists (some of whom, as discussed before, may be funded by the pharmaceutical industry) attempt to scare you away from *all* supplementation. That's ridiculous.

I'm very well aware of the risks associated with supplementation, and I constantly counsel people on the reduction of these risks. But if the uninformed or biased doctors who are trying to scare you away from supplementation want to play that game, I'd love to compare the risks of supplementation with the risks and side effects associated with prescription medications.

Here are just a couple of facts. Some well-known prescription medications are suspected to increase the risk of cancer.[242] Although there were about 960 adverse effects reported to the U.S. government in 2008 from the roughly 65 percent of the total U.S. population that takes some form of supplementation, this compares to 482,154 adverse effects reported for prescription medications in 2007.[243] I could provide many other examples.

The fact that many professionals in conventional or established medicine attack supplement use is surprising because, in the areas of cancer, infectious and inflammatory diseases that are linked, 60-75 percent of the new drugs developed between 1983 and 1994 were based on natural compounds.[244, 245] Why is it OK for conventional medicine to have treatments based on natural plant chemicals that are then modified, but somehow supplementation with natural products is wrong? These scientists need to be consistent.

Many practitioners of conventional medicine also attack supplementation because of the high levels of single nutrients like vitamin C or E used (and I agree that high levels of single nutrients usually aren't the best). But these doctors don't realize that they are doing the same thing by writing prescriptions for single, synthetic chemicals which can have tremendous negative side effects and haven't achieved their touted potential over the last twenty years.[246]

Am I against all prescription medications? Certainly not! Some are wonderful and millions of people are alive today because of them. But for some physicians to imply that all supplementation is dangerous is extremely hypocritical and simply not true. There is a middle ground, and it needs to be reached soon because governments won't be able to afford the cost of health care unless sweeping preventive medicine changes—including the use of supplementation—are made. I strongly recommend intelligent, responsible, controlled supplementation, within the guidelines of the best science and with your private physician's counsel, while avoiding medication interactions. We can find a middle ground, with lower health-care costs and risks, that will benefit everyone.

What Supplements Should I Take?

Let me start with a disclaimer. I am only going to answer this question with regard to reducing chronic disease. A truly exhaustive discussion would fill an entire book! Also, I do not want this chapter to replace discussion with your personal physician. For all the carping I've just done about the medical profession's ignorance on this subject, the fact remains that your doctor knows *you* best. He or she should know whether a certain supplement might be more or less valuable to you personally, or whether it might interact badly with medications you take.

Please discuss supplementation with your doctor and follow his or her recommendations.

My purpose here is to help you understand which supplements might be beneficial to you in reducing your risk of chronic disease and attaining optimal health. Some of my recommendations are stronger than others because of the amount of research available. Before providing a list of selected supplements, I will state a few ground rules.

BLANKET FAD-BUSTER ANNOUNCEMENT!

Most of what you read in the rest of this chapter will constitute Fad Buster statements. There is probably no area of popular health culture more fad-ridden than the issue of supplementation.

Thirteen Rules for Supplementation

1. **More is not better.** There is an optimal amount that you should take of any supplement, and that amount may vary from one person to the next. So just because a certain amount is beneficial—as shown by research—that doesn't mean that two or three times that amount is better. If a supplement has biologically active chemicals, there is a significant risk that you can get too much of it. Don't purchase a supplement just because it has higher levels of the ingredient you're interested in. One of the most common errors I see utilizing this reasoning is with B vitamins. Some people think that since B vitamins are water-soluble, unlimited amounts are fine. This simply isn't true.

2. **"Natural" does not mean "safe."** Marketers sometimes label their products "natural," as if that guarantees wholesomeness and safety. Poison mushrooms and heroin are natural, and they can kill you.

3. **Buying something from a health food store doesn't guarantee it's healthy.** Ma huang, also known as ephedra, was sold in many health

121

food stores long after its dangers became well known. It only stopped being sold in the U.S. when the government banned it on account of its association with abnormal heart rhythms and death. Now available instead is a weight-loss product called bitter orange—which has been shown to have some of the same risks as ephedra. There are other potentially dangerous herbs readily available in stores all around the world, and in some countries their manufacture and sale aren't regulated at all.

4. **Avoid supplements that contain multiple herbs.** Some products contain as many as ten or more different herbs. Herbs are plants that individually have been shown to have some effect on the body. To just throw many herbs together without logical connection is purely a marketing ploy to make the product seem valuable. You'd be using similar logic if you were to grab a lot of products off the pharmacy shelf and randomly take them. Not many of us would consider that a valuable thing to do. Additionally, there is generally no literature that supports the safety of such random combinations. These combinations of multiple randomly selected herbs are completely different than multivitamin/multimineral supplements, which have had a lot of research performed on them.

5. **Check how a supplement is made.** The best supplements are manufactured and packaged under solid manufacturing guidelines that assure cleanliness and purity.

6. **Choose "food" over synthetic chemicals.** The best supplements are those made from pressed or condensed food items, rather than chemicals that are synthesized in a laboratory.

7. **Opt for organic.** Of those supplements that *are* from condensed or pressed food sources, organically grown ones are safer.

8. **Do some research.** Buy your supplements only from companies that can document that the amounts of nutrients in the tablets are equal to what's promised on the label (you can check ConsumerLab.com,

which independently verifies this). Independent studies have shown that some manufacturers have few—if any—nutrients in their supplements. This problem exists especially in the U.S., where there is very little control or regulation of the supplement industry.

9. **Money isn't everything.** *Nutritional* value is the objective, so don't base your purchase on price alone. I have seen x-rays that showed whole, undigested calcium supplements in the lower part of a patient's bowel. That patient probably saved a little money buying a cheap calcium tablet. Too bad her body didn't absorb any of it.

10. **Be cautious of Ayurvedic products.** (This warning comes from even health professionals in India.) Based on a study by Harvard Medical School reported in *JAMA* in 2004,[247] it would be wise to avoid Ayurvedic herbal medicine products—or at least be *extremely* selective in choosing them, especially those manufactured in South Asia. This warning should hold at least until strict testing of those products has become mandatory and the results are published. The Harvard Medical School study reported that one in five Ayurvedic products contained potentially harmful levels of lead, mercury, and/or arsenic. There have been many documented cases of heavy metal toxicity due to these products.[248, 249] There's a reason for this: Traditionally, it was believed by many in Ayurvedic medicine that heavy metals were beneficial. Now we know they are poisonous, but harmful levels are still found in many Ayurvedic supplements.

11. **Listen to the right people.** Infomercials and sales-oriented newsletters are hardly the best sources of information about supplementation. I mean, whom would you ask for advice about buying a used car—a skilled auto mechanic or a used-car salesman? Especially avoid newsletters in which the author portrays the entire medical establishment as an evil conspiracy that is withholding valuable information from you because they have been bought out by the pharmaceutical industry. When an author tells you he is the only guy in the world who is being honest with you, beware, *especially* if he wants your money. Reliable newsletters come from established

academic authorities, like *The Berkeley Newsletter*, *Harvard Men's Health Watch*, *Tufts University Health and Nutrition Letter*, and *Nutrition Action Health Letter* (from the Center for Science in the Public Interest). UC Berkeley, Harvard, and Tufts are highly respected research universities. Harvard isn't in the business of selling dietary supplements; a lot of private newsletter publishers are. Of course, some academic journals have authors with narrow views of supplementation. Overall, though, they usually attempt to be fair.

12. **Beware of drug interactions.** If you are currently taking any prescription medication, check with your pharmacist to make sure that the supplement you are interested in will not interact badly with your medication.

13. **Get smart.** Make informed choices. You need to understand what you are taking and why you are taking it. Read up, and talk to your doctor. (If he or she isn't well informed, get another doctor.) Choose a supplementation plan based on an understanding of your needs and health risks. Focus on the diseases for which you are most at risk instead of taking something because it's in the news or your friend is taking it. You'd be surprised at how often I have to convince our clients to *reduce* their supplement intake, because they believe they should just take everything on the shelf.

Supplements That May Reduce Your Risk of Chronic Disease

Please show this list to your doctor,

You'll find a much wider variety of supplemental products on store shelves than I am going to list here. All I want to present are the supplements that are most likely to help reduce your risk of chronic disease.

Again, please, *please* consult with your physician and pharmacist before you take any supplement. You need to make sure that the supplements you take won't interact negatively with any medications you're already taking.

The list below includes some recommended dosages. Please check these with your doctor and pharmacist as well, since new research may change what are considered safe or effective levels of supplements, especially with regard to interactions with other medications you may be taking. And don't forget to take these precautions in reverse, as well: Any time your doctor prescribes a new medication for you, you need to tell him or her what supplements you're taking to make sure there won't be any problems with the mixture.

The supplements you may wish to consider are:

1. **A good multivitamin/multimineral/multiphytonutrient.** I want you to eat as well as you can, nutritionally speaking. However, there are dozens of essential vitamins and minerals, and many other important phytonutrients. You can't keep accurate track of your daily intake of all of these, or even a few. Moreover, in today's culture, even people who try their best to eat well have diets that are far from ideal. Based on that and the *JAMA* article quoted earlier ("it appears prudent for all adults to take vitamin supplements"), most people should take a good multivitamin/multimineral. A study reported in 2003 revealed that multivitamin use reduced C-reactive protein (CRP).[250] In light of this information and that presented in chapter 3, your doctor would have difficulty disagreeing with this recommendation. And it's never too early to start: Prenatal vitamins have been shown to reduce the risk of pediatric cancers.[251, 252] Remedying simple nutrient deficiencies has been shown to protect DNA from damage.[253] The authors of this study concluded that this could lead to increased longevity at a very low cost.

2. **Omega-3.** A great deal of research indicates that over the last century there has been a great shift in the balance between omega-6 and omega-3 fatty acids in our diets. Traditional Mediterranean or Greek diets included roughly equal amounts of omega-6 and omega-3. But because we're now eating so much processed fat, like partially hydrogenated corn oil, we're now consuming about *twenty to thirty times* more omega-6 than omega-3. Omega-6 fatty acids have a tendency to be inflammatory—that is, to contribute to chronic disease. You can bring this wildly-out-of-whack ratio back into balance by eating foods like salmon and canola oil, which have high levels of omega-3. You can also do it by supplementation. A dose of one gram

of omega-3 per day is usually adequate (for adults in the forms of both DHA and EPA), and capsules that contain fish oil usually have more than that. Omega-3 has many other benefits: it reduces hypertension,[254] insulin resistance,[255] inflammation,[256] death rate from heart attacks,[257] Alzheimer's,[258] and more. It also affects gene expression in the liver, heart, fat, and brain.[259] As mentioned in chapter 4, omega-3 most likely increases lifespan because it controls the same molecule that is associated with increased lifespan during severe caloric restriction.[260, 261, 262] (That means you can get the same longevity with omega-3, but without the starvation!) It slows down a number of auto-immune diseases,[263] decreases the risk of colorectal cancer,[264] and reduces the risk of cancer overall.[265] (See Appendix B.3 for food source guidelines.)

This list only scratches the surface with regard to omega-3 benefits. If you want to read more, I again recommend *The Omega Diet* by Dr. Artemis Simopoulos.[266] Finally, please check with your doctor before taking omega-3.

3. **Calcium supplementation.** We all know that calcium is beneficial for maintaining healthy bone structure, but that's not all. Calcium has been shown to help reduce hypertension. (Coenzyme Q10, garlic, and vitamin C may possibly be effective for hypertension, too.) Calcium has been shown to help reduce insulin resistance.[267] According to the National Institutes of Health in the U.S., there is some evidence that supplemental calcium may decrease the risk of colon cancer. The Dietary Supplement Fact Sheet: Calcium[268] states, "Some studies suggest that increased intakes of dietary [low fat sources] and supplemental calcium are associated with a decreased risk of colon cancer."[269, 270, 271]

4. **Flaxseed** seems to be helpful for reducing elevated cholesterol levels.[272] (Calcium, fish oils, magnesium, and oats may also be.)

5. **Vitamin B complex** reduces elevated homocysteine levels.[273] Folic acid (vitamin B9) may also reduce the risk of colon cancer,[274] but some research is now pointing to the idea that we should not take

unlimited amounts of these vitamins. A good multivitamin will usually contain the amount of folic acid and vitamin B12 necessary to reduce homocysteine, an inflammatory substance associated with heart disease. Supplementing with folic acid also improves blood vessel function.[275, 276]

6. **Actual plant products.** Some manufacturers offer supplements that contain plant material. Certainly these cannot replace actually eating five to nine servings of fruits and vegetables every day, but they can be helpful. Many of these supplements contain phytonutrients that reduce inflammation, including hesperidin, quercetin, resveratrol, ellagic acid, anthocyanins, sulforaphanes, and carotenoids. To list the tremendous benefits of phytonutrients would require another book, but suffice it to say that they can significantly reduce your risk of chronic disease.

7. **Vitamin D** has been shown to reduce many cancers, and recommended dosages are being increased. You should probably get at least 1,000 IU and perhaps 2,000 IU of vitamin D per day. Some research is now pointing to far higher levels as ideal. Vitamin D can also boost heart health.[277] It reduces the risk of osteoporosis, high blood pressure, fibromyalgia, skin inflammatory diseases,[278] diabetes, multiple sclerosis, and rheumatoid arthritis. It reduces the risk of several cancers[279] (see chapter 10), such as prostate cancer, most likely because of its anti-inflammatory effect.[280] If your multivitamin does not contain at least 1,000 IU of vitamin D, consider taking additional vitamin D, especially if you are older, don't get much sun, or live north of 35° N latitude (or, for my friends in New Zealand, Tasmania, and Patagonia, south of 35° S latitude.) Low vitamin D levels are associated with an increased death rate.[281, 282] I prefer that blood levels of vitamin D be at least 37ng/ml (U.S.) or approximately 90nmol/L (outside U.S.).

8. **Chromium** may be effective for reducing insulin resistance when taken orally. It can also be used if you have been diagnosed with type 2 diabetes, but only under the watchful eye of your doctor. Doses of

500 mcg twice daily have been shown to significantly decrease average blood sugar levels (HbA1c) after two months of treatment.[283] (Other supplements that may help reduce the risk of diabetes are omega-3 [only with the guidance of a doctor, please], oat bran, calcium, magnesium, oats, and vitamin D.) Chromium picolinate may also reduce cholesterol and triglycerides.[284]

9. **Fiber** can reduce the risk of insulin resistance,[285] heart disease,[286] and perhaps colon cancer, although its effect on the latter remains controversial.

10. **Magnesium** has been shown to help reduce insulin resistance[287] and inflammation.[288] However, you should already be getting enough magnesium in a good multivitamin.

11. **Coenzyme Q10** has been shown in some studies to help reduce congestive heart failure,[289] but is still somewhat controversial. It helps to lower blood pressure,[290, 291] reduce symptoms of Parkinson's,[292] and improve immune function. It is both an antioxidant and an anti-inflammatory.[293]

12. **Vitamin E.** Most vitamin E research has been in relation to cardiovascular disease. In the past, 300 to 400 IU was usually considered a safe dosage. Some recent studies have questioned vitamin E's cardiovascular benefit, but several of these studies have significant methodological problems.[294] Vitamin E has been shown to have cardiovascular benefit when used in combination with other vitamins and minerals.[295] Unfortunately, most researchers only evaluated vitamin E by itself and apart from other antioxidants. They often didn't control for diet or make sure their subjects were getting enough of other vitamins. Vitamins are team players—they work together with other vitamins. Any study that doesn't control for such basic considerations is poorly constructed.

Vitamin E has been shown to reduce inflammation by reducing proinflammatory cytokines (you'll remember those pesky fellows from chapter 3) and CRP.[296, 297] Therefore, in light of inflammation's contribution to cardiovascular disease, vitamin E is likely to reduce this disease if used appropriately and in combination with other antioxidants. I hope future research is performed with these considerations in mind. (The best sources of vitamin E are those that contain a wide variety of its forms, namely alpha-, beta-, delta-, and gamma tocopherol.)

Some poorly constructed research has even suggested that vitamin E could be damaging. Apparently, these researchers are completely unaware of vitamin E's other benefits. It has also been shown to reduce the risk of prostate[298] and stomach cancer,[299] slow the decline of Alzheimer's disease,[300] and improve immune system functioning in the elderly.[301]

13. **Lycopene** reduces the risk of prostate[302] and lung cancer.[303] It is also associated with decreased risk of stomach, pancreas, colon, rectum, esophagus, breast, oral cavity, and cervical cancers.[304] Not surprisingly, it reduces inflammation.[305]

14. **Green tea (polyphenols)** has been shown to lower cholesterol and triglycerides.[306] It also reduces the risk of breast,[307] bladder,[308] esophageal and pancreatic cancers,[309] and reduces the risk of diseases of the brain like Alzheimer's and Parkinson's disease.[310, 311, 312, 313, 314, 315, 316, 317] In addition, green tea has been shown to have anti-cancer[318, 319] and anti-inflammatory effects.[320, 321]

15. **Garlic** reduces elevated cholesterol,[322] hypertension,[323] and the risk of prostate cancer.[324]

16. **Selenium** reduces the risk of prostate,[325] lung, and colorectal cancers.[326]

17. **Vitamin C** reduces the risk of stomach cancer.[327] It may also reduce the risk of stroke[328] and, in combination with vitamin E, the risk of cardiovascular disease.[329, 330]

18. **Glucosamine** reduces the risk of osteoarthritis[331] and inflamma-

tion.[332]

19. **Resveratrol**, found in grape skins, lowers chronic inflammation.[333]

20. **Pomegranate** contains many plant chemicals that have been shown to not only slow atherosclerosis progression,[334] but also apparently reverse it.[335]

21. **Curcumin** (within the spice turmeric) has been shown to protect nerve and brain function as both an antioxidant and anti-inflammatory.[336, 337, 338] It also has benefit at the nutrigenomic level.[339]

22. **Lutein and Zeaxanthin** may protect the retina from the most damaging chemicals that lead to adult blindness.[340, 341]

23. **Ginkgo biloba.** Though it can interact with several medicines, there is some solid research that indicates that it may reduce development of Alzheimer's disease.[342, 343, 344]

24. **Quercetin** reduces inflammation[345] and has been shown to reduce the risk of prostate cancer.[346]

There is more than enough scientific literature to support the use of these supplements for reducing the risk of chronic diseases. There are always new research projects, and future studies may change some recommendations. But if you have a significant risk of some of the cancers or other diseases mentioned, there is enough research today to support using supplements. With some of these supplements, ten or twenty years may pass before we have definite answers, but waiting for this research may not be in your best interest if you are at risk now.

DR. DUKE'S REVOLUTIONARY SUPPLEMENTATION PLAN

What Supplements Should *You* Take?

You've read the "menu" above, and now you want to know how to apply it to your life. I wish I could tell you! That's like asking, "What medications should I take?" The answer is different for every person. It depends on your medical history, current health problems, current medications, allergies, and the diseases for which you are most at risk.

To find good answers to this question, you might want to consider getting a nutritional assessment. Where do you get one? Start by asking your doctor. He or she may be able to refer you to a good source.

I *can* give solid advice for what constitutes good foundational supplementation for most people. You can modify or add to it based on your personal health needs and risks.

Please keep our thirteen rules for supplementation in mind. Look for a reputable, clinically verifiable, preferably organically grown product from pressed food—or as close to that as you can find. Pressed-food supplements are much more expensive than synthetics, but they're worth it, because they naturally contain many phytonutrients that work synergistically. If you can't afford a condensed food supplement, synthetic is certainly better than nothing.

The recommended foundational supplements are:

1. **A good multivitamin/mutimineral/multiphytonutrient.** These usually include calcium, vitamin B complex, vitamin D, chromium, magnesium, vitamin E, selenium, and vitamin C in dosages similar to those mentioned earlier. Depending on your age, you may need additional calcium to meet the recommendations in the NIH Fact Sheet referred to above. Since vitamins, minerals, trace elements, and phytonutrients work together, it is best to have a balanced multivitamin product rather than taking a few individual nutrients separately. It's easier, too—you only have to swallow one or two tablets (some high-quality "multis" require several tablets for all the nutrients and plant materials in one daily dosage).

    More fun facts in support of your using a multivitamin: Vitamins C and E, beta-carotene, and zinc slow the progression of macular degeneration, a leading cause of blindness, especially in older people.[347, 348] Vitamin E supplementation among male smokers reduces risk of prostate cancer, as does beta-carotene supplementation in men with low dietary intakes of that nutrient.[349] Higher plasma levels of vitamin

B6 are associated with reduced risk of colorectal cancer.[350]

2. **Omega-3.** Supplements usually come in the form of fish oils. Adults generally need 1,000 mg of this kind of omega-3 (of the two types, adults should favor EPA over DHA) daily to help correct imbalance between omega-6 and omega-3 for health benefits. The plant form of omega-3 (alpha-linolenic acid) has been shown to reduce the risk of sudden cardiac death.[351] (See additional information about omega-3 earlier in this chapter, as well as in chapters 2, 3, and 9. See Appendix B.3 for food source guidelines.)

3. **Real fruit and vegetable phytonutrients in supplement form.** This is the ideal way to assure that you obtain a wide variety of phytonutrients (over and above the essential vitamins and minerals) that have been shown to significantly reduce risk of chronic disease. Some phytonutrients to try to make sure you obtain are quercetin, pomegranate, lycopene, and green tea polyphenols.

4. **Calcium and vitamin D supplements** taken together (at mealtime) have been shown to increase bone density and prevent hip and other nonvertebral fractures.[352, 353] Low vitamin D levels are associated with several cancers (see chapter 10). They are also associated with increased risk of hypertension[354] and many other health conditions. Vitamin D and calcium reduce insulin resistance and inflammation in non-diabetic adults.[355] (See additional information about vitamin D and calcium earlier in this chapter, as well as in chapters 3, 9, and 12.) ❖

Any additional supplementation should be based on your own health risks. For example:

- If you have a risk of developing osteoarthritis, add glucosamine sulfate. Glucosamine can delay knee-replacement surgery,[356] most likely due to its ability to reduce inflammation.[357] (Some studies have not shown glucosamine to be beneficial; this was because they used glucosamine hydrochloride rather than glucosamine sulfate.)

- If cardiovascular disease or Parkinson's[358] is a risk for you, then add coenzyme Q10 to your plan.
- If cholesterol is a problem, consider adding flaxseed oil and garlic.
- If you are at elevated risk for cancer, Alzheimer's disease, dementia, or Parkinson's disease, consider adding a green tea supplement (polyphenols).
- If insulin resistance or heart disease is a risk factor for you, add chromium. It not only increases insulin sensitivity in insulin-resistant individuals, but may benefit cholesterol abnormalities as well.[359]

Please ask your doctor before taking any of the above. I want you to have his or her professional consideration, based on your own health and risk factors. However, if all you get is a casual "You don't need them," without a careful review of your list, you need to push your doctor for a more sound, specific response. If he or she refuses to support your efforts with sound counsel, he or she is probably relying on outdated nutritional education and only focused on deficiency diseases, as we discussed earlier. You might want to decide whether that doctor is behind the times on other subjects as well. There are always other doctors.

Supplementation plays a significant role in our game plan for optimal health—to the point that I included it among the eight pillars of optimal health in chapter 6. But please don't make the mistake of thinking that supplements makes up for poor diet or bad lifestyle! You can't smoke like a chimney, drink like a fish, eat like a garbage truck, suffer more stress than an air traffic controller, and then expect supplements to make up for all of it. Supplementation is designed to augment a diet and lifestyle that are already sound. As I said at the outset, supplements are the backup players that ensure there aren't any gaps in your nutritional game plan. The newest research suggests that it's very difficult to win optimal health without them.

Now that we have covered how inflammation is at the root cause of all chronic disease and we have started down the pathway to optimal health, it's time to move on to a more detailed discussion of the first pillar of optimal health from chapter 6—reducing the risk factors of chronic disease. This is absolutely fundamental to joining the Optimal Health Revolution. Lack of knowledge of the risk factors in the next four chapters is probably most responsible for people becoming deceived by fads or experiencing failing health. Our revolution's foundation sits on the next four chapters. Please learn them well and heed the advice given. After that, we will put all the information together for you in a very simple and manageable way.

PART IV:

Risk Factors of
Major Chronic Diseases

CHAPTER 9

Defeating Heart Disease,
Your Toughest Opponent

L eonard is a great guy. He's an extremely successful South Korean businessman in his sixties, the leader of an organization staffed by thousands of people, and his warmth, humility, engaging personality, and high integrity make it easy to understand his success.

When I first met Leonard in 1997, he was overweight and in such poor shape that he was unable to finish a three-minute step test (a test in which one's cardiovascular conditioning is assessed by checking for change in one's pulse rate after stepping onto and off of a step for three minutes).

I talked to Leonard about his health status and the fact that he was deeply at risk for heart disease. His response was indicative of what a great leader he is. He looked me in the eye and said, "Doctor Duke, the next time you see me, I will be a different man."

And so he was. After that visit, Leonard made dramatic changes in his lifestyle and reduced many of his risk factors.

For instance, he began to run. For the most committed people, that usually means taking up jogging and actually sticking with it for life. For Leonard it meant going from being unable to finish a three-minute step test to competing in several marathons a year. I'm not saying *you* have to become a marathoner, but Leonard did. More importantly, because he has changed almost every aspect of his lifestyle (as taught in this book), he now gets top grades in every rigorous health test that we perform.

But Leonard didn't stop at getting himself into shape. He has become an example of optimal health for the thousands of people in his business. His best marathon time is three hours and thirty-nine minutes. However, he keeps a plaque on his wall that records his time in one Honolulu Marathon at over eleven hours. The reason that it took him so long to finish that race is that he repeatedly dropped back from the finish line to run with and encourage people in his business who were also competing that day. Leonard didn't stop running until the last person he knew had finished the race. He probably ran *two* marathons that day!

Leonard is a great example of someone who established a game plan for winning optimal health and carried it out to the nth degree. He has given his best effort to extend his life, and he has led thousands of others to better their own health. If I ever start up an Optimal Health Hall of Fame, Leonard is going to be a charter inductee—as both player and coach.

Heart disease kills more people in the developed world than anything else. I know I have already said that, but I can't emphasize it enough. Heart disease—or, to include strokes, cardiovascular disease—is your most important opponent in the effort to win optimal health. It is the chronic disease *you* are most likely to die of—*unless you have a game plan and follow it.*

I am here to give you that game plan.

It consists of defeating each of the attacks heart disease will throw at you. Doctors and scientists refer to the tactics or weapons of heart disease as risk factors.

Even though it is still the leading cause of death, heart disease is no longer seen as the inevitability it once was. In fact, most of the weapons heart disease uses against you are weapons you gave it.

Risk factors are lifestyle or biological qualities and other characteristics that increase one's chances of getting a given disease. Some of the risk factors I will discuss should be familiar to you, others may not be.

If you are a physician or scientist, you'll note that some of the risk factors I discuss have not been accepted by all medical organizations. However, I will cite the scientific literature that supports their inclusion.

Chapters 9 through 12 of this book are essential to understanding how to reduce your risk of chronic disease. They give you the lifestyle tactics necessary for success with the Optimal Health Revolution. Most importantly, this plan is comprehensive. It doesn't focus on one or two aspects of lifestyle or nutrition. This isn't a fad program for you to try out and throw away. It's a way to live the rest of your life.

Most of the factors listed in this chapter and the three that follow have been confirmed by scientific literature for at least fifteen years. At our institute, we've added a few more, based on recent research. I'm going to talk about that research in the coming chapters, while doing my best to make it easy for readers without scientific training to understand.

Why do we cite more than the standard number or risk factors? Because many heart attacks will occur in people without documented heart disease or without the cardiovascular risk factors commonly accepted by established medicine.[360]

At our institute, we teach that there are fifteen risk factors for heart disease. They are not listed here according to any priority; they are all important. Since an entire book could be written about each risk factor, the descriptions below are presented in a condensed form. My aim is to help you determine how many risk factors you have.

So let's get started on beating heart disease. We'll go through the risk factors one by one, and talk about how you can defend yourself against them.

1. Family history and genetic predisposition

We've known for many years that family history was a risk factor for cardiovascular disease.[361, 362, 363] When I worked in emergency rooms, one of the first questions I asked patients who complained of chest pain was whether heart disease ran in their families. If one of your parents has or had heart disease, your own risk of having it is higher than normal. If a brother or sister also has it, your risk is higher still.[364]

Until recently, nobody understood how this genetic predisposition worked. But the recent mapping of the human genome has given us a much better understanding, even though further research is needed. Sir

Gordon Duff, M.D., Ph.D., at the University of Sheffield in the United Kingdom, and Dr. Ken Kornman at Interleukin Genetics in Waltham, Massachusetts, have done excellent research that helps explain the genetic predisposition to heart disease.[365]

Duff and Kornman have shown that if a person has a genetic characteristic associated with the inflammatory marker interleukin-1, his or her risk of heart disease is increased more than three-fold. Some combinations of genetic abnormalities increase the risk seven-fold.

Let's suppose you have such a tendency—that your beloved mom and dad, who gave you love, food, shelter, education, and a sense of right and wrong, also gave you a genetic predisposition to heart disease. Does that mean your fate is sealed and your days numbered? No, it doesn't. It just means the odds are higher. Tendency is not fate. Even if your genetic makeup predisposes you to heart disease, the expression of your genes can be influenced by environmental factors. And the nice thing about environmental factors is that you have some control over them.

Remember these two words from a few chapters ago? Your *genotype*, as modified by environmental influences, determines the end result, your phenotype. The exact relationship between genetics and environment is still an area of mystery. We're working on it. But we already know that testing for genetic predisposition is important, because a positive test means you have to work even harder at the things you *can* control to offset the tendency you were born with.

Genetic predisposition is a bummer. It's like finding out that your opponent has scored on you before the game even started. And of all the players heart disease has on its roster, this is the one guy you can't knock out of the game.

However, genetic predisposition is only one player, one risk factor. If you have it, you just need to work on knocking out the other ones, which is something you want to do anyway.

Many patients tell me they don't worry about heart disease, because several of their relatives lived to be over ninety years old. The fallacy in that thinking is that you do not have the exact genetic makeup of your older relatives. You don't look exactly like your grandmother or your Uncle Fred, do you? Thank heavens, no! You are a unique combination of genetic traits that you have received from your parents, and you have lived a different life from theirs in a different environment. Their risk of heart disease is not the same as yours. It may be lower or higher, but it is uniquely yours.

Nonetheless, if you have a family history of heart disease, especially among your grandparents, parents, and siblings, then you have one of the risk factors for heart disease.

DR. DUKE'S GAME PLAN

- Tell your doctor about your family's history of heart disease and stroke.
- If possible, get tested for genetic predisposition. ❖

2. Diabetes

Diabetes mellitus significantly increases the risk of cardiovascular complications and death.[366]

We have known for a long time that one of the complications of diabetes is damage to small blood vessels in the kidneys, eyes, and extremities, often leading to kidney failure, blindness, and amputations. This damage to small blood vessels is called microvascular disease.

However, there is a growing epidemic of macrovascular disease— damage to larger blood vessels—that is also associated with diabetes. This growing problem is especially common among people who have type 2 or "adult" diabetes.[367]

The World Health Organization now states that there is a worldwide epidemic of type 2 diabetes. And the condition that commonly leads to type 2 diabetes, called metabolic syndrome, is also associated with an increased risk of heart disease.

This epidemic of insulin resistance and type 2 diabetes is discussed thoroughly in chapter 12. Millions of people who have insulin resistance and metabolic syndrome don't even know it. So please, carefully read this chapter and the section below on elevated cholesterol to determine if you might have insulin resistance, metabolic syndrome, or type 2 diabetes. If you test positive for any of these conditions, you have another risk factor for heart disease.

DR. DUKE'S GAME PLAN

- Get tested by your doctor to see if you have insulin resistance or diabetes (see chapter 12).
- If you have diabetes, follow your doctor's treatment program carefully and make the lifestyle changes discussed in chapter 12 to help reduce its severity.
- If you are insulin resistant, follow the recommendations in chapter 12 for reducing insulin resistance and the risk of type 2 diabetes. ❖

3. Smoking

When it comes to winning optimal health, smoking is like throwing the game. It is lying down and letting your opponent score at will. As a health risk, smoking is not as dangerous as jumping out of an airplane without a parachute, but it comes close.

Cigarette smoking has been widely accepted as a major risk factor for cardiovascular disease for many years.[368] It increases risk for several kinds of cancer (see chapter 10). And it damages blood vessels, leading to heart disease.

All kinds of smoking increase the risk of heart disease: pipe smoking,[369] cigar smoking,[370] cigarette smoking,[371] marijuana smoking,[372] and even passive or secondhand smoking.[373]

Both the number of years you smoke and the amount of tobacco you smoke per day increase your risk of developing heart disease.

One in every ten cardiovascular deaths in the world during the year 2000 was due to smoking.[374] According to the World Health Organization, tobacco is the second major cause of death in the world.[375]

Many review research papers have affirmed that passive smoking is associated with both heart disease[376] and sudden infant death syndrome.[377] A few review articles in scientific publications have concluded that passive smoking is not harmful to health,[378] but nearly all of these studies had suspected affiliations or financial conflicts of interest.[379]

The United States Environmental Protection Agency,[380] the Surgeon General,[381] and the National Research Council of the National Academy of Sciences[382] have all concluded that passive smoking increases the risk of diseases. Secondhand smoke increases the risk of coronary disease by 30 percent, and even brief exposure—hours or minutes—can have effects that are 80 to 90 percent as strong as those due to active smoking.[383]

According to the Surgeon General, secondhand smoke annually kills 46,000 adult nonsmokers via heart disease, 3,000 adult *nonsmokers* via lung cancer and 430 newborns from sudden infant death syndrome in the United States alone.[384]

I hope my theme here is not too subtle. In case it is, I will state it more directly:

DO NOT SMOKE!

If you do smoke, do *anything* you have to in order to quit. If nothing works, including prescription assistance from your physician, then reduce your smoking as much as you can. Any amount of smoking is terrible, but even cutting back on your smoking will reduce your statistical risk of death from heart disease. A study that looked at California's tough tobacco-control program concluded that it was associated with a reduction in deaths from heart disease.[385]

And if you must light up, please don't do it where others have to breathe your smoke. Exposing others to your smoke isn't as criminal as firing a gun in random directions in a crowded room, but the morality of it leans in that direction.

DR. DUKE'S GAME PLAN

- Stop smoking.
- If you can't stop on your own, ask your doctor for help.
- If you still can't stop, cut back as much as you can.
- Do not smoke around others.
- Get adequate vitamin C. I recommend at least 100 mg per day. ❖

4. High blood pressure

About 50 million people in the United States and 1 billion people worldwide have high blood pressure, which is also called hypertension.[386]

Here is why hypertension is a risk factor for heart disease and stroke.

Think of your blood vessels as pipes or hoses. If the pressure of the fluid inside is too great, small cracks will form. These are called microfissures, and they lead to vascular disease because cholesterol in your blood collects in these fissures, forming the plaque deposits of atherosclerosis.

These deposits can shut down blood flow in the arteries that supply the heart muscles, causing heart attacks. Plaque deposits can also break off and flow to the brain, where they cause strokes by blocking smaller arteries, thus cutting off the blood supply to brain tissue.

The latter risk is especially prevalent in China, Japan, and other eastern Asian countries, where stroke is a principal cause of death.[387]

Interestingly, hypertension has a vicious-cycle relationship with chronic inflammation. Inflammation increases hypertension[388] and hypertension increases inflammation.[389]

Surely you have had your blood pressure measured at some point in your life—when a doctor or nurse straps a cuff around your upper arm, inflates it, and then listens to your blood flow with a stethoscope while the cuff pressure is slowly released. Your blood pressure is read in terms of two numbers, which represent millimeters of mercury displaced. The higher one is the *systolic* blood pressure; the lower is the *diastolic*. I should point out, though, that a *proper* blood pressure measurement is the average of two separate blood pressure readings taken while you are sitting down.

The National High Blood Pressure Education Program (NHBPEP) Coordinating Committee has issued blood pressure prevention, detection, evaluation, and treatment guidelines for more than thirty years. The most recent committee report (2003)[390] contains some important things for you to know about hypertension:

- There is a consistent relationship between increased blood pressure and development of cardiovascular disease.
- For people forty to seventy years old, the risk of developing heart disease doubles for every 20 mm in systolic blood pressure or 10 mm in diastolic pressure above 115/75.
- In people over fifty, a systolic blood pressure of more than 140 mm indicates a higher risk of developing heart disease than elevated diastolic blood pressure does.

- People who have normal blood pressure at age fifty-five have a 90 percent chance of developing high blood pressure sometime in their lives, usually because of atherosclerosis, which is hardening of the arteries.
- People with systolic blood pressure of 120 to 139 mm or diastolic blood pressure of 80 to 89 mm of mercury are now considered prehypertensive. They, too, need to change their lifestyles to reduce the risk of heart disease. Many physicians don't treat unless the blood pressure is above 140/90. Remember that a systolic blood pressure of over 136 or a diastolic blood pressure of over 86 doubles the risk of heart disease. Discuss treating these numbers with your doctor, especially if you have other risk factors.

Do you take your own blood pressure regularly? Good for you! Just two notes of caution. First, make sure you understand how to use the cuff and stethoscope properly. Second, the NHBPEP report suggests that home devices should be calibrated regularly by comparing your home cuff with one in your doctor's office.

DR. DUKE'S GAME PLAN

- Have your blood pressure checked regularly, or check it yourself. Hypertension is a "silent killer": you can't feel it. You have to test for it.
- Blood pressure above 115/75 increases risk of developing heart disease and may need to be treated if you have other risk factors.
- High blood pressure can often be reduced by reducing your other risk factors, including smoking, stress, and excess weight.
- Talk to your doctor. If lifestyle changes don't help, medication may be a good choice. ❖

5. Lack of exercise
In 1990, a research paper reported that physically active people are half

as likely to suffer heart attacks as those who are sedentary.[391]

That was fantastic news! You wanted to do something simple, easy, and dramatic to avoid having a heart attack, you could get off that sofa and into the gym, thus reducing the statistical likelihood of your having a heart attack by 50 percent.

However, many early studies reported that only vigorous exercise yielded coronary benefit, and that was a problem for a lot of people.[392] Doctors and health experts told everyone to train like Olympians. Most people didn't bother, because they didn't have the time or didn't want the pain that went with the gain.

Then came even better news. New studies showed that even less-vigorous activity can result in very significant cardiovascular benefits. One study[393] reported that light to moderate activity was associated with lower heart disease rates in women; just one hour of walking *per week* resulted in lower risk. Another study[394] reported that total physical activity, whether it involved running, weight training or walking, was associated with reduced risk of heart disease. Both vigorous exercise and mere walking are associated with significant reduction in heart disease among postmenopausal women.[395]

Don't get me wrong. I want you to get all the exercise you reasonably can. And while fairly rigorous exercise is best (as long as it is approved by your doctor and age-appropriate), any form of regular exercise is far better than none. Does your concept of "exercise" entail $100 running shoes, an expensive membership at a gym populated by chiseled bodies wrapped in bright leotards, and a two-hour-a-day obsession you don't have time for? That's the paradigm we need to shatter.

The best definition of exercise for most people is this: any activity that involves moving your body.

Even if you don't have a formal exercise program, you can still benefit from adding exercise to your normal daily activities—even in short quick episodes throughout the day. For example, park your car a block or two from your destination and walk the rest of the way. If you commute to work, get off the train or bus one stop early. Do a few squats or lunges while talking on the phone or watching TV. Some studies have shown that even making simple changes—such as using stairs instead of elevators—will help reduce your risk of heart disease.

In one study involving obese women, a program of healthier diet combined with increased lifestyle activity yielded similar health benefits to a program of healthier diet combined with structured aerobic workouts.[396]

Another study reported that in previously sedentary healthy adults, a lifestyle physical activity program was *as effective as a structured exercise program* in improving physical activity, cardiorespiratory fitness, and blood pressure.[397] According to one researcher's data, walking briskly for fifteen minutes per day was associated with a 16 percent reduction in heart disease.[398]

Daily activity levels are one of the most dramatic changes between the way people lived one hundred years ago and today. Then, most people worked at physically active jobs and walked to work and back. Now we drive or ride to work, sit all day in front of computer screens, drive home again, and spend the evening sitting in front of the computer or TV with our brains on standby and our bodies in energy-saver/sleep mode. With regard to cardiovascular health, that isn't progress.

If you don't exercise or lead a physically active life, you have another risk factor for heart disease.

Exercise has many benefits in addition to reducing heart disease. It has been shown to be effective in helping people to:

- lose weight[399]
- reduce the risk of type 2 diabetes[400]
- improve sugar control in type 2 diabetics[401]
- reduce the risk of some cancers

That said, here is a warning.

Before you start any exercise program, *get your doctor's approval*. If you already have heart disease that has progressed too far, exercise may not be safe right now. The last thing I want to do is to get you so fired up about changing your life that you drop dead in your driveway on day one. Once you have your doctor's blessing, then get moving.

Exercise as much as you can, but remember that any physical activity is better than none. Running two miles three times a week is better than walking those two miles while playing nine holes of golf. But walking nine holes is better than riding in a golf cart. And playing nine holes out of a cart is far better than watching someone else play them on TV while you gobble chips and dip. (The repeated motion of lifting a beer or soft drink to your lips is not what I mean by the "exercise of daily living.")

Exercise shouldn't be a chore or a bore, so choose something that's fun. Ride your bike. Walk by a river instead of a highway. Reward yourself at the health club by shooting baskets or relaxing in the sauna after you get off the treadmill. Play your favorite music or work out in front of your favorite TV show. Instead of shooing your kids and dog out of the house, go out to the park with them. Playing catch, Frisbee® or hide-and-seek is great for building healthy bodies, not to mention stronger family ties. Even your dog will like you more.

Whether you engage in special exercise activities or not, you can easily add exercise to your day. Take a walk in your neighborhood. Push your lawnmower. Take the stairs. Carry your luggage instead of rolling it. Or roll your luggage instead of taking the moving sidewalk. Just find any way you can to keep in motion. Soon you'll begin to feel better and want to do more.

And finally, here's what not to do.

Don't think that you have to buy in to the latest fad. Any regular physical activity is a step in the right direction. If you join a gym or club, don't be ashamed if you can't pedal as fast or lift as much as someone next to you. Start out doing what you can without being miserable or injuring yourself. You'll get better faster than you think.

And don't feel that you have to join a gym or club to get healthy. Just do things you enjoy that keep you moving.

Remember Dr. Duke's First Law of Motion: A body in motion will stay in motion longer; a body that stays at rest will rest in peace sooner.

Finally, don't become an exercise freak while ignoring all the other risk factors. Remember the example of Jim Fixx, the running guru who died prematurely of heart disease. In fact, some extreme-endurance athletes may be overtaxing their hearts, resulting in arrhythmias.[402] This chapter lists fifteen risk factors for heart disease. Exercise alone cannot make up for deficiencies in all the other fourteen. (You can find the most recent U.S. government recommendations for exercise at

www.health.gov/PAguidelines and the World Health Organization recommendations at www.who.int/dietphysicalactivity/factsheet_recom-
mendations/en.)

DR. DUKE'S GAME PLAN

- Add more of the "exercise of daily living" to your life.
- With your doctor's approval, start an organized exercise program, such as the 10,000 Steps program, which uses a
  pedometer to help you meet the goal of walking five miles a
  day.
- Keep moving! Any increase in daily movement is better than
  none. ❖

6. Obesity

Obesity is a risk factor for heart disease.[403, 404, 405, 406] Moreover, the risk of
death from heart disease increases 500 percent if obese individuals are
also unfit,[407] so regular exercise, good diet, and all the other aspects of
this game plan are important to follow even if you never become as
svelte as a model or as chiseled as a bodybuilder.

In order to determine if obesity is a risk factor for you, you must first
understand the criteria for making the diagnosis. The definition of obesity isn't as simple as popular culture leads you to think.

The criteria for obesity are explained very carefully in chapter 11.
They involve far more than your ratio of height to weight. They include
factors such as body fat percentage and waist-to-hip ratio.

Please see chapter 11 for a very thorough discussion of this important
and much-misunderstood subject. Many people who fit the criteria for
obesity as a risk factor are unaware of it.

DR. DUKE'S GAME PLAN

- Determine if you are overweight or obese by reading chapter 11 carefully. Therein is a feast of solid scientific information on the cause of obesity and how you can reduce it.
- Good news. When you reduce the risk factors for obesity

and live the optimal health lifestyle, you will lose weight. ❖

7. Elevated lipids

Sorry, but I have to throw some science at you here. Knowing your opponent is a key part of our game plan. So please bear with me—I'll make it as brief and painless as I can.

Many studies have shown that an elevated blood cholesterol level is one of the major risk factors for heart disease.[408] There are several types of cholesterol, and not all cholesterol is bad. A quick review:

- HDL (high-density lipoprotein) cholesterol is good.
- LDL (low-density lipoprotein) cholesterol is bad.
- VLDL (very-low-density lipoprotein) cholesterol is bad.

How to remember: high-density, good; low-density, bad.

Managing levels of blood lipids (fats), especially cholesterol, has become the cornerstone of heart disease prevention and treatment for most physicians. This strategy is based on extensive research that demonstrated that lowering cholesterol slows the progression of heart disease and even promotes its regression.

One project, called the 4S study, revealed a substantial reduction in death rate and heart attacks in people with documented heart disease who received medication to lower their cholesterol.[409] Another large study revealed a 32 percent reduced risk of death from all causes related to the heart in patients treated with a class of medications called statins.[410] Some studies used angiograms—a method of literally looking at the insides of arteries—to confirm the benefits of these medicines.[411] The research and the treatment results have been so convincing that many physicians neglect other risk factors. However, recent guidelines issued by the most respected advisory group on lipid control have started to change this trend.

In 2001 the National Cholesterol Education Program of the National Institutes of Health introduced a new Adult Treatment Panel (NCEP-ATP III), which expanded the list of risk factors for cardiovascular disease and placed new emphasis on prevention.[412] Prior to this report, the major heart disease risk factors were listed as cigarette smoking, hypertension, low HDL cholesterol, family history of heart disease, and age. ATP III added obesity, lack of exercise, and poor diet.

The report also acknowledged possible emerging risk factors such as lipoprotein (a), insulin resistance, homocysteine, increased tendency to form clots, underlying undetected heart disease, and inflammatory factors such as CRP. Apolipoprotein B (apoB) will probably be added to this list soon, since it has been shown to be a better predictor of heart disease than LDL.[413]

Sorry for all the scientific jargon, but I want you to understand that there are many more risk factors than cholesterol.

That said, let's go back to talking about cholesterol. Or more specifically, testing for it.

Almost all physicians around the world use a lab test that doesn't actually count LDL molecules, but uses a mathematical formula to estimate LDL levels, based on measurement of HDL and total cholesterol levels. However, almost half of all people who have heart attacks have normal LDL levels.[414] Even the new NCEP guidelines are based on the old laboratory technology; they merely require that LDL cholesterol be controlled to a lower level.

I think there's a better way.

For my patients' best interest, I measure cholesterol levels with technology that can actually "see" cholesterol molecules, rather than just estimating their number. It is a far more accurate way of measuring lipid levels.

The current norm for starting patients on medication to lower cholesterol is a total cholesterol level greater than 200 mg/dl. Appendix A.2 outlines better, more meaningful criteria.

However, even the current standard lab calculations are reasonably good predictors when we look at the ratio of total cholesterol to HDL (the good kind.) Generally, you want your ratio of total cholesterol to HDL to be below 4.0 and ideally less than 3.5.

Next question: Is medication the only way to control high cholesterol?

Answer: No.

Diet has a major impact on cholesterol levels. Unfortunately, there has been a lot of controversy over how to eat for cholesterol control, resulting in a lot of confusion for consumers.

For a generation or more we have been exhorted from all quarters to eat a low-fat diet. Now the latest fad diets are high in fats and low in carbohydrates! Remember this nursery rhyme:

> Jack Sprat could eat no fat.
> His wife could eat no lean.
> And so, between the two of them,
> They licked the platter clean.

With all the conflicting information, who knows whether Jack or Mrs. Sprat had the right idea? I do: The answer is neither.

As usual, the discussion has been oversimplified and has too much to do with fad marketing.

I'll talk about food and eating habits at length in chapter 11. Also, I've included an example of an optimally healthy diet in Appendix B. However, I'll add a few specific comments here about diet and the risk of heart disease.

There are bad fats and good fats. I am not talking now about the different kinds of cholesterol, but about fats in the food you eat. Also, there are good and bad sources of carbohydrates and proteins.

Omega-3 fats are very good for you. They help reduce your risk of heart disease (see risk factor 14). Extremely low-fat diets rob you of the levels of anti-inflammatory omega-3 fats you need for optimal health and have even been shown to result in increased inflammation.[415] Extremely low-fat diets are based on outdated science and are not recommended.

On the other hand, extremely high-fat diets are associated with increased cancer risk (see chapter 10). And the high-fat, low-carb fad diets ignore the tremendous benefits of "good" carbohydrates, i.e., higher-carb foods that are also rich in fiber and phytonutrients. Worse yet, high-fat fad diets include too many partially hydrogenated or trans fats, which increase your risk of heart disease. (A 2 percent increase in caloric intake of trans fats is associated with a 23 percent higher risk of heart disease.[416, 417])

Although omega-6 fats (found in dark meats and cheap oils) are required in our diet, we are getting too much of them and they are harmful for us because they worsen the bad fats in the blood.[418]

The popular DASH diet has been shown to be beneficial for reducing the risk of heart disease,[419] especially if you tweak it with slightly more monounsaturated fat or protein.[420] But later in this book I'll present a diet that is even better.

In 2006, a huge study called the Women's Health Initiative[421] created a lot of confusion when it concluded that low-fat diets didn't reduce the risk of heart disease. There were many problems with the study, however. First, the researchers attempted to get the subjects to reduce their fat intake to 20 percent of calories but were only able to get them down to 29 percent. (As an aside, this illustrates the problem with many low-this and high-that diets: People can't stick to them in real life.) Second, the researchers didn't control for the *types* of fat, so some subjects may have been eating more "good" fats than others. In short, this study is not an excuse to eat more fat than Mrs. Sprat.

Finally, regular exercise is also proven to help control or reduce cholesterol levels. If you need to lower yours, it's generally better to try diet and exercise first, before resorting to medication.

DR. DUKE'S GAME PLAN

- Have your cholesterol and lipid panel checked, preferably obtaining a specialized cholesterol test like the one described in Appendix A.2.
- If your level is elevated, consult with your doctor and then begin reducing the risk factors of chronic disease and following the pillars of optimal health.
- Following these steps should help reduce your cholesterol, so that you may need less medication or possibly even none.
- However, never stop taking a medication unless advised to by a doctor.
- Reduce the saturated, omega-6, trans, and other harmful fats in your diet. ❖

8. Not enough fruits and vegetables

Listen to your mother: Eat your fruits and vegetables. She might not have known why, but she was right.

There is no substitute for eating adequate amounts of fresh fruits and vegetables. These foods contain hundreds of antioxidants and phytonutrients, many of which we haven't even named yet, that reduce the risk of cardiovascular disease.

Many studies show that eating fruit and vegetables can reduce the risk of heart disease. A study in Finland showed that men who consumed higher amounts of fruits, berries, and vegetables had a 34 percent lower risk of heart disease than those who didn't.[422] In another study, those who ate higher amounts of dietary fiber contained in cereal, fruit, and vegetables had a 27 percent lower risk of death from heart disease.[423]

One interesting study looked at the combined effect of saturated fat, fruits, and vegetables on heart disease.[424] They followed 501 healthy men over eighteen years old and found that those who ate more than five servings of fruits and vegetables daily and got less than 12 percent of their calories from saturated fat were 76 percent less likely to die from coronary heart disease than men whose diets were low in fruits and vegetable and high in saturated fats. What's more, the men who ate more than five servings of fruits and vegetables but had higher saturated fat intake still had a 64 percent lower risk of death from heart disease.

So there's no doubt: Fruits and vegetables are among the most valuable players in your efforts to beat heart disease.

The global burden of disease related to low consumption of fruits and vegetables, as revealed in another recent study by the World Health Organization,[425] is astounding. The researchers estimate that 2.63 million premature deaths occur yearly worldwide because people aren't eating enough fruits and vegetables. If people could consume the baseline of 600 g (or 1.3 lbs.) per day of fruits and vegetables, the total worldwide burden of disease would be reduced 1.8 percent and of heart disease by 31 percent.

DR. DUKE'S GAME PLAN

- Eat at least five to nine servings per day of fruits and vegetables.

- Better yet, eat nine servings per day.
- Make them a part of every meal.
- Eat them for snacks—junk that junk food.
- "Think color." Different antioxidants and phytonutrients give plants their colors, so vary the color of fruits and vegetables you eat from day to day. Wider variety gives you broader protection from more diseases.
- Consider adding antioxidant supplements, like vitamin C.[426] ❖

9. Depression

Depression is a proven risk factor for heart disease.

Scientists studying this phenomenon believe that depression stimulates two hormonal pathways that accelerate heart disease. More research is needed,[427] but the statistical correlation is clear. Depressive symptoms increase not only the risk for heart disease in men, but also the mortality rate.[428, 429] Among people with coronary heart disease, those who have been depressed for more than two years have twice the risk of dying, compared to those with coronary heart disease who aren't depressed.[430]

The studies that have connected depression to heart disease have been quite consistent. So there are some important things to know about what depression is and how to spot it in yourself or a person close to you.

Depression not simply a state of mind; it's a disease, and it can be fatal in ways other than promoting heart disease. Moreover, the symptoms go far beyond chronic sadness or crying. Symptoms include changes in eating habits, changes in sleeping habits, difficulty making decisions, worsening self-image, short temper, avoidance of people, decreased motivation, decreased interest in those things one formerly found stimulating.

If you are struggling with several of these symptoms, please contact your doctor, religious counselor, or a trained professional. Do the same if you see these symptoms in someone close to you. Chronic depression is a miserable way to spend one's life, and it's miserable for people close to the depressed person as well. And as if all that isn't bad enough, depression also significantly increases one's chances of dying from heart disease.

So I can't stress enough the importance of actively dealing with depression.

Too often people are in denial about their own depression, or else ashamed of it. Please don't let that happen. Depression is *not* a sign of weakness; usually it is a sign of chemical or psychological imbalances that can be treated.

DR. DUKE'S GAME PLAN

- If you have three or more of the symptoms described above, see a doctor, a religious counselor or a qualified professional.
- In addition to other therapies, and with clearance from your doctor, consider an exercise program.[431] ❖

10. Stress

When you think about it, it's hard to understand why stress should be so prevalent a problem in modern civilization. On the list of things to worry about, job deadlines, family finances, social calendars, meal planning, and getting the kids to soccer practice don't seem quite as serious as our ancestors' chronic problems—famine, pestilence, and war, for example.

And yet stress is endemic to modern life and, unfortunately, it is a risk factor for heart disease.

Many research investigations have confirmed relationships between coronary heart disease and psychological factors such as stress. We've known it's a risk factor but only recently have begun to understand why. There are obvious lifestyle factors—people under stress have a greater tendency to smoke, drink excessively, lose sleep, and eat poorly, which are all risk factors for heart disease. But new research technologies have demonstrated that acute stress itself can cause low oxygen levels for the heart and stimulate abnormal heart rhythms.[432] Another recent study found that some people have uneven brain stimulation during stress, which increases the likelihood of abnormal heart rhythms.[433] Anxiety has even been shown to be an independent predictor of heart attacks in men.[434]

The physical effects of chronic stress have great impact on cardiovascular disease. These effects include increased blood pressure[435] and the risk of metabolic syndrome,[436] which I'll cover in chapter 12. In chapter 3, we already talked about yet another critical consequence of chronic stress.

So how do you tell if *your* stress level amounts to a risk factor? After all, everybody feels stressed from time to time. Are you bound for the cardiac unit if you don't find a way to live in constant bliss?

It is fairly easy to determine if stress is a risk factor for you. **If you feel significant stress almost every day, then you have another risk factor for heart disease.**

Also, please do not rationalize your stressful life by noting that everyone around you is as stressed out as you are. Chronic stress *is* endemic to every industrialized nation on the planet. We see it in our clients from Asia, Europe, and the Americas. It is easy to conclude that your level of chronic stress is normal, and therefore not a risk factor. But the chronic stress that is normal today *is* a risk factor.

The good news, though, is that we can reduce the stress we feel in our lives. That's because much of our stress is self-imposed. We worry too much about the little stuff, or about things we can't control. We find it hard to forgive and forget, to live and let live. We are angry, bitter, resentful, selfish, quick to engage in conflict. We take on too many responsibilities. We harbor irrational fears. We try to manage too many things. If you are beginning to see yourself in at least part of this paragraph, then the way you are living may be shortening your life, not to mention robbing you of the joy of living.

The stress-reduction program I created was implemented over ten years ago, and I'm very blessed that the feedback from my clients has been wonderful. Most stress-reduction programs focus on temporary relief. I think we can do better. This shouldn't be about feeling better for a week or getting past a rough patch; it is about reducing a risk factor for heart disease and living a better life.

So if chronic stress is a significant part of your life, please follow the guidelines in chapter 7 carefully for beating stress long term.

DR. DUKE'S GAME PLAN

- If you have a problem with stress, see chapter 7.
- If that isn't enough, please contact your doctor, religious counselor or qualified professional for help. ❖

11. Lack of intrinsic faith

The understanding that spiritual and religious factors influence health goes back centuries. Sir William Osler, the founder of modern cardiology, wrote a series of articles in the early 1900s about religious factors in medical care.[437] The interest in this topic has increased dramatically over the last thirty years.

The National Institutes of Health has held conferences on the topic,[438] and there are prominent programs for its study at Harvard and Duke Universities. (Duke's Center for Spirituality, Theology, and Health is probably the leader in this field.) Many medical schools now teach classes on the integration of faith and health care.

There are now over 1,200 studies showing that people who have a committed religious faith are more likely to enjoy better health. However, in our age of reason and skepticism, this is the most underreported and misunderstood of all the risk factors. I can understand some degree of healthy skepticism, because a few studies have shown benefits or even slightly negative tendencies. However, to ignore the topic after 1,200 studies have indicated it is a positive factor is not good science or good medicine.

Also, I want to insert a few disclaimers here. Of the hundreds of studies I have seen that suggest a significant correlation between faith and health, none has compared one religion to another, although health benefits have been shown in the practice of many different religions.

What the studies have in common is conclusions about the effect that a committed religious faith has on health. The particular religion is inconsequential; the effect is nondenominational and nonsectarian. A committed religious faith, also termed "intrinsic faith," is defined in terms of regular attendance at one's place of worship on a regular basis, regular reading of sacred scriptures, and faith being very important in one's life.

The alternatives are "extrinsic faith" and no faith at all. Extrinsic faith applies to people who profess some religious affiliation, but don't practice and live it in the committed, daily manner of those with intrinsic faith. People of extrinsic faith, along with atheists and agnostics, have been shown by research to have poorer health than people of intrinsic faith.

Studies have even shown benefits in praying for the sick. Probably the first modern landmark research studied recovering heart patients.[439] Three hundred and ninety-three patients who were admitted to a coronary-care unit were randomly assigned to two groups. One group was prayed for by a group outside the hospital, while the control group was not prayed for. None of the patients knew whether or not they had people praying for them. Those being prayed for required less use of ventilators, fewer antibiotics, and less medicine to remove fluid. Overall, their recovery was much better. A later, duplicate study found similar results;[440] of 990 coronary care unit patients, those who were prayed for had a much less complicated hospital course.

People who have intrinsic faith have been shown to have lower blood pressure,[441] a 60 percent reduced risk of dying from heart disease for men and 50 percent for women,[442] fourteen times lower likelihood of dying after cardiac surgery,[443] shorter hospital stays,[444] lower levels of the damaging chemical interleukin-6,[445, 446] lower C-reactive protein levels,[447] and longer lives.[448]

The data in that last category are fairly spectacular. **The increased longevity attributed to intrinsic faith by some studies is approximately seven years.**[449] That's about the same as the lifespan advantage that nonsmokers have over smokers.

There are scores of other health benefits linked to intrinsic faith. It amazes me that, because of our intellectualism and our hesitancy to discuss religion, many of us in the health-care field have overlooked something so obvious and important.

Why does intrinsic faith, or the lack of it, affect our health? It's still a mystery. But mystery is a component of faith. It's how we deal with the vast areas of existence beyond what we know. Scientists are studying the topic at a physiological level. Perhaps it's related to the hormonal pathways associated with having a positive attitude or reduced depression discussed in chapter 6. Perhaps we'll never completely understand how or why it affects our health.

I'll let you know if science finds an answer. In the meantime, suffice it to say that practicing your faith is good for your heart and your general health.

DR. DUKE'S GAME PLAN

- Practice the faith of your choice with serious commitment.
- Don't let anybody tell you that his "brand" of religion is healthier than yours. ❖

12. Homocysteine

If this is the first time you've ever seen that word in print, I'm not surprised. Cholesterol is the stuff in your blood that gets all the publicity. But homocysteine is a rising star among risk factors for heart disease, and it's gaining more and more attention from scientists. Dealing with it has to be an important part of our game plan.

There are several essential amino acids. ("Essential" in this context refers to nutrients that the human body requires.) Our bodies metabolize one essential amino acid called *methionine* into a molecule called homocysteine. About 10 percent of people have a genetic tendency to create excessive amounts of homocysteine.

The pathologist Kilmer McCully recognized over thirty years ago that people with elevated homocysteine levels in their blood had increased risk of heart disease, and subsequent research has supported this connection. For example, one study published in the medical journal *Lancet* has shown that homocysteine is an independent risk factor for heart disease, especially among Indians.[450] Two studies have shown that residents of India and South Asia have higher homocysteine levels generally, compared to Caucasians, East Asians, West Africans, and Caribbean populations.[451, 452]

In 2006 two studies reported that lowering homocysteine among people with significant heart disease did not reduce their risk of additional heart attacks.[453, 454] These studies have caused some to conclude that homocysteine should not be considered a risk factor but rather an "associated" factor for heart disease. The problem with both of these studies is that they were done on patients who already had severe heart disease and other health conditions. (Please see further support of this position in chapter 8.) Until further research comes out that looks at homocysteine from a truly preventive point of view—that is, in patients who, at the outset, have not yet developed significant atherosclerosis—I will continue to consider it a risk factor because of its association with inflammation (see chapters 2 and 3). It has been shown that increased homocysteine is associated with reduced heart function.[455]

Among the known treatments for reducing homocysteine levels are folic acid (which improves blood vessel function),[456] vitamin B$_{12}$, and omega-3 fatty acids. One study showed that supplementation with folic acid in healthy siblings of patients with heart disease decreased their risk of potential coronary events.[457] This is an example of how appropriate supplementation may be used to reduce the risk of chronic disease (see chapter 8).

DR. DUKE'S GAME PLAN

- If you do not have established heart disease, have your homocysteine level checked.
- If it's elevated, start taking a good vitamin B supplement, then have your homocysteine level rechecked.
- If vitamin B supplementation doesn't reduce your homocysteine level in a fairly short time, you may be insulin resistant. Get tested for this. (See chapter 12.) ❖

If you already have established heart disease, forget about homocysteine for now. New research is needed to find whether there is any benefit to you in lowering it.

13. Hypothyroidism

Many studies have established that that low thyroid function—hypothyroidism—increases the risk of heart disease. A study from France reveals that hypothyroidism is commonly associated with cholesterol abnormalities, elevated C-reactive protein, elevated homocysteine, and other risk factors associated with heart disease.[458]

Hypothyroidism causes your metabolism to slow down. It has more than a dozen symptoms, starting with fatigue, weakness, and aching muscles. However, according the study just cited, as many as 10 percent of us have low thyroid function that hasn't been diagnosed because we haven't shown any symptoms of it. This is called *subclinical hypothyroidism*, and it is important to know whether you have it or not, because even subclinical hypothyroidism increases the risk of elevated C-reactive protein.[459] A study done recently in Japan reveals that subclinical hypothyroidism is also associated with increased deaths from heart disease, as well as increased total death rate.[460]

The only way to know whether you have this disorder is by getting a blood test from your doctor, especially one for TSH level.

DR. DUKE'S GAME PLAN

- If you haven't had your thyroid level, including TSH, checked recently, do so.
- If your TSH is too high or too low, work with your doctor to manage it. ❖

14. Lack of omega-3 in your diet

As I wrote earlier, some of the fats that we eat are very good for us. One of these is the polyunsaturated fat called omega-3. Foods that are rich in omega-3 include salmon, canola oil, flaxseed oil, and walnuts.

Many studies have shown that omega-3 reduces heart disease risk[461, 462, 463] and death from abnormal heart rhythms.[464, 465] It affects the electrical and physiological activity of the heart.[466] Omega-3 also reduces many risk factors associated with heart disease. For example, it lowers LDL cholesterol production,[467] lowers blood pressure,[468] and enables the interior of blood vessels to work better.[469]

As previously mentioned, one of the world's leading authorities on omega-3 research is Artemis Simopoulos, M.D., president of the Center for Genetics, Nutrition, and Health in Washington, D.C. She has written an outstanding book, *The Omega Diet*,[470] that I highly recommend.

We check omega-3 levels in our clients with both a red blood cell level test[471] and a new complete fatty acid panel, because we think it's critical for our clients to know whether or not their omega-3 intake is adequate.

While it isn't always easy to get optimal amounts of omega-3 in your diet, supplements are widely available. (IMPORTANT NOTE: Be sure to check with your doctor before taking omega-3 supplements, especially if you are on blood thinners like Coumadin® or warfarin.) Guidelines for obtaining omega-3 from fish are provided in Appendix B.3.

A LOW-FAT FALLACY

Some diet marketers have gone way overboard on the low-fat thing, recommending diets in which less than 10 percent of calories come from fats. These diets generally came out prior to the major research on omega-3. They are dangerously outdated, because you can't get enough omega-3 if you are eating so little total fat.

Such diets rarely lead to permanent weight loss, and they rob you of an important player in your game plan to beat chronic heart disease. As noted earlier, extremely low-fat diets are associated with increased inflammation.[472]

DR. DUKE'S GAME PLAN

- Make foods rich in omega-3 an important part of your diet.
- For great sources of information on how to do this, read *The Omega Diet* and see Appendix B in this book.
- Take an omega-3 supplement—but only after getting clearance from your doctor. ❖

15. Elevated inflammation

You know what inflammation is. You'll see it on your skin if you get a cut or a splinter. The skin turns red, swollen, painful, and warm.

Inflammation also occurs inside our blood vessels. This is a critical factor in the development of atherosclerosis, or heart disease. Inflammation is a factor in other diseases, as well. Chapter 3 contained a thorough discussion of how inflammation contributes to chronic disease.

C-reactive protein (CRP) is a molecule in the blood that is a signal for inflammation.

The Centers for Disease Control and the American Heart Association workshop on markers of inflammation and cardiovascular disease concluded that high-sensitive C-reactive protein is an independent risk factor for heart disease.[473] Many studies have shown that elevated C-reactive protein is strongly associated with heart disease.[474, 475] Other studies have shown that CRP and other markers for inflammation, such as IL-6 and ICAM-1, are associated with atherosclerosis and its progression.[476] When CRP is elevated in older men and women, it increases their ten-year incidence of heart disease.[477] As mentioned in chapter 3, a large study completed in 2008 called the Jupiter study[478] showed that people with normal cholesterol but elevated CRP had their risk of heart disease and stroke cut in half after two years on the medicine. The medicine reduced both LDL cholesterol and CRP but as discussed earlier, the benefit was most likely from the medicine's ability to lower CRP.

We have been checking our clients for high-sensitive C-reactive proteins for several years. Sometimes C-reactive protein can be elevated merely because of a recent infection or a chronic inflammatory condition like arthritis. But in the absence of those factors, it indicates elevated risk of heart disease.

DR. DUKE'S GAME PLAN

- Ask your doctor about a high-sensitive C-reactive protein level test.
- Review chapters 2 and 3 to see why elevated C-reactive protein is a risk factor.
- Learn how to reduce elevated C-reactive protein in chapter 3. ❖

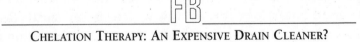

CHELATION THERAPY: AN EXPENSIVE DRAIN CLEANER?

Chelation refers to the method of removing heavy metals from the body using a chemical called EDTA. It has been approved only for heavy metal poisonings.

Since atherosclerosis is made partially of calcium, some groups like the American College for Advancement in Medicine (ACAM) claim that chelation is effective for many diseases, including heart disease. It is estimated that 100,000 people in the U.S. get chelation therapy each year at an average cost for all treatments adding up to $4,000 U.S. I don't recommend this practice because there are no quality studies which prove its effectiveness over placebo.[479, 480] Even if calcium could be removed, plaques that cause heart disease are made up of more than calcium. Risks involved in chelation therapy include kidney failure, irregular heartbeats, and death. A U.S. government study called Trial to Assess Chelation Therapy (TACT) will be completed in 2009, and that should provide more information, but even that study is controversial.[481] Obviously, it would be much safer and more scientifically sound to simply reduce your risk factors and follow the recommendations in this book.

Your Risk factors: What's the Score?

Our game plan for beating heart disease identifies fifteen risk factors—factors we have to neutralize in order to be successful in obtaining optimal health. And we've laid out a plan for beating those risk factors.

So let's start by adding up the risk factors you actually have. Let's see which players are the biggest threats in *your* life.

Also, let's understand that those players are a team. They work together. In terms of the power they have to make us sick or shorten our lives, they don't merely add up—they *multiply*. In other words, if you have two risk factors for heart disease, you don't just have twice the risk—typically your risk is between two and four times greater.

As bad as that news may be, the flip side is good news: If you reduce just one risk factor, you can dramatically reduce your total risk for heart disease. Any improvement in risk factor reduction is a step in the right direction.

Next, take another look at that list of risk factors. How many of them are beyond your control?

The answer is just one: heredity.

You can't change the genes you inherited from your parents. When it comes to beating heart disease, heredity is the one factor you can't stop, but you can try to contain it. Following all the recommendations provided in this book will reduce the expression of your genetic tendency.

There are fourteen other risk factors, and you now have a plan for beating every one that applies to you.

The word "victim" is often applied to people who have heart attacks. But having read this chapter, you now know that your behavior, your lifestyle, and your choices determine the strength of your defense against heart disease. It's the number one cause of early death in industrialized nations. It's time we started beating it.

Beating heart disease can only happen one person at a time. And now you have the plan for slowing the process down, and perhaps even beating it.

You have the power, because you have a choice. You don't have to meet me in the emergency room suffering from chest pain long before your time. I passionately want to protect you and your loved ones from heart disease. But this plan is only words on paper. It's up to you to follow it.

You're the one who has to go out there and win this revolution.

CHAPTER 10

Checkmating Cancer

CHESS IS A THINKING PERSON'S GAME.

A chess game isn't won with bursts of speed or strength or with physical skill and agility. It's all about strategy. Moreover, winning strategies are necessarily complex, because of the different ways in which the pieces are moved on the board. Rooks move only forward or sideways, bishops diagonally, knights in an L-shape. Pawns and kings can move only one space at a time. Queens can move in any direction.

The game is about taking out the other guy's pieces, stymieing his attack and foiling his strategy, all while protecting your king from being checkmated.

Battling cancer is a lot like that. Getting cancer is like having your king in check. It doesn't mean you've lost, but at that point you're completely on the defensive.

However, this chapter isn't about fighting cancer once you have it. It's about prevention. Just because you don't have cancer doesn't mean you don't have to fight it. Cancer is trying to beat you whether you have it or not—it started playing the game before you were born. Its chess pieces are moving against you, trying to knock yours out one by one.

Also, there is a special clock rule in this game: Cancer gets to keep making moves whether you do or not. So you'd better be actively in the game and playing with a winning strategy.

Like any other chess player, cancer starts the game with sixteen pieces—the sixteen risk factors for cancer.

Let's review each one and talk about how to take them out of the game.

The Sixteen Risk Factors for Cancer

Cancer is one of the two leading causes of early death in every industrialized nation. In many cases our own behavior or lifestyle increases the risk of cancer—it's as if we resign that chess game without even trying. We can give ourselves the best chance of winning by understanding the sixteen risk factors and how to counter them.

When you read the previous chapter about heart disease, you saw that many of those risk factors have been thoroughly studied and are well understood. This is less true with cancer. Several important risk factors are still not clearly understood; science is still trying to find out how they work. But careful statistical research shows that each of these sixteen factors do indeed increase your risk of cancer.

1. Family history and genetic predisposition

Some people have a significant family history of cancer. Unfortunately, they begin the chess match by spotting cancer an important piece.

Many cancers do not seem to be hereditary. But some kinds of cancer do tend to run in families. Breast cancer is one of these; there are two chromosome abnormalities that increase its risk, at the BRCA1 and BRCA2 gene.[482]

Prostate cancer is another example: a man's chances of getting it rise if his father or brother has had it.

DR. DUKE'S GAME PLAN

- As they become available, take advantage of reliable, well-studied genetic tests to see if you are at an increased risk for certain cancers.

- Talk to your doctor about any cancer in your family history.
- Read the rest of this chapter and follow the game plan—the strategy that will help you capture cancer's other chess pieces.
- Start now. Cancer won't wait on you. ❖

2. Smoking

Smoking is cancer's queen. It is the most versatile and deadly chess piece that cancer can use against you. And while everyone knows about the link between smoking and lung cancer, you may not know that smoking is also associated with many other cancers, affecting almost every organ of the body.

According to the Centers for Disease Control (CDC),[483] smoking causes about 90 percent of lung cancer deaths in men and almost 80 percent in women. It also increases the risk of cancers of the mouth, throat, esophagus, bladder, stomach, cervix, kidney, and pancreas, as well as a type of leukemia. Other cancers are also suspected of being related to smoking. It is estimated to have caused some 57,000 new cases of bladder cancer in 2003 in the U.S. and 30,000 new cases of pancreatic cancer.

Secondhand smoke was designated as a known human carcinogen by the U.S. Environmental Protection Agency in 1993. The EPA reports that secondhand smoke causes 3,000 lung cancer deaths each year among Americans *nonsmokers*. So it isn't just your game to lose. Your smoking endangers the health and lives of those around you.

Also, how much you smoke makes a difference. One study revealed that the risk of lung cancer significantly decreased when smoking was reduced by 50 percent.[484]

I've used chess as a metaphor in this chapter, but when it comes to smoking, I think a stronger comparison is called for. Let's say smoking is like playing Russian roulette, and playing it with two or three bullets in the gun instead of the customary one.

DR. DUKE'S GAME PLAN

- In case you missed this in the previous chapter, I'll repeat it here:

DO NOT SMOKE!
- If you do smoke, do whatever it takes to stop. See your doctor about getting help.
- If all your attempts to stop smoking fail, smoke as little as you can. Cutting back from a pack a day to half a pack or three-quarters can reduce your risk.
- Make sure you get adequate vitamin C if you do smoke. I would recommend at least 100 mg per day. ❖

3. Lack of exercise

Exercise is an important chess piece. Take it off the board and it becomes significantly harder to outflank cancer.

Regular exercise has been shown to reduce the risk of several types of cancer. According to the National Cancer Institute, physical activity has been shown by research to lower the risk of getting colon cancer by 50 percent.[485] Physical activity appears to lower the risk of breast cancer,[486] and possibly prostate and uterine cancer as well. Over twenty large epidemiological studies have looked at the relationship between exercise and breast cancer; on the average, risk was reduced 30 to 40 percent for women who exercised for three or four hours a week at moderate to vigorous levels.[487] There are several studies currently looking at physical activity and the reduction of other cancers. Even moderate levels of physical activity appear to reduce the risk of cancer.

In 1997, the U.S. Surgeon General's Report on Physical Activity and Health and a report issued by CDC and the American College of Sports Medicine recommended participating in at least thirty minutes of moderate physical activity four or more days a week in order to obtain health benefits that include reducing one's risk of cancer. Other groups have recommended at least sixty minutes of moderate to intense physical activity to achieve additional health benefits, including weight loss and maintenance.

This is not to say that you have to train like an triathlete to reduce your risk of cancer. What you need is a realistic exercise program. One that you have time for. One that you can stick with and make a normal part of your life.

"Exercise" means nothing more than moving your body. According to the National Cancer Institute, even physical activity at work contributes to lowering the risk of colon cancer. Brisk walking is a great form of exercise, and if you work it into your daily routine, it doesn't take much time at all.

There are lots of little things you can do to elevate your metabolism and burn more calories. Take a flight of stairs instead of the elevator. Two or three evenings a week, take the family for a walk instead of turning on the TV. Park on the outer edge of the parking lot at the mall or your workplace. Mow your own lawn. Rake your own leaves. Push your own snow blower.

Exercise your imagination. There are thousands of things you can do to increase physical activity and reduce your risk of cancer and other chronic diseases.

DR. DUKE'S GAME PLAN

- Add more of the "exercise of daily living" to your life.
- With your doctor's clearance, start an organized exercise program, such as the 10,000 Steps program, which uses pedometer to help you meet the goal of walking five miles a day.
- Keep moving! Any increase in daily movement is better than none. ❖

4. Obesity

There may be more confusion surrounding obesity than any other health concern—and more cynical profiteering as well. Much of the confusion has to do with a culture, especially in the U.S., that regards obesity as a cosmetic or social problem.

We need to stop expressing contempt for obese people—nobody really chooses to be seriously overweight. And overweight people need to stop feeling shame. Instead, we need to address the health issues, and we need to do that based on the best science, not on social hysteria or the marketing of fad diets, phony remedies, and exercise gadgets.

Obesity is associated with very dangerous chronic diseases. We need to take the problem seriously and base our solution on the best science.

This is why I have carefully documented the science on which this book is based. I want you to approach any weight problem you have with a strategy that is effective and safe. I want you to avoid the thousands of ineffective and often dangerous quick-fix, single-focus products, and programs. This is a multibillion-dollar industry, and most of the players in it are much more effective at reducing your wealth than your weight.

Even the definition of obesity is obscured in a dust cloud kicked up by all the hot air that surrounds the subject. Making an accurate diagnosis of obesity isn't quite as simple as it seems, which I'll explain very carefully in chapter 11.

Obesity increases the risk of several cancers.[488] It's like forfeiting a bishop and a rook to your opponent. Obesity can double a woman's risk of developing breast cancer.[489] Weight loss after menopause is associated with a decreased risk of breast cancer.[490] The Agency for Research on Cancer reported that obesity and inactivity account for up to 33 percent of breast, colon, endometrial, kidney, and esophagus cancers.[491] It also increases the rate of prostate cancer, the second most deadly cancer among men in the United States, by 39 percent.[492]

DR. DUKE'S GAME PLAN

- Read the next chapter to learn the proper diagnosis for obesity—many people don't realize they fit the criteria.
- Then read the rest of this book. You'll learn how adopting an optimally healthy lifestyle will result in weight loss. ❖

5. Stress

The effects of chronic stress on health are difficult to study. The symptoms are subjective, and most people living in industrialized nations worldwide are under fairly constant stress, so it's difficult to find a control group.

However, a great deal of research has shown that psychological stress weakens our immune systems. A 2004 study in the scientific journal *Lancet Oncology*[493] showed that people under chronic stress had decreased levels of two kinds of cells, cytotoxic T-cells and natural killer cells. The function of these cells is to attack and eliminate abnormal cells. In other words, they are important chess pieces your body uses to ward off cancer. The authors concluded that chronic stress response probably impairs the immune system, contributing to the development of some types of cancers.

Although there is still debate as to whether or not psychological stress increases the risk of breast cancer, one recent study concluded that there was indeed a connection.[494]

So chronic stress is another one of cancer's chess pieces. We discussed the best ways to reduce stress in chapter 7.

DR. DUKE'S GAME PLAN

- If you live with chronic stress, don't assume it's normal or acceptable. See a qualified professional or your religious counselor about ways to reduce it.
- Read chapter 7 of this book. ❖

6. Animal fat

We've talked about the fat in your body, now let's talk about the fat in your diet. And contrary to what many voices in the diet-fad industry tell you, these are two very separate issues. For example, just because you are thin doesn't mean that eating the wrong kinds of fats won't increase your risk of cancer.

I've said this several times throughout this book, but allow me to repeat myself: *Not all fats are bad.* There are fats that you need to support good heart health that do not increase the risk of cancer. These include monounsaturated fats, like olive oil and omega-3 fats.

However, there are fats that do increase your risk of cancer, including the high-saturated fats found in red meat, which appear to increase the risk of colon cancer.[495, 496] Red and processed meats are associated with the risk of stomach cancer,[497] breast cancer,[498] and pancreatic cancer.[499] One study reported that there was an increase in colorectal cancer with red and processed meats, but an inverse association with fish intake.[500] According to the National Cancer Institute, some studies have also linked high-fat diets to cancer of the prostate, lung, and uterus. They report that saturated fatty acids are thought to be the most harmful kind.[501] The Harvard School of Public Health reports that high intake of trans fats increases the risk of non-Hodgkin's lymphoma.[502]

In 2006, the Women's Health Initiative Study raised a lot of eyebrows, including both of mine, when it reported that a low-fat diet didn't reduce the risk of invasive breast cancer[503] or colorectal cancer.[504] There were some problems with this study, and even though the results weren't reported as statistically significant, there *were* some very important trends. (The main problem was that the subjects were asked to reduce their fat intake to 20 percent of their total calories, but they only reduced it to 29 percent on average.) For example, the group with lower-fat diets had a tendency for reduced risk of breast cancer, so the trend was definitely there. Moreover, women in the lower-fat group who had cut their fat the most had a 22 percent lower risk of breast cancer—that number is indeed statistically significant. Women in the lower-fat group also had fewer precancerous colon polyps, which would suggest a reduced risk of colon cancer over time.

When it comes to colon cancer risk in women, the traditional Japanese diet is no better than the Western diet at reducing the risk of the disease.[505] In fact, a healthy diet emphasizing fresh produce and low-fat protein sources was better than either normal American or Japanese diets.

High-Fat Diets

One of my greatest motivations to write this book is the recent over-hyped high-fat diet craze (also discussed in an earlier sidebar). Many people have achieved short-term weight loss on these high-fat diets. But at what long-term cost?

It is well established that certain high-fat diets increase the risk of cancer, but our cultural obsession with weight loss has led many to ignore that risk. But let's be clear: The marketers who promote high-fat diets are urging you to lose weight at the risk of getting cancer. It's not much different from telling you to start smoking in order to lose weight. It just doesn't make sense.

Also, it has been proven that high-fat diets don't work any better after one year than more traditional diets like Weight Watchers.[506]

DR. DUKE'S GAME PLAN

- Reduce your intake of animal fats as much as possible, except the omega-3 fats in salmon and some other cold-water fish.
- If you have been on a high-fat diet for more than a few months, back off from it, even if you have lost weight. Long-term, a diet high in animal fats increases your risk of cancer. ❖

7. Not enough fruits and vegetables

By now you may be noticing some similarities between this chapter and the last. It's true, many of the risk factors for cancer are the same as those for heart disease. That's a good thing, since it makes winning optimal health a little simpler. You don't need a completely different plan for each opponent.

Fruits and vegetables are enormously important chess pieces in your defense against cancer (and, unlike other chess pieces, they're very tasty!). They are loaded with antioxidants and phytonutrients that provide tremendous protection against chronic disease, including cancer. (We talked about how these phytonutrients interact with gene expression in chapter 4.)

The World Health Organization estimates that if people ate the minimum of 600 g (1.3 lbs) of fruits and vegetables per day, stomach cancer rates would drop 19 percent, esophageal cancer 20 percent, and both lung and colorectal cancer 2 percent worldwide.[507] The National Cancer Institute reports that people with diets rich in fruits and vegetables are also likely to have a lower risk of getting colon, mouth, throat, and prostate cancers.[508] Some of these benefits may be partially due to the low glycemic load of most raw fruits and vegetables. Low-glycemic foods are associated with protection from developing obesity,[509] colon cancer,[510] breast cancer,[511] ovarian cancer,[512] and stomach cancer.[513] (See Appendix C for the definition of low-glycemic load and a reference for where you can find a list of low-glycemic foods.) Phytoestrogens (isoflavons, lignans, and cumestrans) are compounds found in many fruits and vegetables, which have been shown to reduce the risk of lung cancer.[514]

People who eat more than five servings of fruits and vegetables per day live longer. One study from the U.S. Department of Agriculture Human Nutrition Research Center on Aging at Tufts University reports that men who consumed more than five servings of fruits and vegetables per day while getting less than 12 percent of their calories from saturated fat were *31 percent less likely to die of any cause.*[515] A study from Finland reported that men who ate the most fruits, berries, and vegetables reduced their non-heart-related causes of death by 32 percent.[516]

There is absolutely no doubt about the tremendous benefits derived from fruits and vegetables. So why do so many people not get enough of them, despite being affluent members of modern societies? Well, some people just don't like 'em. Even a recent president of the United States risked losing the truck-farmer vote when he proclaimed his dislike of broccoli. In fact, some people may have a genetic aversion to the taste of fruits and vegetables. For most of us, though, the avoidance of fruits and vegetables is simply a matter of personal history. We weren't fed enough of them as children. We never acquired the taste or the habit of eating them. At dinner, we fill up on yummy meats and starches. When we want a snack, we reach for a candy bar, cookies, or a bag of starch-laden salty snacks instead of an apple or some carrot sticks.

So here's a suggestion. Fruits and vegetables can be an "acquired taste." Yes, I know. That's a phrase one usually associates with things like liquor, beer, cigars, or Wagnerian opera. But if people can acquire a taste for scotch whisky, *you* can acquire a taste for things that are good for you, like fruits and vegetables.

Give your taste buds a chance to adapt. They will. And soon you will look forward to your daily doses of nature's best preventive medicine.

DR. DUKE'S GAME PLAN

- Eating seven to nine servings of fruits and vegetables daily is like adding a queen to your side of the chess board.

- Make fruits and vegetables part of every meal, and eat them for snacks.
- When you choose fruits and veggies, "think color." Eating a wide variety of colors will provide a wide variety of antioxidants. That means more protection against a wider variety of cancers and other chronic diseases.
- Consider taking additional vitamin E and carotinoids, which have been shown to reduce the risk of abnormal cells in the stomach.[517] ❖

8. Excessive alcohol

Drinking red wine is a good way to support heart health. Right? It *must* be right because it's the conventional wisdom, supported by research. Even people living in isolated villages in the Arctic and the upper Amazon basin know this.

Wrong. In reality, the greatest benefits of red wine come from the antioxidant (resveratrol) in the grapes, not the alcohol. So we *could* just eat the grapes. But then we wouldn't have a rationalization for drinking wine.

It is human nature to pay attention to research that supports what we want to do and ignore research that indicates we should do something else in order to be optimally healthy.

Nonetheless...

According to the National Cancer Institute,[518] drinking alcohol increases the risk of cancer of the mouth, esophagus, throat, breast, and liver. Two drinks a day increases women's risk of getting breast cancer by 25 percent. Heavy alcohol use may also increase the risk of colorectal and ovarian cancer. These risks increase after approximately one drink daily for women and two for men.

Alcohol attacks the body oxidatively. Overall, the negative health effects of alcohol outweigh any benefits.

DR. DUKE'S GAME PLAN

- If you have a strong family history of cancer, it would be wise not to drink alcohol at all. If you choose to drink, you should not have more than one drink (for women) or two (for men) four or five days per week. Your liver needs those days of rest to recover from the oxidative attack of alcohol. (By the way, a drink is defined as a shot of hard liquor, a 5 ounce glass of wine, or a can of beer. Those enormous German beer schooners exceed the definition of "a drink.")

- Don't save up your "weekly allowance" of alcohol and drink it in one day.
- If these guidelines seem unduly oppressive or impossible to follow, then perhaps alcohol has a greater influence in your life than it should. Consider speaking to your doctor or a counselor qualified in screening for addictions. ❖

9. High salt intake

A few years ago I spoke with the head of the National Cancer Institute in Japan. I asked him why he thought that the stomach cancer rate was so high in his country. He said they believed it was related to the high salt intake in the average Japanese diet. Several studies have reported this relationship, including one conducted in the Netherlands.[519] The exact mechanism isn't known, but it appears that high amounts of salt in the diet irritate and erode the stomach lining, making it more susceptible to carcinogens.

The lead author of a study referred to earlier[520] that compared Japanese and western diets is quoted as saying that their group believes the traditional Japanese diet is associated with increased risk of colon cancer because of nitrosamines, which are substances in salt-preserved foods such as those common in the traditional Japanese diet.[521]

DR. DUKE'S GAME PLAN

- Use salt moderately. ❖

10. Pollution

Many studies report a connection between air pollution and upper respiratory cancers. The International Agency for Research on Cancer reports that 2 percent of all work-related cancers in the world and 1 percent of all environment-related cancers worldwide are due to air pollution.[522] These cancers, of course, are more concentrated in regions with the highest pollution levels.

Does that mean I'm going to tell you to stop breathing? Well, don't hold your breath.

While atmospheric air pollution is a political, economic, and technological problem that is difficult for an individual to combat, there are important of sources of air pollution that are extremely local, as in inside our own homes and offices. Secondhand smoke is one of these. Radon is another. Radon gas comes from disintegrating rock and can penetrate into homes through the basement or foundation. It is odorless, colorless, and tasteless; one has to test for it specifically. Radon dramatically increases the risk of lung cancer among smokers and recent ex-smokers. A European study[523] reports that radon increases the risk of lung cancer among smokers twenty-five times. Radon increases the risk of lung cancer among *nonsmokers* less than 1 percent. (You still have an urge to light one up?)

DR. DUKE'S GAME PLAN

- Have your home checked for radon.
- Reduce exposure to carcinogenic chemicals, pollution, and cigarette or cigar smoke as much as possible.
- Consider buying an air treatment system for your home or office. ❖

11. Smoked or grilled foods

I know this will bring grief to many, especially my friends in the Southern United States, but I have to say it.

It has been reported for years that smoking or grilling foods, especially over charcoal, increases the risk of colon cancer. This is probably because the smoke that rises from the heat sources has many carcinogens in it. Recent studies, though, seem to show that the increased risk may be more related to high cooking temperature, and especially superheated fat.[524] Barbecuing meat creates dangerous chemicals called *heterocyclic amines*, which increase the risk of cancer[525, 526] and increase inflammation.[527]

DR. DUKE'S GAME PLAN

- Cook as little as possible over charcoal or professional-style infrared grills.
- Use gas as a heat source for your outdoor cooking.
- Cook foods that are low in fat.
- Keep your grill clean.
- Don't cook on your barbecue grill more than once a week. ❖

12. Excessive sunlight

Skin cancer is the most common type of cancer in people with light complexions everywhere in the world. And no, I'm sorry, but getting a good tan doesn't help. Quite the opposite.

Ultraviolet light is the culprit. According to the National Cancer Institute, research suggests that reducing long-term exposure to sunlight, sun lamps, and tanning beds can reduce the risk of non-melanoma skin cancer. Avoiding sunburn, especially during childhood and teen years, may reduce one's lifetime risk of getting melanoma skin cancer.[528]

Most people don't know that artificial tanning beds and sunlamps are listed as carcinogens by the U.S. government. Some studies have even linked tanning bed use to development of melanoma.[529] Another study reports that ultraviolet radiation from sun exposure is the leading cause of skin cancer.[530]

So protect yourself. I know it is discouraging to hear that cancer has the sun on its side. But today we have great ways to cover up and still enjoy the outdoors.

DR. DUKE'S GAME PLAN

- Avoid tanning beds like a vampire avoids the sun.
- When you are out in the sun, always wear sunscreen that protects from both UVA and UVB radiation. The SPF should be at least 30.
- Use hats, umbrellas, and long-sleeved shirts to reduce prolonged exposure to the sun. If you spend a lot of time outdoors—fishing, hiking, boating, golfing, etc.—shop for out-

door clothing that has a rated sun-block factor. Try to avoid the sun between 10 a.m. and 2 p.m. especially. Morning and afternoon rays are safer. ❖

13. Certain infections

There are many viral infections that increase the risk of cancer. Human papillomavirus (HPV) is a sexually transmitted disease that causes venereal warts. More than 99 percent of cervical cancers contain HPV segments in the cancer's DNA.[531] Unfortunately, many people who choose to have sex with multiple partners, especially adolescents, think that they don't need worry about venereal disease. It won't happen to me, and if it does, there's a cure, right?

No. Wrong. Some sexually transmitted diseases that have very serious long-term consequences and are difficult or impossible to cure. HPV is one of them.

Other viruses have been associated with increased risk of cancer. Both hepatitis C and hepatitis B increase the risk of liver cancer.[532] Hepatitis B is spread through body fluid contact, including sexual contact. It is believed that some cases of hepatitis C may be sexually transmitted as well.

DR. DUKE'S GAME PLAN

- Monogamy. Having sex with more than one person in your life significantly increases the risk of venereal disease, including infections that elevate cancer risk.
- Avoid contact with other people's blood and body fluids as much as possible.
- Ask your doctor about the vaccine for HPV and whether or not it's right for you. ❖

14. Vitamin D deficiency

You would think that in modern civilization vitamin deficiencies would be as rare as hand-copied parchment books or smallpox. The truth is that they are fairly prevalent, and some are the result of our modern culture.

Take vitamin D. Please. You probably need more of this essential nutrient than you're getting.

Vitamin D deficiency has reached alarming rates in both the United States and Europe. And this deficiency is a risk factor for several cancers. Here's why.

First, exposure to sunlight regenerates vitamin D in our skin through the reaction of a vitamin D precursor to UVB radiation. For this reason vitamin D deficiency is more common in extreme northern and southern latitudes, where people get less exposure to sunlight. Another reason is that people in developed nations are constantly exposed to people like me haranguing them to stay out of the sun or use sunscreen in order to avoid cancer. In reducing our risk of non-melanoma skin cancer, we're *increasing* our risk of other cancers through vitamin D deficiency. What's a body to do? Keep reading.

Another common cause of this deficiency is reduced intake of dairy products, which are commonly fortified with vitamin D. The diet industry strikes again.

Vitamin D deficiency raises your risk for several kinds of cancer. It doubles the chance of developing colon cancer[533] and significantly increases the risk of prostate cancer.[534] Conversely, adequate amounts of vitamin D reduce the risk of prostate cancer and are anti-inflammatory.[535] One study concluded that lack of sun exposure accounts for perhaps 25 percent of the breast cancer death rate in northern Europe.[536] Another study revealed that women with the highest levels of vitamin D would have a 50 percent reduction in breast cancer compared to women with the lowest levels.[537] To obtain these levels, though, would require a vitamin D intake of 2,700 IU daily, while the National Academy of Sciences has set the safe upper limit at 2,400 IU. There are discussions that perhaps this upper limit needs to be readdressed because the most recent research indicates that supplementation with higher levels is most protective.[538]

Other cancers associated with vitamin D deficiency are ovarian and non-Hodgkin's lymphoma.[539] This same study reported that other cancers may be related to vitamin D deficiency, including cancers of the bladder, esophagus, kidney, lung, pancreas, rectum, and stomach. Low vitamin D levels may be associated with increased digestive system cancers and increased mortality in men.[540]

DR. DUKE'S GAME PLAN

- Have your vitamin D level checked. Some studies seem to indicate that the blood level of 25-hydroxy vitamin D necessary to be protective is over 37 ng/ml.
- Get about ten minutes' exposure to the sun daily; this is enough to meet vitamin D needs without significantly increasing the risk of skin cancer.
- Consider regular vitamin D supplementation if your levels are low. You should probably take in at least 1000 IU per day and some newer research is even suggesting more. ❖

15. Inflammation

Some cancers have been associated with elevated C-reactive protein, which is a marker for inflammation. One example is colorectal cancer.[541] An interesting study reported that use of nonsteroidal anti-inflammatory drugs is associated with a decreased incidence of lung cancer.[542] Inflammation has also been shown to play a role in the development of prostate,[543] liver, and pancreatic cancer,[544] as well as digestive system cancers.[545, 546, 547, 548, 549] Natural anti-inflammatory nutrients like omega-3 have been shown to reduce the risk of colorectal[550] and other cancers.[551] In fact, researchers have even identified an inflammatory molecule which probably causes a lot of cancer.[552]

DR. DUKE'S GAME PLAN

- Talk to your doctor about getting a high sensitive C-reactive protein level test—a measure of inflammation.
- Follow the recommendations in chapter 3 and the rest of the book concerning how to reduce inflammation. ❖

16. Insulin resistance and type 2 diabetes

This chapter ends with what for many people will be a bit of a surprise. Insulin resistance and diabetes aren't just risk factors for cardiovascular disease. They play on cancer's team as well.

Insulin resistance is a syndrome of several cardiovascular risk factors that increase the risk of heart disease, diabetes, and other health problems.[553] Among those are liver and colorectal cancer.[554, 555] I'll explain it in detail in chapter 12.

Type 2 diabetes is also associated with increased risk of colon, endometrial (uterus), kidney, pancreatic, and liver cancer.[556] Both diabetes and liver cancer are increasing rapidly in many countries, and the former may be a contributing factor to the latter.

There is much we don't know yet about the relationship between insulin resistance and diabetes and increased cancer risk. It is being studied. But that doesn't mean you should wait to do something about it. If your house is on fire, you grab the fire extinguisher first and figure out how it started later.

And of course, the first step is to find out if you have this risk factor. Many people do and don't know it.

DR. DUKE'S GAME PLAN

- Read chapter 12 and talk to your doctor about testing for these conditions.
- If you have insulin resistance or type 2 diabetes, please follow your doctor's advice carefully, and ask him or her about following the suggestions to reduce insulin resistance presented in chapter 12. ❖

Playing to Win

Cancer starts with a full complement of chessmen, and it's a wily opponent. Chess strategy isn't simple. You have to defend against a lot of pieces, moves, and tactics.

But you do have control of your own pieces. You can counter every risk factor, every move cancer can make against you. The exception is heredity, but even then you can significantly control whether or not a gene is expressed by your lifestyle.

This game will last as long as you live, too. And I can't guarantee you'll win, even if you play the game as well as possible. What's more, I know that after reading this chapter, the idea of putting up a complete defense may seem intimidating. It takes strategy, focus, and a thinking person's approach to the disease.

That's another reason why I want this book to change your lifestyle, not just one or two habits. And in the end that's an *easier* way. As we gradually incorporate changes into the way we live, rather than taking up fads and then dropping them, the changes become second nature to us.

You weren't born smoking tobacco or refusing to eat your vegetables or spending all your free time in front of a television. These habits are not in your genes. Healthy eating, regular exercise, and annual checkups with your doctor may seem like a drag now, but given a chance, they will become parts of your life you will look forward to.

Even the part about seeing your doctor.

Before reading on, please take a minute to scan the list of cancer risk factors again. How many chessmen does cancer have over which you have no control? The answer is the same as for heart disease: one, genetics. But even that piece can be limited by capturing the enemy's other chess pieces. An opponent who is down to nothing but his king and one other piece isn't likely to beat you. And living the lifestyle we teach is like capturing or severely outnumbering all of cancer's other chessmen.

It's much better to change your lifestyle now before a cancer is diagnosed.

CHAPTER 11

Deflating the Balloon of Obesity

LOVE CAN MAKE YOU STUPID.

I have acrophobia, the fear of heights. I don't like climbing ladders. I am grateful not to be taller than I am. But when you are in love your head is in the clouds, so my desire to find the most romantic way to ask my sweetheart to marry me, to create a moment she would never forget, led me on a strange journey one day.

It involved getting up at 4 a.m., driving through the dark into the Southern California countryside, stepping at dawn into an oversized Easter basket and allowing a complete stranger to take us hundreds of feet into the air suspended from a hot-air balloon.

And for the first minute or two it *did* seem romantic.

Then I looked down.

Cars below me seemed like little beetles, and I don't mean the Volkswagens. Then I realized there were questions I had neglected to ask the pilot prior to takeoff. Like, who was he and what kind of brain damage led him to do this for a living? Was the brain damage incurred in a balloon crash? What happens if a sharp-beaked bird flies into the balloon? Why am I doing this? Will my beloved be more or less likely to accept my proposal after she sees me whimpering like a frightened child? Is what I'm feeling love or impending incontinence? If the latter, can I be sued for damages by people on the ground?

I took a good look at the balloon's pilot. He seemed different from the clean-shaven, confidence-inspiring guy I had met in his office. Now he looked like a pirate who'd had a long, rum-soaked night ashore and hadn't had time to sleep it off. I could only hope he hadn't lost his will to live.

Of course, we went up and then down again without incident, except that my wonderful wife accepted my proposal. Perhaps she thought my abject, cold-sweat fear was inspired by the possibility that she might say no. I have always thought it best not to ask.

Anyway, I do have a point. Most people who go up in balloons do so because they enjoy it. The health risk of hot-air ballooning is extremely low. On the other hand, people throughout the developed world are themselves ballooning in size, at considerable risk to their health. The level of anxiety about this ought to be similar to mine that day in the balloon, and in some quarters it is. But nothing seems to be effective, so far, in bringing this ballooning public-health problem back down to hearth.

That is mostly because there is enough hot air being generated from all sides of the obesity issue to keep every balloon in the world aloft indefinitely.

Everybody has an opinion, and almost everybody has a cure for sale. Thousands of companies offer diets, drugs (both prescription and over-the-counter), exercise programs and equipment, food and beverage products, books, videos, classes, surgical processes, and magical charms, each touted as the true path to weight control. We are obsessed with being thin, and yet obesity rates continue to rise.

There is so much confusion that most people don't even have a clear idea how to define the problem. For instance, even though many of us will admit to being a few pounds overweight, we're reluctant to accept a diagnosis of obesity. That's understandable, given the social stigma attached to obesity in modern cultures, but it's also a shame. We don't make derisive wisecracks about people who have diabetes or heart disease or cancer. We don't blame those victims for their own diseases, even though lifestyle choices probably contributed. But many of us think that even morbidly obese people choose to be that way and could easily drop one or two hundred pounds just by saying no to Twinkies® and soft drinks.

But let's be realistic: If it were that easy to lose weight, would anyone choose to be obese?

Also, many of us think of obesity only in terms of being extremely fat. That's another misconception. The medical issues are more complex than that; I'll explain why presently.

Finally, too many people, both fat and thin, regard obesity as a cosmetic problem. People are literally dying to be thin, trying one diet or drug "cure" after another in order to conform to society's standards of beauty, all while damaging their health through poor nutrition and worse. Obesity is a *health* problem. There are many documented ways in which it elevates our risk for chronic disease. We have to address obesity in ways that make us healthier.

It's time to abandon the shame, prejudice, and misconceptions surrounding obesity and look at realistic ways to deal with this problem. People are spending billions of dollars trying to get thinner, yet obesity rates keep rising.

There has been a great deal of research over the last five years concerning both obesity and fat-cell metabolism. Any book written prior to this time lacks significant understanding of this worldwide problem. The information in this chapter differs from many popular diet books, but I've backed it up with references to the research on which it is based so that you can examine the data for yourself.

Not surprisingly, this is the fattest chapter in this book (if you'll pardon the pun). It has to be, in order to counter all the misconceptions. There are more lies circulating around the world concerning weight loss than any other aspect of our quest for optimal health. Information is the key component of our game plan for winning your best life.

Reading this chapter will help you understand the following:

- The definitions: obesity, overweight, Body Mass Index, and more.
- Whether or not you qualify as overweight or obese.
- The association between chronic inflammation and obesity.

- The extent of the worldwide epidemic of obesity for both adults and children, including the alarming statistics.
- The causes, effects and reversibility of many of the health problems associated with obesity.
- The problems with some of the most popular fad diets.
- How to lay the foundation for optimal health and successful weight loss.

Obesity Defined: A Formula That Makes Sense

Let's begin clearing up the misconceptions by defining both obesity and overweight. It's important to know which category you're in (if either), because there are significant differences in chronic disease risk between the two. You need to be properly motivated and make the right choices. Of course, this issue isn't quite that simple; later on, we'll talk about the different types of fat in the body and their physiological significance. But first things first.

The most common method for defining obesity is the Body Mass Index, or BMI (see Appendix A.3). BMI is calculated by dividing your body weight in kilograms by the square of your height in meters. If you use the English system of measurements (the system still used in America, but long abandoned in England and everywhere else), you can multiply your weight in pounds by 703, then divide this number by the square of your height in inches.

BMI formula using the metric system:
(body weight in kilograms, height in meters)
weight ÷ height^2

BMI formula using the English system:
(body weight in pounds, height in inches)
weight × 703 ÷ height^2

Example using metric system:
Let's calculate the BMI for a person weighing 90 kilograms and standing 1.75 meters tall.

$$1.75 \times 1.75 = 3.06$$

90 ÷ 3.06 = 29.41
This person has a Body Mass Index of 29

Example using the English system:
Using the English system of weights and measures, that same person is 198 pounds and 5 feet, 9 inches, or 69 inches.

200 × 703 = 139,194
69 × 69 = 4,761
139,194 ÷ 4,761 = 29.23

Again, the BMI works out to 29.

If you ever find yourself needing to calculate someone's BMI and you don't have this book with you, just type "body mass index" into any Internet search engine, such as Google, and you will get links to online programs that will calculate BMI for you.

IMPORTANT NOTE: While BMI is the most widely used scale in scientific literature for measuring overweight and obesity, it is too simplistic to be accurate for diagnosis in all cases. It doesn't account for the size of one's skeletal frame or for the ratio of fat to muscle tissue. That is why our institute has developed a more comprehensive diagnostic formula that includes BMI as one of three factors.

BMI is used to classify body weights in four general categories. For adults of European descent, it breaks out this way:

Under 19 = underweight
19 to 24.9 = normal
25 to 29.9 = overweight
30 or above = obese

Since it has been shown that excess weight gain in Asians is associated with greater health risk than an equivalent weight gain for people of European descent,[557] the BMI scale for Asians is a bit different:

Under 19 = underweight
19 to 22.9 = normal
23 to 24.9 = overweight

25 or above = obese

The "obese" end of the scale is further subdivided. For adults of European descent, it breaks out like this:

Class 1 obesity: BMI 30 to 34.9
Class 2 obesity: BMI 35 to 39.9
Class 3 obesity: BMI 40 or above[558, 559, 560]

Class 3 obesity is also called morbid or extreme obesity; this designation is clinically significant, because the morbidly obese have twice the risk of early death, compared to obese individuals with a BMI of 30 to 31.9.[561]

BMI is also the most widely used measure of obesity in children and adolescents.[562] The Centers for Disease Control (CDC) has issued pediatric growth charts that help to determine acceptable weight ranges by age and gender. (See Appendix A.4 and A.5 for the BMI recommendations for boys and girls, respectively.)

A BMI above the 95th percentile qualifies for obesity in children. A BMI between the 85th and 95th percentile indicates increased risk of obesity, and these children should be screened for other complications associated with obesity. An increase in BMI of three to four units per year should be taken seriously, because the normal increase for growing children is only one BMI unit per year.[563]

As noted above, BMI is a somewhat simplistic formula. Used alone, it is prone to error with regard to diagnosis. For example, a person with a delicate frame, relatively little muscle tissue and a high percentage of body fat might register "normal" on the BMI scale but in fact have the elevated health risk of an obese person. Such a person is designated "metabolically obese normal weight" (MONW).[564, 565]

Conversely, a muscular athlete with a very low percentage of body fat might be incorrectly designated as obese. Being built like an American football linebacker isn't a risk factor for chronic disease, unless you got those muscles by taking steroids.

So—body fat percentage is another factor that needs to be added to the formula for defining obesity.

You should consult your health-care provider about the amount of body fat that should be considered elevated for you, based on your specific body type. (Ask your doctor or a personal trainer at your gym about measuring your body fat percentage.) Here are the general ranges, given as a percent of total body weight.

Body fat, men:
> 12% to 20% = ideal
> 20.1% to 25% = overweight
> over 25% = obese

Body fat, women:
> 15% to 22% = ideal
> 22.1% to 30% = overweight
> over 30% = obese

Another problem with BMI is that it doesn't take into account *where* you are fat. Believe it or not, the way fat is distributed on your body is critically important. Men tend to have fat deposits around the waist region near the major internal organs (viscera). Women tend carry fat on the buttocks and thighs. Fat cells near the abdomen and viscera tend to be of a different type, and they present increased health risk compared to fat elsewhere in the body. Therefore, we need to consider the distribution of fat on the body when we calculate health risk.

In other words, even if a BMI measurement classifies your weight as normal, you may still have an elevated health risk based on your body fat ratio and the distribution of fat on your body.

The best and least expensive way to determine fat distribution is to figure your waist-to-hip ratio. All you need is a tape measure and third-grade math skills. Measure the distance around your waist at the umbilicus (belly button) and around your hips—right at the hip joints. Then divide waist by hips. That gives us a ratio, so it doesn't matter if you measure in centimeters or inches. Here are the ideal ratios:

Men:
> waist ÷ hips should equal 0.95 or less

Women:

> waist ÷ hips should equal 0.88 or less

The importance of the waist-to-hip ratio was validated in a study in Sweden involving 1,400 women over twelve years.[566] **That study showed that waist-to-hip ratio is actually a better predictor for heart disease, stroke, and death than are BMI and skin-fold thickness.** (Some studies are even showing a predictive risk for chronic disease based on waist measurement alone.)

None of these three methods of diagnosing obesity is perfect, but they are all useful. Some older methods are less so. For instance, the charts used by insurance companies are inaccurate, because they are simplistic and biased toward lower weights. This bias benefits insurance companies, making it easy for them to categorize large swaths of the population as obese. These companies have been reluctant to use the better, if less simple, methods now available.

We need an accurate system for designating obesity, so that we can determine whether a person is at risk for chronic disease that can lead to early death. The most accurate method combines BMI, body fat percentage and waist-to-hip ratio.

At the institute where I consult, we have developed a formula that incorporates all of these measurements for determining a Body Composition Health Risk Score. We call it the BCoR Score.

The formulas for adults other than Asians are as follows (the formulas for Asians are the same, except divide the BMI by 24, not 25):

Men:
(BMI ÷ 25) + (% body fat ÷ 21) + (waist-to-hip ratio) ÷ 3 = _____

Women:
(BMI ÷ 25) + (% body fat ÷ 27) + (waist-to-hip ratio ÷ 0.85) ÷ 3 = _____

Example:
A woman has a BMI of 24, 29% body fat, and a waist-to-hip ratio of 0.85.

BMI: (24 ÷ 25 = 0.96)

% body fat: (29 ÷ 27 = 1.07)
waist-to-hip ratio: (.85 ÷ .85 = 1.0)

0.96 + 1.07 + 1.0 = 3.03 ÷ 3 = **BCoR score of 1.01**

This woman would fit into the increased-risk category, even though she would look fine and not be considered at risk under two of the three methods. She is apparently a woman with a delicate frame, so even though her BMI and waist-to-hip ratio were good, her body fat percentage made the difference.

We have categorized BCoR scores according to the following table:

BCoR Scores

	MEN	WOMEN
Underweight	< 0.64	< 0.74
Ideal (low risk)	0.64—0.84	0.74—0.87
Normal	0.85—1.0	0.88—1.0
Increased risk	1.0—1.13	1.0—1.13
Significant risk	> 1.13	> 1.13

Men should not have a score that is less than 0.64 and women should not be below 0.74. At the other end of the scale, a score of 1.0 to 1.13 indicates a moderate increase in risk of chronic disease for both men and women. A score over 1.13 indicates significantly increased risk. We are accumulating research data to further validate these score guidelines over time.

These parameters should help you set goals for how much weight you should lose. If you are in the obese category, start by getting down to overweight. If you're overweight, then shoot for normal. Once your score is below 1.0, stop worrying about your weight and focus on other risk factors since further weight loss won't reduce your risk of chronic disease.

FB

Lose Fat, Not Weight

Most fad diets want you measure success on your bathroom scale, but that's the wrong focus. If you change your lifestyle to include a better diet and regular exercise, you will probably lose fat while gaining muscle. Your weight might not change much, and yet you're getting healthier by the week.

Fad diets define this as failure. That's a dangerous lie.

Once you start losing weight, it's easy to become obsessed with reaching some ideal. Your goals need to be realistic and based on optimal health. Forget about what you weighed in high school. Forget about losing those "last five pounds." With that kind of focus, you'll get discouraged and give up on your healthier new lifestyle. Or else you'll lose *too much* weight. Often those "last five pounds" are lost muscle, not lost fat. Muscle is good.

In most industrial societies, popular culture focuses on scale weight. That's wrong. Please throw your scale away, and focus instead on the values given above. Fad diets focus on scales because that lets them show quick results. Unfortunately, the five or ten pounds you lose on these diets are usually just water weight. They're charging you money to show you how to get dehydrated, rather than help you to lose fat.

Real and safe loss of fat tissue doesn't happen overnight. It takes a while. But wouldn't you rather live a lifestyle that will cause you to lose fat and keep it off? Quick-loss diets give you a temporary, false sense of success. But they aren't healthy, and they can make it harder to lose fat in the future.

In the Optimal Health Revolution, we're talking about a permanent lifestyle change, with lifelong health benefits.

The Missing Link Between Obesity and Chronic Inflammation

Can inflammation be at the root cause of essentially every chronic disease known to man but not be involved with weight gain and obesity? I think not. Nevertheless, many researchers and physicians aren't convinced that there's a correlation. They know inflammation increases with weight gain but see inflammation as a result rather than a cause of obesity. I believe inflammation is the cause of the worldwide obesity epidemic and will attempt to explain it here. This correlation is a critical point because we are in the midst of a worldwide obesity epidemic, and health-care systems globally have been powerless to stop it. If we are truly missing the real cause, then we will continue to be doomed to failure. How can anyone win a battle when you don't know who your real opponent is?

My insight was again purely by accident, though anyone in my position would have suspected the same thing. While obtaining statistics from the World Health Organization for upcoming programs at the center where I consult, I noted that increased obesity perfectly paralleled industrialization in every country, no matter where they were in the world. Even in poorer countries like Brazil, where a high percentage of the population doesn't have the money to gorge themselves (many people only spend $1.00 U.S. per day on food), obesity is rising significantly. I also know of many morbidly obese people who don't eat the vast quantities of food you would assume they would be eating. There must be something going on at the cellular level. Certainly restricted caloric intake and exercise helped these people, but only temporarily. Why does seemingly everyone rebound after dieting? It was time to look deeper.

The first research that was beneficial to see inflammation as causing the obesity epidemic involved inflammation's role in insulin resistance and type 2 diabetes (see chapter 12). The obesity and diabetes epidemics have been almost simultaneous, and inflammation disrupts normal sugar metabolism, often leading to type 2 diabetes. But there have been some more studies that have pointed to the direct link between inflammation, type 2 diabetes, and obesity.[567, 568] The absolute inflammatory link that causes overweight and obesity is still under investigation, but I suspect that it's related to a protein called adiponectin, which is made by fat cells and regulates normal metabolism. Inflammation lowers this protein even in people who aren't overweight, and it doesn't take long for overweight problems to begin.[569, 570, 571, 572] Therefore, obesity wasn't only increasing inflammation, it was also caused by it. Evidence of a vicious cycle.

Armed with this understanding, I helped create a weight-loss program that focused on inflammation reduction. We have also incorporated good eating practices and exercise (both of which reduce inflammation), and have had very good success.

What does this mean for you? All you have to do is focus on reducing inflammation and weight loss will happen. The reason that many people have failed to lose weight is because they have been recommended to also include things into their weight loss program that increase inflammation. The teaching here will consistently reduce inflammation for you, and it works.

Worldwide Obesity: The Weight of Numbers

Obesity and overweight are now reaching epidemic proportions around the world, and the condition continues to worsen.[573, 574] Check out the table below, which gives the percentages of people who are either overweight or obese in eleven countries around the world, according to the North American Association for the Study of Obesity.[575]

Rates of Overweight/Obesity[576]

	MEN	WOMEN
Australia	63%	46.8%
Canada	71%	56%
China	16%	23%
Italy	47%	35%
Japan	26%	22.6%
Mexico	56.3%	60.7%
Romania	60%	59%
Russia	45.3%	56.4%
Samoa	58%	77%
United Kingdom	62.8%	53.3%
United States	60%	50%

The most recent (2006) China Health and Nutrition Survey reports that 26 percent of the Chinese population is overweight, and that overweight is climbing faster in China than in all developing countries

FIGURE 11.1

Obesity Trends* Among U.S. Adults
BRFSS, 1990
(*BMI ≥30, or 30 lbs overweight for a 5'4" person)

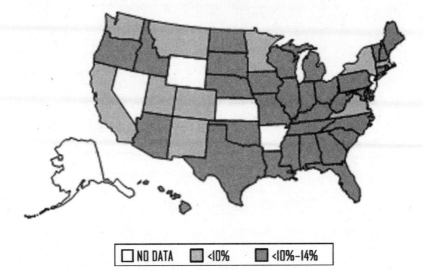

| ☐ NO DATA | ▨ <10% | ▪ <10%–14% |

Source: Behavioral Risk Factors Surveillance System, CDC.

except Mexico.[577]

The weight of the average American is growing by two pounds a year.[578] Class 3 obesity (BMI > 40) has increased 300 percent between 1990 and 2000.[579] Class 3 obesity is associated with twice the risk of death from all causes, as compared to class 1 (BMI 30 to 34.9).[580] There are over 120 million people in the U.S. who are overweight or obese. The obesity rates in the U.S. are even worse for African American and Hispanic women, whose obesity rates are worsening 2.1 and 1.5 times faster, respectively, than those of Caucasian women.[581]

Figures 1 and 2 show obesity trends among U.S. adults from 1990 to 2003. And this phenomenon isn't exclusive to the U.S., as the numbers above suggest. A more recent study has shown that increases in weight are continuing to rise among children, adolescents, and men, but have leveled off among women.[582]

The World Health Organization estimates that 1.2 billion people

FIGURE 11.2

Obesity Trends Among U.S. Adults, 2003

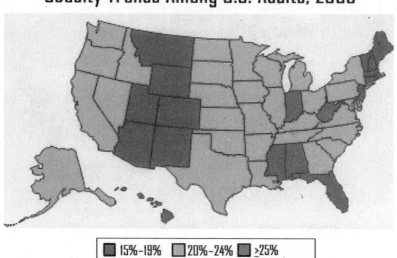

| ■ 15%–19% | □ 20%–24% | ■ ≥25% |

Source: http://www.cdc.gov/nccdphp/dnpa/obesity/trend/maps/index.htm.

worldwide are affected by overweight and obesity, with numbers increasing at an unprecedented rate.[583] The World Health Organization, commenting on data from worldwide surveys, stated, "Obesity's impact is so diverse and extreme that it should be regarded as one of the greatest neglected public health problems of our time, with an impact on health which may well prove to be as great as that of smoking."[584]

The director of the U.S. Centers for Disease Control and Prevention stated, "Obesity is an epidemic and should be taken as seriously as any infectious disease epidemic."[585]

The Worldwatch Institute released a report stating that for the first time in history, there are as many overweight people as there are underfed.[586]

Obesity rates are large and ballooning in every industrialized nation, as well as many poorer ones. But the problem becomes even more ponderous when we realize that *the numbers are probably underestimated.* Most of our data are based on telephone surveys that ask people to give their height and weight. In what scientists call validation studies, overweight people tend to underestimate their weight, and all participants tend to overestimate their height, which, of course, causes BMI numbers to skew low.[587, 588, 589] According to one recent source, the proportion of U.S. adults who are obese has increased 7 percent, to a national average of 25.6 percent according to the U.S. Center for Disease Control.[590]

The problem of obesity is not restricted to adults. In fact, we are seeing unprecedented obesity rates in children and adolescents worldwide. This means we can expect a far greater problem in the future, because obesity at an early age is predictive of overweight and obesity in adulthood.[591, 592, 593, 594]

In case the weight of the numbers hasn't convinced you, here are a last few, concerning the changes in obesity rates in recent years. Obesity rates have increased:

- 230 to 333 percent over the last twenty-five years in the United States[595, 596]
- 200 to 280 percent over the last seventeen years in England[597]
- 180 to 230 percent over the last seventeen years in Scotland[598]
- 140 percent over six years in China[599]
- 250 percent over twenty-six years in Japan[600]
- 390 percent over eighteen years in Egypt[601]
- 342 to 460 percent over ten years in Australia[602]
- 380 percent over six years in Ghana[603]
- 360 percent over seventeen years in Brazil[604]
- 270 percent over fourteen years in Costa Rica[605]

The epidemic among children affects a wide age range, most ethnic groups, and every socioeconomic stratum, if sometimes in different proportions.[606, 607] In developed nations, children in lower socioeconomic strata are more likely to have diets that are poor in general nutrition but high in calories.[608] Though the rise in obesity in children may be leveling off in the U.S.,[609] the American Academy of Pediatrics now recommends that some children as young as eight years old be started on cholesterol-lowering medication.[610] The lower socioeconomic children also tend to have limited access to physical fitness opportunities.[611] Childhood obesity in developing nations is more common in more affluent socioeconomic strata, apparently because these people are adopting Western diets and lifestyles along with the rest of Western culture.[612, 613]

In 1998, the American Heart Association issued a "call to action" as a response to the rapid growth of obesity in the U.S.[614] Almost a decade later, the authors' statement still holds true: "The sad reality is that the call seems to have fallen on deaf ears. Not only has little progress been made in addressing and treating obesity, but we must have lost ground to the epidemic."[615]

I think there are several reasons why obesity rates continue to grow:

1. **Ignorance.** Too many people don't understand the severe health problems that obesity presents.
2. **The fad diet industry.** Over forty years of misinformation and ill-conceived approaches to weight loss, while profits are the only thing growing fatter than people's waistlines.
3. **Surrender.** The various fad diets confuse people with conflicting recommendations, not to mention that none of them really work for most people. So many people have stopped trying.
4. **The food industry.** This industry, especially the food-service segment, basically denies that they are part of the problem. They could change the food they sell in ways that would slow this epidemic down, but they haven't. They have even cherry-picked statistics to deny, in an ad campaign, that an obesity epidemic exists.[616] In light of the research that I have presented here, this action by the food industry is reprehensible and immoral. It's like the erstwhile denials by the cigarette industry that smoking is harmful to health. If you doubt an obesity epidemic exists, go people-watching anywhere the general public gathers.
5. **Lifestyle.** People are busy. People are stressed. People think they don't have time to eat well and exercise. Don't believe it. I have a family and an incredibly busy schedule that includes a great deal of travel, and yet I find it easy to live a healthy lifestyle. So will you! Yes, you'll need to change the way you live, but I'll show you how.

There are still more causes of obesity. We'll get to those soon enough. Right now I want to pose this question: Would you rather take a little time out of your schedule to get healthy now, or would you rather save the time now and lose it—and maybe a lot more—off the end of your life?

Seems like an easy choice, doesn't it?

Obesity Is a Disease

Another reason this problem keeps ballooning is that people don't take it seriously as a *health* problem.

Let me tell you something you won't hear from fat-fad promoters. I don't care how your clothes look on you. I don't care how good you look in your swimsuit. I don't care about six-pack abs or sculpted thighs. All I care about is how long and how well you live.

Obesity is not a cosmetic problem. It isn't a social problem, except to the extent that fools make it so. This has nothing to do with how good you want to look at your class reunion. It has to do with how many class reunions you will live to attend.

In short, we need to see obesity as a disease.

Obesity is a disease in the truest sense of the word. It is responsible for over 300,000 deaths per year in the United States alone[617] and **has probably surpassed smoking as the leading preventable cause of death**.

We lie awake at night worrying about epidemics like SARS, West Nile virus, and "bird flu." In reality, the deaths caused by these diseases are a tiny fraction of the deaths caused worldwide by obesity.

What if it were something else? Suppose 300,000 people died every year in your country on account of a virus, a defective product or drug, a cruel dictator, a war? There would be widespread outrage or panic. But we don't see obesity in that light. Instead, we avoid exercise, we stuff our faces with the wrong foods, and we allow our children to do the same. The result is that our bad diets and sedentary lifestyles are killing us before our time and often causing debilitating health conditions while we live.

More American children are killed by obesity than by gun violence.[618] And somehow we accept that.

The World Health Organization declared in 1997, "Obesity is a chronic **disease**, prevalent in both developed and developing countries, and affecting children as well as adults."[619] The Institute of Medicine at the National Academy of Sciences published a report stating, "These figures [regarding the prevalence of obesity] point to the fact that obesity is one of the most pervasive public health problems in this country, a complex, multi-factorial **disease** of appetite regulation and energy metabolism involving genetics, physiology, biochemistry, and the neurosciences as well as environmental, psychological, and cultural factors."[620] The vice chairperson of the Nutritional Committee of the American Heart Association has declared, "Obesity itself has become a lifelong **disease**, not a cosmetic issue, nor moral judgment—and it is becoming a danger-ous epidemic."[621] (All emphasis in this paragraph is mine.)

Now that we know that we are facing a serious disease, to combat it most effectively we must understand the effects and causes of the disorder.

Health Effects of Obesity and Overweight

Now comes the part that will really scare you—the part where I list all

FIGURE 11.3

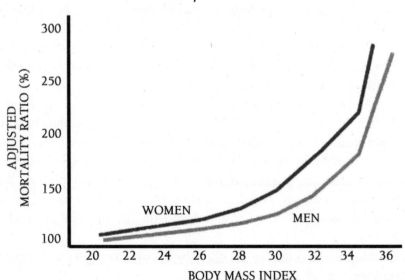

Source: Van Italle T. In: Stunkard AJ and Wadden TA, eds. *Obesity and Therapy*, 2nd ed. New York, NY; Raven Press; 1993.

the disorders and diseases that you are more likely to have if you are obese.

Disclaimer: While I want you to be scared, I don't want you to be discouraged. The *great news* is that many of these effects are reversible. You'll see how at the end of the chapter.

The first health effect I want to talk about is death.

Overweight and obesity are associated with increased death rate.[622] As BMI increases, so does the death rate—dramatically. (See Figure 3.)

Obesity increases the mortality rate 50 to 100 percent over that of nonobese individuals.[623, 624] Overweight people have a 10 to 25 percent higher death rate.[625] The same trend in mortality and obesity is seen among Chinese as it is in all racial and ethnic groups.[626]

As I noted in chapter 9, obesity increases the risk of heart disease, which is the current leading cause of premature death in virtually every industrialized nation around the world.[627, 628, 629] In one study, the risk of death from heart disease increased 500 percent if the obese individuals were unfit,[630] so even if you don't lose weight, regular exercise and a healthy diet are important. Obesity also is associated with abnormal functioning of the coronary blood vessels.[631] It increases the risk of heart failure,[632] affects heart structure,[633] heart function,[634] and heart rhythm.[635]

Obesity also increases many of the risk factors for heart disease discussed in chapter 9. It increases the prevalence of hypertension up to 300 percent,[636] diabetes up to 300 percent,[637, 638, 639] metabolic syndrome (insulin resistance),[640] cholesterol abnormalities,[641] kidney abnormalities,[642, 643] platelet activation (which increases clotting and is the event that rapidly causes heart attacks)[644] and markers of inflammation like C-reactive protein and interleukin-6.[645, 646, 647]

Obesity has also been shown to increase heart disease in children.[648] It also increases the risk factors for heart disease among youth, such as hypertension,[649] cholesterol abnormalities,[650] and insulin resistance.[651] In fact, the past president of the American Diabetes Association states that twenty years ago, 2 percent of children diagnosed with diabetes had type 2, but today it accounts for 30 to 50 percent of all new diagnoses among children nine to nineteen years old.[652] Severely obese children have significantly lower quality of life (QOL) scores compared to healthy children. The scores of obese children are similar to children diagnosed with cancer.[653] Obesity also accelerates puberty in children, causing it to begin in children as young as eight years.[654] It also increases sleep apnea[655] and skeletal development disorders.[656]

Obesity increases the risk of many cancers.[657] It can double the risk of developing breast cancer.[658] A study in the *American Journal of Epidemiology*[659] reported that obesity increases the risk of all cancer deaths in women by 5.9 percent and those in men by 9.7 percent. The Agency for Research on Cancer reported that obesity and inactivity account for up to 33 percent of cancers of the breast, colon, endometrium, kidney, and esophagus.[660] Obesity increases the rate of prostate cancer, which is the number two cancer killer of men in the United States, by 39 percent.[661] It also significantly increases the risk of pancreatic cancer, which is the fifth leading cause of cancer deaths in the United States.

As they say on TV: Wait, there's more. Obesity also increases the risk of gallbladder disease,[662] osteoarthritis,[663] nonalcoholic fatty liver,[664] and impotence.[665] The obesity and diabetes epidemics are not coincidental to the dramatic increase in the need for performance medications like Viagra.

Obesity isn't a joke. It's time we got serious about it.

And while fad diets and fast food are a big part of the problem, so are you. Spending all your free time in front of a TV or computer screen isn't a fad somebody sold you. It's a choice you make every day. You could choose instead to get more exercise, buy healthier foods, and set an example of optimal health for your children.

Your children. If you don't change your lifestyle for your own sake, will you do it for theirs? As parents, you're the ones who set the pattern for your children's lifestyle. The pattern you choose can add years to their lives—or subtract them.

I know these are hard words, but I write them out of love. I want you to understand the need for change now, not later when you or someone you love is on life support in an emergency room.

The Financial Weight of Obesity

If knowing how obesity threatens you or your family doesn't move you to change, then a quick review of the economic costs probably won't either. But you're going to get one anyway. I want you to know how obesity contributes to bloated health-care spending in industrialized countries.

In a study estimating the financial costs of obesity for a population of one million people between the ages of thirty-five and eighty-four, researchers concluded that obesity would account for 132,000 cases of hypertension (45 percent of all cases), 58,500 cases of type 2 diabetes (85 percent of all cases), 51,500 cases of increased cholesterol (18 percent of all cases), and 16,500 cases of heart disease (35 percent of all cases). The study estimated the obesity-related health-care costs for eight diseases—coronary heart disease, hypertension, hypercholesterolemia, gallbladder disease, stroke, type 2 diabetes, osteoarthritis of the knee, and endometrial cancer—at $345.9 million annually. Remember, that was for a population of only a million people. The extra cost imposed by obesity was 41 percent of the total cost for these eight diseases.[666]

Another study shows that the average lifetime cost for medical treatment for hypertension, elevated cholesterol, type 2 diabetes, and heart disease is $17,000 more for obese people.[667] So if you're a person who can't find time to live a healthier lifestyle, maybe saving a lot of money (and the time you lose getting medical treatment) will sway you. You can also save money on insurance—both health and life—if you're healthier. Total lifetime medical costs are almost doubled if you are obese, according to the study in Appendix A.6.[668]

The medical costs of obesity in China are estimated to be 21.11 billion Yuan (RMB) (approximately $2.74 billion U.S.) and could increase to 37 billion Yuan (RMB) (approx. $4.8 billion U.S.) if the obesity epidemic continues.[669]

How Did We Get This Fat? The Risk Factors for Obesity

When a public health problem gets this big this fast all over the world, it's worth asking why.

H.L. Mencken wrote, "There is always an easy solution to every human problem—neat, plausible, and wrong." There are thousands of such "solutions" for sale, but the real solution to the obesity problem isn't simple, and at first it won't seem easy.

The physiological causes of obesity are complex in the extreme. I could take you through a discussion of the biochemical and hormonal factors that influence fat metabolism. I could present the latest research on neuropeptide Y, melanin concentrating hormone, recombinant human variant ciliary neurotropic factor, adiponectin, leptin, ghrelin, interleukin 6, interleukin 18, tumor necrosis factor alpha, and more. But that would cause you to put down the book, turn on the TV, and reach for a bag of chips—not my intended outcome.

In any case, the biochemistry is beside the point. The obesity balloon didn't go up all over the world on account of rapid changes in our DNA or biochemistry. Genetic characteristics don't change that fast.

We need to get out of this problem the same way we got into it, which is to change the way we live. Our ancestors didn't spend all day sitting on their behinds guzzling carbonated sugar water and munching super-sized orders of French fries.

Yes, it would be nice if we could just take a pill, or follow a diet for a few weeks, or squeeze some spring-loaded gadget between our knees while watching TV, but that isn't the way to get to optimal health. You don't win any kind of game on a single play. And this game lasts all your life. So does my game plan.

It's only natural to resist change, especially when it requires you to expend some energy. But we're going to take this one step at a time, so it doesn't seem forbidding, and so that the changes you make can become normal parts of your lifestyle—habits you don't even have to think about, activities you even look forward to.

In fact, the changes that you will need to make *won't* require a lot of time and energy. They will involve many aspects of your life in order to address all the risk factors associated with chronic disease. They will improve your health *and* help you lose weight.

What virtually every previous diet book or plan has missed is that **the risk factors for chronic disease contribute both to our worsening health *and* to obesity**. Temporary change provides only temporary benefit. Permanent changes in behavior and lifestyle caused obesity rates to balloon. Only permanent behavior and lifestyle changes can solve the problem.

For that reason, I will concentrate this discussion on the behavioral and lifestyle characteristics that have caused the obesity epidemic. There are additional risk factors, as we discussed in chapters 2 and 3, and any risk factor that increases inflammation will also impair metabolism and increase the risk of obesity. Since essentially every risk factor we teach increases inflammation, thus contributing to obesity, this is why programs that neglect to reduce inflammation don't work for the long-term.

The primary behavioral causes of obesity are:

1. Ignorance

This is the big one. You can't control the risk factors for chronic disease until you know what they are. I gave you the risk factors for heart disease and cancer in chapters 9 and 10. I'll list more later on and lay out a game plan for controlling them. One reason that my game plan addresses your whole lifestyle is that the risk factors for chronic disease gang up to induce an inflammatory response by the body. This response not only leads to most chronic diseases, but also affects insulin resistance.

I'll discuss insulin resistance at length later. Right now I just want you to understand that insulin resistance promotes weight gain and vice versa. It's a biochemical vicious cycle, a synergy. To break it, you have to address virtually all risk factors. This is why narrow-focus diets are doomed to fail.

2. Excess calories

A calorie isn't a substance; it is a measurement, a unit of energy. If your diet contains more calories than you burn, your body stores those calories for future use, in the form of fat. **If you want to lose fat, you need to burn more calories than you take in.**

In an excellent study by the U.S. Department of Agriculture (USDA) comparing popular diets,[670] the researchers actually documented what people in their study ate, rather than what they *said* they ate. They concluded that "the key to weight loss is energy [calorie] restriction."

Sadly, most of us couldn't guess our daily intake within 500 calories. And that doesn't matter, because nobody takes the time to do accurate daily calculations anyway. My game plan for calorie management is very simple to learn and easy to follow. I'll show you a way to estimate calories so that after a couple of days of planning reasonable meals you'll hardly ever have to do calculations again. Basically, you'll just know how to plan meals for calorie control.

FB

CALORIE IS A CALORIE IS A CALORIE

Some fad diets teach that you can eat as many calories as you want as long as they come from fat. While there may be some differences in the way our bodies metabolize dietary fat versus carbohydrate, the bottom line involves very simple math. If you consume more calories than you burn, you're going to get fatter.

Conversely, if you want to shed fat, your weight-loss program has to include burning more calories than you consume.

The average person in the developed world needs roughly 1,800 to 2,500 calories a day, but eats 3,100 to 3,700. Since 100 excess calories a day can lead to a ten-pound weight gain in a year, you can see where the problem lies.

So the first big question is: How many calories do *you* need per day? What is your break-even point? There are two easy ways to figure this.

One way is to use this formula.

Step one: Multiply your body weight in pounds by 11 (men) or 10 (women). (Metric system: Multiply your weight in kilograms by 24.2 [men] or 22 [women].)

Step two: Multiply that number by a factor that accounts for your normal level of daily activity:

- sedentary—1.25
- lightly active—1.5
- moderately active—1.65
- highly active—2.0
- exceptionally active (e.g., athlete in training)—2.3

The result of step two will be the approximate number of calories you need per day to *maintain* both your health and your current weight. To *lose* weight, you should subtract 500 to 1,000 calories from that number. With that daily caloric intake, you should be able to lose a pound or two a week.

A pound a week? Does that sound chintzy compared to the promises you hear on TV? Sorry, but I want you to be healthy. If you're racing to make weight for a Caribbean vacation, I'm not your coach. This isn't about the way your bikini fits. It's about your health and longevity. That means changing your lifestyle for good, not damaging your health to drop ten pounds in a week.

Another way to calculate the calories you need is to look at a chart prepared by the USDA,[671] which I have included in Appendix A.7. It shows the calories you need based on your age, sex, and activity level.

We should probably manage calories the way we do money. Only a neurotically obsessive person accounts for every penny he or she spends every day. But we do plan, budget, and keep prudently careful track of how much we're making, saving, and spending. That's how we keep from bouncing checks, maxing out our credit cards, or going broke.

Likewise, if we eat either impulsively or compulsively, without generally monitoring the caloric numbers, we can't expect to manage our weight.

3. Obsession over fats and carbs

For a generation, we were taught that eating fat made us fat. We bought books and gimmicks to help us count fat grams in out diets. We spent billions on low-fat and no-fat food products. We even bought potato chips made with an indigestible fat substitute, despite the disclaimer on the package that the product might cause "anal leakage."

Then we learned that dietary fat was really our friend and that we needed to cut all possible carbohydrates from our diet. We stopped stuffing our faces with low-fat cookies and swilling no-fat, all-sugar beverages. And we stopped eating stuff we really need, like fruits and vegetables and whole grains.

The diet industry was wrong about that, too.

The USDA study to which I referred a few paragraphs ago[672] also found that "weight-loss is independent of macronutrient composition of the diet." This means that those popular books that prescribe very specific percentages of fat, carbohydrates, and protein are completely wrong. The study's author, E.M. Kennedy, and her group found that *the most obese people were on low-carbohydrate diets*. Diets moderate in fats and higher in carbohydrates were associated most consistently with weight loss, and the participants consumed fewer calories overall. None of these extremely prescriptive diets has the metabolic advantage that it claims.

A recent study comparing the most popular fad diets revealed that there was very little difference in weight loss between one diet and another.[673] This may surprise those of you who have in fact lost weight on one of these diets. But there are reasons why they fail in the long run for most people, which I'll discuss later. Suffice it to say that short-term weight loss is different from permanent weight loss.

We need to stop worrying about the ratios of fats, proteins, and carbohydrates. Instead, we must learn to eat the *right* fats, proteins, and carbohydrates.

Ratios do have some meaning—I'll supply you with reasonable ranges later on. However, the *types* of fats, carbohydrates, and proteins are far more important. For instance, there are good and bad carbohydrates. On the bad side are simple sugars, processed sugars, high-fructose corn syrup, and others. Some carb-rich foods that are good for you are those vegetables and whole grains with low glycemic indexes. Basically, glycemic index is the degree to which a gram of carbohydrate in food increases the level of sugar in the blood. (See Appendix C for the full explanation of glycemic index and load.)

It's time to stop our cultural "carbophobia." There are good and bad fats, good and bad proteins, and good and bad carbohydrates. The best research shows that we probably should be taking in more protein than we normally do, but that, too, is something I'll explain later.

4. Lack of exercise

Not all change is progress.

It is estimated that changes in technology have shaved about 700 calories off our daily calorie burn in the last fifty years. That means you now have to spend about an hour a day in the gym to burn the calories your grandparents burned in their normal lives.

Or maybe not. What in fact was different about life in the 1950s?

With technological advances, physical labor keeps getting engineered out of our lives.[674] Modern airports worldwide have moving walkways and golf-cart courtesy vehicles. We don't carry our bags or briefcases anymore, because they have wheels. We drive instead of riding bicycles or walking. We sit for long hours at computers or desks and e-mail our colleagues down the hall or upstairs. We call our neighbors instead of walking down the street and knocking on their door.

The same is true for our children. We live in subdivisions bounded by highways, so they seldom walk or ride bikes any distance. We drive them to soccer, baseball, or softball games where they might spend a good deal of time on the bench before going home to their computer games. Modern conveniences mean they have fewer household chores. Schools have reduced or eliminated physical education programs; daily participation among high school students in the U.S. declined from 42 percent in 1991 to 25 percent in 1995.[675] Electronic games and media players hold children rapt, glassy-eyed, and motionless for many hours that former generations spent in physically active play.

I know what you're thinking: Dr. Duke is about to start yapping about the "exercise of daily living" again. Yes, I am.

Health clubs are great. But with or without them, *we don't move our bodies enough*. Most of us would find it far easier to control our weight if we added more movement to our daily routines. Take the stairs instead of an escalator or elevator. Buy a lawnmower that doesn't have a seat and push it yourself. Park farther away from stores. Replace a half hour a day of television with a leisurely stroll. Spend time with your family outdoors rather than glued to the tube. Buy your kids computer games that involve moving their whole bodies, rather than just their thumbs. (There are some very cool ones that you can enjoy, too.) These things take little of your time, but add up to hundreds of calories a day.

5. Narrow focus

Another problem with the way we approach weight management is that we tend to focus on a single remedy. It's no wonder why. It's hard to make money marketing a whole-lifestyle change. So weight-loss profiteers sell us what's easy to sell.

A health club membership. An exercise gimmick. A diet food. A diet menu. A pill. And we buy these things because we want a magic bullet—a simple, easy way to melt off those pounds. However, it should be obvious there is no simple, single-focus miracle cure. If there were, the inventor would be richer than Bill Gates, and we would all have healthy body types.

But here's the truth. You can't shed excess fat by changing only one aspect of your life. **To manage your weight successfully, healthily, and for life, you have to change your lifestyle.**

I can think of only one for-profit industry that really understands this concept. I qualify for a low preferred rate on my life insurance because I changed my whole lifestyle. Insurance companies make money literally by betting on whether you're going to die prematurely. Actuaries are the handicappers of the insurance industry; they are paid big salaries to set the odds accurately. If I get a super-low rate, that's because they have to give me very good odds to get my bet, in the form of insurance premiums.

You know by now how I feel about exercise. I have cited many studies touting its profound benefits. If exercise is the only change you make in your life, you'll be better off. But even the most extreme exercise regimen will not alone lead to optimal health. Remember the story of Jim Fixx? Being a dedicated marathon runner couldn't save him from his other risk factors.

You may have already discovered for yourself that exercise alone won't get you to a healthy weight and enable you to stay there. It isn't just you. The National Weight Registry is a University of Pittsburgh study that follows people who have lost a significant amount of weight and kept it off for more than five years. The data[676] show that 90 percent of long-term weight maintainers share three characteristics:

- they get 20 to 30 percent of their calories from fat
- they restrict total calorie intake
- they participate in regular physical activity

According to a study from the former acting Undersecretary of the USDA,[677] only 9 percent of people in the National Weight Registry were able to maintain weight loss by diet alone, and only 1 percent maintained weight by regular exercise alone. Optimal health is total lifestyle management, and not single-issue management.

6. The TV, the PC, and the WWW

Next time you pick up the remote control, take a moment to consider which end of that transaction is really running the show—you or the TV.

For far too many of us, television controls our free time. Over the last fifty years, many technological advancements have reduced the labor we perform daily, but none has contributed more to obesity rates worldwide than television. (Although I have to think that the personal computer and electronic gaming are gaining.) A great deal of scientific research supports that statement.

In a 1997 survey, the average adult American male spent twenty-nine hours per week watching TV, the adult female thirty-four hours per week.[678] Over the last several decades, the rise of obesity has paralleled the increase in the number of homes with multiple TVs, as well as the hours spent watching TV.[679] Many other studies have linked obesity with television viewing time in both adults[680, 681, 682] and children.[683, 684] A study involving children in Mexico City showed that the percentage of obese children increased 12 percent for each hour per day of television viewing.[685]

Television viewing contributes to the obesity epidemic in several ways.

First, watching TV seems to lower one's metabolic rate more than other sedentary activities such as sewing, playing board games, reading, and writing.[686] One study concluded, "TV watching has the highest risk for obesity and diabetes among the several sedentary behaviors."[687] The authors estimated that 30 percent of obesity cases and 43 percent of type 2 diabetes could be prevented by reducing TV watching to less than ten hours per week and using some of that time to walk briskly thirty minutes per day. They found that each two-hour increment of television watching per day increased the risk of obesity by 23 percent and diabetes by 14 percent.

Second, TV watching replaces physical activity for many people.[688]

Third, most people tend to eat while watching TV, which leads to significant imbalances in energy intake versus energy use.[689]

Fourth, food marketers know a golden opportunity when they see it. The foods we eat while watching TV are a reflection of the unhealthful foods advertised on the TV itself.[690, 691] British and U.S. children see approximately ten food commercials per hour of television viewing time, and these are mainly for sugar-sweetened cereals, soft drinks, fast food, and similar products.[692, 693] Moreover, TV viewing during mealtime was inversely associated with consumption of healthy foods, such as fruits and vegetables, that weren't advertised.[694]

In light of the nauseating statistics linking obesity and chronic disease to television viewing, you'd think that millions of people would want to increase their metabolic rates by carrying their television sets out to the dumpster. The hours we spend watching TV may be hurting us more than air pollution. Unfortunately, the research has not affected our behaviors. Many people around the world show greater loyalty to their televisions than they do to their religions.

I don't really want you to carry your television set out to the curb for trash pick-up—if you're out of shape from TV watching, you might hurt yourself. But scientific research shows that restricting our viewing time—in favor of almost any other activities, even sedentary ones—is an obvious step to take.

Why do we have such devotion to television? Please don't tell me it's a good way to spend time together as a family. Just because you're all in the same room doesn't mean you're spending time "together"! Playing a board game, a card game, a lawn game, or taking a family walk constitutes togetherness. Watching TV is a solitary activity, whether or not other people are in the room.

So why are we addicted to television—and more recently electronic gaming and Internet surfing? I think it has to do with escape from the daily pressures and stresses of our modern world. By tuning in the television, we tune everything else out. Which leads us to...

7. Coping with stress by eating

Everybody everywhere lives with stress. In poor and developing nations, stress often has to do with daily struggles for survival. We who live in developed nations seldom worry about hunger, thirst, acute disease, or violence, and yet we live with more stress than we want to admit.

Technology allows the average person to do work that required several people just a few years ago. It also makes it impossible for many of us to leave our jobs at the office at 5 p.m. Cell phones, e-mail, and text messaging make us accessible twenty-four hours a day almost anywhere in the world. "Downsizing" and "lean" business strategies leave us working nights and weekends, often just to keep up with the communications we didn't have time for during the regular business day. With changing technology, population growth, global economic pressures, and international conflicts, stress levels are high everywhere in the world.

At our institute, we have an unusual view of the global extent of the problem. We see stress in our clients from India, Thailand, Malaysia, Indonesia, China, Japan, Brazil, Mexico, Australia, Europe, the U.S., and elsewhere. The impact has been so great that we found it imperative to develop a stress-reduction program. It has been very effective for thousands of people.

With stress levels high and rising, it is natural that most of us are looking for release or escape. Unfortunately, many of us choose escape routes that damage our health. The "smoke break" at work was once commonplace; now laws and building rules leave smokers wrought up in withdrawal. (That's far better than actually smoking, but it doesn't relieve stress.) Some of us cope with stress by using alcohol or drugs. Alcohol is a major source of "empty" (nutrition-free) calories, and both can become major sources of human misery.

One popular way of dealing with stress is through the pleasure of eating. We learn at an early age to cheer ourselves up by eating something tasty. (Grandma: "I'm so sorry you got your feelings hurt. Here, have a nice piece of pie.") Snack foods are always close at hand, and we can enjoy a tasty treat without slowing down the pace of our work.

The problem is that using snack food for stress relief makes us fat. So it is very important to understand the difference between eating for nutrition when we are hungry and eating for pleasure when we are stressed. That difference is both physiological and psychological.

The urge to eat arises from several sources. Eating can be a release from anxiety. It can supply immediate gratification of our desire for pleasure rather than of hunger pangs. ("Chocoholics" take note: There are components in chocolate that affect the nervous system; it stimulates pleasurable feelings in general, not just on your tongue.) Further, stress can make you think you're hungry when you aren't. Stress often increases the secretion of stomach acid, and the subsequent discomfort is easy to interpret as hunger pangs.

Also, anxiety and depression often go hand in hand. One of the criteria for diagnosing depression is change in eating habits. It's not surprising that depressed adults and adolescents have nearly twice the risk of developing obesity.[695]

When overeating is a response to stress, we need to either reduce the stress or change the response—or both.

If you have trouble handling the stress in your life, seek professional or religious counseling, and read my chapter on stress. If you have persistent hunger pangs, talk to your doctor about whether these could be related to stomach acid; medication might be in order. I've seen many of my patients lose weight after they realized the difference between hunger pangs and excessive gastric acid secretion.

Finally, explore healthy ways of dealing with stress. A brisk half-hour walk during your lunch break or right after work can do wonders. It gives you a little time to withdraw and reflect and put things in perspective. Also, exercise releases endorphins, which make you feel good. That brisk walk is a lot like having a chocolate bar or a beer, except that it's good for your health and your waistline, not bad.

8. Snack foods

This is a completely separate issue from stress-induced eating. It has to do with the massive amounts of processed snack foods and sugar-sweetened drinks we consume.

There's nothing wrong with snacking, as long as you eat nutritious, natural (preferably organic), unprocessed food. You can eat lots of fruit and vegetables, because many such foods are very filling but not dense in calories. A small candy bar generally has more calories than a whole plate of nutritious vegetables. And a handful of those vegetables will keep you feeling full until your next meal, while you'll likely be hungry again soon after you eat the candy bar.

But it isn't just the calories. I wish it were! There are many other physiological and biochemical reasons why processed snack foods are harmful. Virtually all processed snacks and sweetened drinks have chemicals that harmfully affect hormone secretion and even DNA expression. Unfortunately, this problem is economic. Processed snack foods are a worldwide multibillion-dollar industry. Competition encourages manufacturers to hold down their prices by using inexpensive but unhealthy chemicals and modified oils. However, a tremendous amount of research now shows these additives make significant contributions to chronic disease.

Corn oil is a conspicuous example. (I'm referring here to what we call corn in North America, i.e., maize.) Prior to 1950, corn oil was not commonly used for cooking or in mass-produced foods. Our ancestors never used corn oil because it was too difficult to produce in substantial amounts. It's hard to squeeze the oil out of corn.

Then came industrial technology. Hydraulic presses, heat extraction, and new solvents made corn an inexpensive source of cooking oil. Hydrogen ions are usually added to corn oil to change its texture and increase its shelf life. This process creates trans fats, which have been shown to increase heart disease,[696] type 2 diabetes,[697] and other chronic diseases.

And yet, if you read ingredients label of the great majority of manufactured foods, you'll find that they contain "partially hydrogenated" corn oil or soybean oil. Fortunately, new laws in the U.S. and around the world require that manufacturers list the amount of trans fats on their labels, so the use of trans fat is beginning to decline.

The problem with many processed foods is not that they contain oil, but that they contain the cheapest, most dangerous kinds of oil. When you are cooking at home, the choice of what oils to use is easy. Unprocessed canola or extra-virgin olive oils cost more but provide great, protective health benefits. But when it comes to mass-produced, processed foods, the cost of these oils is prohibitive, or so the manufacturers tell us.

Processed foods, especially snack foods, also contain simple sugars. They are referred to as high-glycemic-index carbohydrates, because eating them induces a rapid rise in the level of the sugar glucose in our blood. These foods tend to stimulate hunger, rather than satiate it, which results in overeating.[698, 699] Carbohydrates with high glycemic indexes have been associated with heart disease,[700] diabetes,[701] chronic disease risk,[702] and inflammation.[703]

In Appendix C you'll get a reference for where you can find the glycemic indexes and load values of a fairly comprehensive list of foods. Please review it carefully for carbohydrates only. Weight management and optimal health require that you reduce your intake of high-glycemic foods. Appendix C carefully explains why I recommend low-glycemic-index and load carbohydrates but don't recommend a completely low-glycemic-index diet or menu.

Another bad component of processed foods is high-fructose corn syrup (HFCS). High-fructose corn sweeteners were introduced into the food industry around 1970, exactly the same time that obesity began to rise dramatically in the U.S.[704] Almost every sweetened drink contains high-fructose corn syrup, even those whose labels tout them as health elixirs. HFCS increases insulin resistance, inflammation, triglycerides, obesity, and the harmful LDL cholesterol.[705, 706, 707]

Sugar-sweetened drinks are probably the greatest source of "empty calories"—excess calories unaccompanied by nutritional value. You might as well eat white sugar by the spoonful and wash it down with water. At least you'd avoid the excess sodium and phosphorus in most junk foods.

According to the USDA, soft drink consumption has increased almost 500 percent in the past fifty years.[708] More than half of all Americans and most adolescents (74 percent of boys and 65 percent of girls) consume soft drinks daily,[709] of which most are sugar-sweetened.[710] Soft drinks are the leading source of added sugars to the diet.[711, 712] All sugar-sweetened drinks (not just soft drinks) increase the risk of obesity. One study monitored the consumption of sugar-sweetened drinks by 548 ethnically diverse schoolchildren for nineteen months. The researchers found that the risk of obesity increased 160 percent for every additional can of sugar-sweetened drink they drank per day; children in this study who drank artificially sweetened soft drinks did *not* gain excess weight. But even diet soft drinks increase the risk of metabolic syndrome (see chapter 12), and diabetes.[713, 714]

One reason sugar-sweetened drinks are like instant fat is that they don't satiate hunger as well as solid food does. Most people who snack on solid food compensate by eating less at subsequent meals.[715] But it's easy to consume hundreds of empty calories a day in liquid form without satisfying your hunger at all. This is a major reason why many obese people around the world are overfed but still undernourished. Interestingly, preschool children who consumed excess calories in liquid form compensated well at the next meal by eating less,[716] but by age nine or ten, children seem to lose this ability.[717]

How about artificial sweeteners?

A ten-week study[718] that provided either sucrose (sugar) or artificial sweeteners to overweight people as they desired found that those who consumed large amounts of sucrose had increased calorie intake, body weight, fat mass, and blood pressure. These effects were not noted in the group that consumed artificial sweeteners. Overall, sweeteners that contain calories, such as high-fructose corn syrup or sucrose, should be avoided as much as possible. (See Appendix B.1 for ingredients to avoid.)

For many people, switching to diet sodas will slash hundreds of calories from their daily intake, resulting in significant weight loss. Artificial sweeteners *are* processed foods, so your use of them should be moderate. But if sweetness is your thing, artificial sweeteners are worlds better than sugar. (Though artificial sweeteners have been shown in some studies to possibly stimulate appetite,[719, 720, 721] other studies have not shown this effect.[722, 723] However, the former tended to be short-term studies, which is probably not as reflective of how such sweeteners will affect weight long-term.)

Some of the bad stuff in processed foods has received little media attention. Many processed foods, including cheese, contain substances derived from food proteins that stimulate the opioid (pleasure) receptors in the brain. They have names like alpha-, beta- or kappa casein, casomorphin and beta-lactoglobulin, and lactotransferrin.[724] Studies, mainly on animals, show that these substances can stimulate the immune system,[725] which may affect inflammation, increase the desire to eat more fat,[726] and increase insulin release after a meal.[727] Obviously, there is potential harm just from these substances alone.

While that last item may seem a bit obscure, there is no shortage of well-publicized scientific information about the problems with snack foods. And yet not enough people are listening.

So please listen to this.

A recent study shows that the average person gets nearly one-third of his or her calories from "junk food"—that is, from food that is high in calories and low in other nutritional value. Though this study was done in the U.S.,[728] utilizing national surveys,[729, 730] the trend of eating foods with higher calories and lower nutrition is increasing around the world. The prevalence of snacking in children rose from 77 percent in 1977 to 91 percent in 1996.[731] Teenagers drink 40 percent less milk today than their counterparts did in the 1960s, and they have nearly tripled their intake of sweetened juice and soft drinks.[732]

One of the insidious things about snack foods is that they are generally high in sugar or other carbohydrates but low in fiber, which means they don't satisfy hunger, especially since they are often eaten as treats when you aren't hungry in the first place. So you wolf down a lot of calories without feeling full, and are soon hungry again.[733]

With sweets, desserts, salty snacks, alcoholic beverages, soft drinks, and fruit-flavored drinks providing up to one-third of our calories, is it really any wonder that there is a growing worldwide epidemic of obesity? Many pop diets provide special, complex formulas that are next to impossible to follow. And yet the most important, effective thing we can do is simply to replace junk-food snacks with healthier alternatives. And I'm not talking about total abstinence. If I asked to eliminate all "treats," you'd ignore me, and I'd be a hypocrite. But many of us can make a huge difference by switching *most* of our between-meal intake from unhealthy, sugary, high-calorie, processed snacks to healthy ones.

9. Feeding our emotions

We often live in denial about why we eat. Many of us have developed psychological needs concerning food that exceed our biological needs.

Eating is one of life's great pleasures. You're supposed to enjoy it. And, as with other worldly pleasures, it's common to reward, comfort, or console ourselves with food. That's understandable, but it can also get out of control.

This pattern is often ingrained in childhood. Your parents promised you a burger and a milkshake after a trip to the doctor. Your mom gave you a piece of cake or some ice cream when you finished your chores. You didn't make the cheerleading squad? Let's bake some brownies. Feeding our fears and sorrows can become a deep-seated aspect of one's psychology, and our relationship with food can become complex and damaging.

The other side of that coin is parents forcing children to clean their plates at every meal. Making your child feel guilty for not finishing his or her meal is wrong. A child's stomach will tell him or her when it's had enough. Yes, it is terrible to think that children in some parts of the world are starving. But that's not a good reason to push your child toward obesity! I know many overweight adults who still feel they must eat all the food on their plate, even if they are full. They were brought up to think it is wrong to waste food.

So please understand this: Children are not garbage disposals. Once they've had enough to eat, the remaining food on their plates isn't "wasted." You can save it or throw it out. Children need balanced diets, and I think it's fine to ask them to try a little of each item on their plates. But forcing them to always eat it *all* can shape their psychological relationships with food in ways that will harm them for the rest of their lives.

Our psychological associations with food can become so strong that we are very reluctant to give them up. One study provides a good example of what I mean. Obese men were requested to record their food intake, though they were not asked to restrict eating. The men began eating 26 percent fewer calories than prior to the study, but they still under-recorded the foods they were eating by 12 percent. They knew how they should eat, but lied about what they did eat.[734]

If your psychological or emotional relationship to food is making you physically ill, you need to face that issue honestly. Don't feel hesitant about getting professional or religious counseling.

10. Quitting on your new lifestyle

This game plan for optimal health won't work if the players give up. And what makes me sad is that often people get discouraged and give up for the wrong reasons.

Here's the scenario. You start eating well and getting some kind of exercise every day. You lose a few pounds. Then you stop losing weight.

And then you give up. If you're not losing any more weight anyway, why deprive yourself of corn chips and television reruns?

Here's what nobody explained to you. When you took up exercise, your body started to build muscle to handle the increased work. Bodies do that. Muscle weighs more than fat. That's why many would-be weight-losers hit a plateau—their muscle gain has offset their fat loss. And that's good. As muscle mass increases, the body's metabolic rate increases, too, and that helps you lose more weight faster. Stay with it and you *will* begin to lose weight again, as the increase in your muscle mass levels off.

I'll say it again. This game plan isn't about losing weight. It's about losing fat. Work the whole plan and you *will* lose weight (assuming you needed to in the first place). Just don't be discouraged if your fat loss is temporarily offset by muscle gain. This phenomenon has discouraged millions who gave up too soon.

THE EASY WAY ISN'T

Many people who get discouraged too soon with their healthy diet and exercise plans look to pills as an "easier" way. Many of those people get sick. Some die. The Phen-Fen fad was hugely popular, and too many people stayed with it even after it became well known to increase the risk of heart valve abnormalities. Brazilian diet pills have been found to contain substances that are either prescription medications or controlled substances in the U.S.[735] Heart problems and drug abuse don't fit into any sane concept of optimal health.

11. Restaurant food, both fast and slow

At work, at school, in city centers, at shopping malls, in airports and ground transportation terminals, even traveling by car on country highways, we are seldom more than a few minutes from food, quickly and easily obtainable. We're surrounded by vending machines, street vendors, convenience stores, and every kind of restaurant.

That food is almost literally at arm's reach everywhere we go is both a blessing and a curse in modern society. It's a blessing compared to the way some of our ancestors had to live, and the way a billion or more malnourished people around the world live today. And it's a curse for those of us in the developed world, because so much of that fast food is bad food.

Fast foods are generally high in the harmful food components and additives I've discussed throughout this book, including saturated or trans fats, high glycemic index, high energy density with low nutritional value, low fiber, high-fructose corn syrup, sucrose, and the rest. The growth in fast food outlets throughout the world corresponds to the rise in obesity rates, especially among children.

Here are some research statistics.

Adolescent girls who eat fast food four times a week consumed about 260 calories more per day than those who didn't.[736] Not only do children eat in restaurants more than ever, they eat more per meal when they eat out than when they eat at home.[737] On an average day in the United States, nearly half of adults eat at a restaurant and 21 percent of households use some form of takeout or delivery.[738]

Since both husbands and wives now work outside the home in 60 to 70 percent of households in industrialized nations, it's understandable that reliance on fast food and other restaurants has increased over the last thirty years. Single parents are squeezed for time even more. But here's the good news:

It is possible to eat out and eat well. Even at fast food restaurants.

Our family chooses restaurants, fast food and otherwise, that offer salad bars or sandwiches. That way we can control what goes onto our plates. My wife and I guide our children by letting them choose one of three healthy meals on the menu. We have taught our children the importance of healthy eating, and they now choose the healthier meals on their own without guidance (or nagging, threatening, or cajoling) from us. Believe it or not, we don't have battles over food choices.

Planning ahead just a little is another good way to optimize both time and diet. For example, you can make fruit salads or healthy casseroles on the weekend and portion them out during the week.

Fast food franchises and many other restaurants commonly use the cheapest ingredients in order to keep their prices competitive. Unfortunately, the cheapest ingredients—like lard and corn oil—are usually the unhealthiest.

Fast food marketing is part of the problem, too. It's tempting to spend just a few cents more to get the giant-size French fries and soft drink. Who doesn't want to get more for their money? The question, though, is more of what. When it's more sugar, more starch, and more trans fat, the nutritional value is less, not more.

Value increases when we spend our money on good nutrition, and on foods that are high in vitamins, minerals, phytonutrients, fiber, and protein. Those last two items especially help us feel full and satisfied while meeting our needs for nutrients and calories. Fast foods are typically low in fiber and protein, so we have to eat more of this high-calorie junk to satisfy our hunger pangs.

And finally, there are two reasons we call it "fast" food. Not only is it served up in a hurry, but as time-stressed people we tend to eat it in a hurry. We don't allow time for our body's feedback mechanisms to tell us to stop eating.

High-fiber diets are associated with better weight control. All fast food chains now provide brochures that explain the components of their meals offered. So take control. Read the brochures, and make better choices. The last chapter of this book also provides guidelines help you choose wisely. You *can* buy meals at restaurants and take-out places that accommodate your busy schedule and satisfy your appetite and palate without gorging on calories or skimping on healthy nutrition. All you have to do is make informed, healthful decisions rather than caving in and buying today's special.

Order food on *your* terms. The fast food industry has proven over the last fifty years that your good health is not their primary goal.

When one of my daughters was nine years old, she saw a news program that investigated the McDonald's process for deciding which new foods to offer. When the McDonald's executive was unable to respond to a reporter's question concerning the fact that children's health had not been not a major factor in developing new products, my daughter turned to me and said, "Daddy, I don't ever want to eat at McDonald's again."

She has held strongly to that position ever since. Fortunately, McDonald's is offering some slightly healthier foods today, but the whole fast food industry needs to do far better. An article in the *New England Journal of Medicine*[739] reported that the French fries McDonald's sells in the U.S. contain far more trans fats—23 percent of total fat, or 10.2 grams—than the fries they sell in most other countries. For example, in the fries they sell in Denmark, trans fat is only 1 percent of total fat.

This is shocking in light of the fact that just 5 grams of trans fats per day can increase the risk of heart disease by 25 percent. Fortunately, in September 2002, McDonald's promised to cut their use of trans fats in half.

The fast food industry is not unlike the tobacco industry, which denied for years that cigarettes were addicting and unhealthful. Historically, these companies have made billions at the expense of the health of children. I hope some will have the courage to improve nutritional value, even at the risk of affecting their profits.

But in the end, we can all change what the fast food companies do by making healthy choices about where we eat and what we order. The one thing you can count on is that these companies will react to the demands of the market.

12. Genetic predisposition

Genetics can also play a role in obesity. Leptin, a hormone secreted by fat cells, sends a signal to the brain to curb appetite. Obese people are not as sensitive to leptin. The cause of this tendency could be environmental, but it can also be genetic in origin.

The dreaded "sweet tooth"—an unusual craving for sweets—may have a genetic basis. Sucrose (the chemical name for table sugar) stimulates a release of endorphins, which are chemicals in the brain that reduce pain and provide a general good feeling. Sucrose has even been shown in studies to relieve pain in newborns.[740] We taste sweetness in varying degrees from one person to the next. This variation is genetic in origin; the location of one responsible gene has recently been discovered.[741]

Scientists suspect that there are many other ways in which we are genetically predisposed to obesity, but no one really knows how these factors contribute to the obesity epidemic. This is an exciting new field of study that may someday yield advances in the treatment of obesity. However, genetic predisposition is unlikely to be a major cause of the ballooning growth in obesity rates. Genetic change in humans takes place very slowly, over many thousands of years. The obesity epidemic has arisen in the last thirty. Human behavior is the problem. It's a matter of economics and lifestyle choices.

But what about individuals who are dealing with their own genetic heritage?

Our genes are expressed through a combination of genetics and environment or personal history. It's obvious that our environment and lifestyles have changed recently. That is why the greatest emphasis in this book is placed upon changing our lifestyle.

13. Lack of adequate sleep

As noted in chapter 6, the importance of adequate sleep shouldn't be underestimated. Among the many benefits of getting seven to eight hours of sleep a night is weight loss. Inadequate sleep is a risk factor for obesity.[742] I have had obese patients with sleep disorders (like sleep apnea) who were put on breathing machines to help them sleep better, and they began losing weight. I have had some absolutely swear that they didn't change anything else in their life and they just began to lose weight when their sleep improved.

This list of thirteen risk factors for obesity is not comprehensive. There are others. However, the list does cover the major factors—the ones that account for nearly all of the global imbalance between the energy we take in via food and drink and the energy we burn.

Most important, this list gives you a clear understanding of why virtually all other weight-loss diets are unsuccessful in the long haul. They typically focus on just one issue, like "low-carb" or "low-fat," while neglecting overall lifestyle.

A game-plan analogy: Suppose you are the owner of a really bad soccer team. You're trying to hire a new manager to turn things around. One applicant for the job says he can make your team a winner by greatly improving the technique of your goalkeeper. The guy is a wizard goal-

FIGURE 11.4

Reduction in Mortality Rates Due to Various Causes With Weight Loss

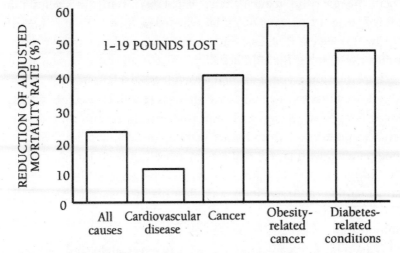

Source: Williamson DF, et al. Am J Epidemiol. 1995; 141: 1128–1141

keeper coach. Everybody says so. Are you going to hire him? No, you're not. You can't turn around the fortunes of your side by improving play at only one position. You send eleven players out onto a soccer pitch. You need the best players at each position. They all need to be fit. The necessary skills vary from one position to the next, so you need a strategy that optimizes your team's strengths and compensates for its weaknesses. You need a game plan that can be adapted to each new opponent.

And there's the good news. I realize this long chapter has painted a pretty grim picture. But the last word is that many of the consequences are reversible. There is great hope for reversing this epidemic if we are willing to change. There is great hope for reversing your risk factors if you are willing to change.

All you need is to be part of a revolution that you can adopt, step by step.

Letting the Air Out of the Balloon

It's true. Many of the adverse health effects of obesity are reversible.

One study showed that weight loss of any amount from one to nineteen pounds was associated with a 20 percent reduction in the mortality rate from all causes[743] (see Figure 4).

Another notable study associates fat loss with decreased death rate.[744] Diabetic people who reduce their weight by twenty to twenty-nine pounds (10 to 15 percent of initial weight) reduce their risk of early death by 33 percent.[745] A sustained moderate weight loss (10 percent) significantly reduces the number of years that an obese person would have hypertension, type 2 diabetes, or elevated cholesterol.[746, 747] One study showed that the same lifestyle changes that decreased obesity also reduced C-reactive protein and improved insulin sensitivity.[748] Positive lifestyle changes also reduced other markers of inflammation.[749] Survival among patients with type 2 diabetes increased three to four months for each kilogram of weight lost.[750] According to the American Gastroenterological Association, a modest planned weight loss of 5 percent can improve many of the medical conditions related to obesity.[751] Weight loss also decreases hypertension.[752]

This is great news for anybody who is overweight and frustrated with attempts to lose fat. It's not too late to do something to improve your health. Any step you take toward optimal health will help.

And if you are obese, please remember this: You didn't get that way overnight and neither will you lose your excess fat overnight. As a population we have become increasingly obese because of lifestyle changes. Lifestyle changes are the only healthy way to lose fat and keep from regaining it. There are many changes we need to make. But we can make them one at a time, and they all reap benefits. The size and shape of your body may change slowly, but the changes will be long-lasting.

This book outlines those changes for you. Start making them, and you'll be walking briskly down the road to optimal health.

Understanding the global epidemic of diabetes is also critical. It's another area where you need to be protected from fads, take action to avoid devastating chronic diseases, and know which lifestyle changes to make.

And that's the next chapter.

CHAPTER 12

Sweet and Lethal—
The Worldwide Epidemic
of Insulin Resistance
and Type 2 Diabetes

E verybody's job has its good and bad points, but the job of a food
taster in the royal courts of yore was special in its extremes. The
good side was that you got to dine in the best company and sample
the finest fare in whatever realm your liege was lord of—not to mention
being the first one served. The downside was that if somebody tried to
kill the sovereign by poisoning his meat, meal, or mead, *you* were the
one who shuffled off this mortal coil on his behalf. That was the catch
in the job description, along with the lack of a retirement plan.

Most of the dangerous food we eat today is not fast-acting enough for
a food taster to be of any use, which is unfortunate for everyone but food
tasters. But bad diet is one of the key risk factors for two closely related
diseases that are growing exponentially in the modernized world.

Diabetes and insulin resistance are diseases that involve elevated
sugar levels in the blood. That might sound sweet, but in fact these disorders are associated with increased risk of death. And the bitter truth is
that these diseases are increasing rapidly all over the world.

Diabetes is a chronic disease caused by an inherited or acquired deficiency in the amount of insulin the body produces. In type 1 diabetes,

the body fails to produce insulin. With type 2, the body is unable to respond properly to the insulin it does produce.[753]

According to the World Health Organization, a worldwide epidemic of type 2 diabetes has arisen in the last two decades. The human and financial costs of this epidemic are staggering, so it is critical that every person in every industrialized nation understand these diseases.

What caused this epidemic? It's a matter of changing lifestyles. And of course, that means the epidemic is reversible, just like the obesity epidemic. In fact, these two phenomena are closely related.

According to the World Health Organization's Noncommunicable Disease Prevention Fact Sheet on Diabetes,[754] at least 180 million people worldwide currently suffer from diabetes; that figure is likely to be 360 million by 2030. Worldwide, around 4 million deaths every year are directly attributable to complications from diabetes. The top ten countries in cases of diabetes are India, China, United States, Indonesia, Russia, Japan, Bangladesh, Pakistan, Brazil, and Italy.[755] According to the World Health Organization, India is home to about one-fourth of the world's diabetics.[756]

The epidemic has grown rapidly. In 1985 an estimated 30 million people worldwide had diabetes. As of 2008, the estimated number of people globally with type 2 diabetes is 180 million, and the disease accounts for 90 percent of all cases of diabetes around the world.

In industrialized nations, about half of diabetes sufferers die of cardiovascular disease, but diabetes is responsible for other disorders, too. It damages blood vessels throughout the body, both large vessels (macrovascular damage) and small (microvascular damage). Diabetic neuropathy (nerve damage) is probably the most common complication, with 50 percent of diabetics affected to some degree. Neuropathy can lead to sensory loss, damage to the autonomic nervous system (which controls functions like breathing, digestion, and heart rate) and is the major source of impotence in diabetic men. Diabetic retinopathy, or damage to the eye's retina, is a leading cause of blindness. Diabetes is also among the leading causes of kidney failure, and is the most common cause of nontraumatic amputation of the lower limbs.

In the eastern Mediterranean, diabetes is the fourth leading cause of death, afflicting 17 million of the region's 220 million people. The prevalence of diabetes ranges from 7 to 25 percent of the adult population.

The epidemic of type 2 diabetes is as bad in the United States as the rest of the developed world, affecting 6.3 percent of the U.S. population, or roughly 19 million people. And those numbers are based on *diagnosed* cases. It is believed that as many as 5 million Americans have diabetes and don't know it. These people are at increased risk of severe complications, including blindness, amputations, and death, because they aren't getting treatment for their disease. According to the American Diabetes Association, of those who receive treatment for diabetes, 63 percent are not receiving care that corresponds with the American Diabetic Association standards.[757] The American College of Endocrinology has recently recommended lowering the HbA1c (a test to monitor long-term control of diabetes), which indicates that that medical society believes there are even more Americans who should be getting treatment but are not.

While type 2 diabetes was once thought of as an adult disease, the epidemic now widely afflicts children, too. According to one study,[758] "Among…Japanese schoolchildren, type 2 diabetes has increased more than thirty-fold in the past 20 years." In the United States nearly 20 percent of all newly diagnosed type 2 diabetes is in children between the ages of nine and nineteen. According to the International Diabetes Federation,[759] one in three Americans born today will develop type 2 diabetes as a consequence of overweight and obesity.

The financial costs of diabetes are staggering. It is estimated that the direct and indirect costs attributable to diabetes for 2002 in the U.S. alone totaled $132 billion, with hospitalization and treatment of complications making significant contributions to the national bill. Direct medical expenses were $92 billion, and indirect expenses—such as lost workdays, restricted activity days, and disability—totaled $40 billion. Per capita medical expenses were $13,243 for individuals with diabetes, compared to $2,500 for people without the disease—more than five times as high.[760]

But here's the good news: **The worldwide diabetes epidemic can be slowed down and even reversed.** According to the World Health Organization's diabetes report mentioned earlier, "Large population base studies in China, Canada, USA, and several European countries suggested [that] even moderate reduction in weight and a half an hour of walk-ing each day reduces the incidence of diabetes by more than half in over-weight subjects with mildly impaired glucose tolerance." One of these studies was from the *New England Journal of Medicine*.[761] This study ran-domly assigned 522 middle-aged, overweight people with impaired glu-cose tolerance to either an intervention group or a control group. Each subject in the intervention group received individual counseling about reducing his or her weight, reducing total intake of fat and of saturated fat, and increasing fiber intake and physical activity. These people were followed for 3.2 years, and the study concluded, "during the trial, the risk of diabetes was reduced by 58 percent in the intervention group. The reduction in incidence of diabetes was directly associated with changes in lifestyle."

This is another example of why the best way to improve your health, reduce weight, and reduce the risk of heart disease, cancer, and diabetes is through **lifestyle change**—not through quick fixes, gimmicks, "mira-cle" products or diets alone. We have always taught this and always will. Fad diets and single-focus weight-loss programs don't work in the long run, and they may even *increase* your risk of other chronic diseases.

The Optimal Health Revolution is not a fad or a quick fix. I want to protect you from fads and quick fixes.

Our best chance for slowing this epidemic is to nip type 2 diabetes in the bud—to block it before it gets started. People commonly have some degree of insulin resistance before developing type 2 diabetes—so that is the best time to reverse the progression of the disease.

Insulin is like a key that opens the door to a cell to allow glucose (sugar) to go inside. We used to think that the only problem with type 2 diabetics was that the patient's pancreas wasn't making enough insulin. Now we know that, early in the disease process, the problem is not with production of the insulin "key," but rather the "lock"—the receptor in the cell wall. These receptors become resistant to insulin. This causes the body to sense that not enough glucose is getting into the cells, and it responds by sending an order to the pancreas for more insulin. And having too much insulin your blood is not a good thing.

As noted above, there are many reasons why insulin resistance has increased so rapidly during the last several decades, and they all have to do with changing lifestyles.

Presently, I'll explain what you can do to help reduce the risk of type 2 diabetes for yourself and your family. But first, I want you to understand a little of the science, including the difference between type 1 and type 2 diabetes. I'll make it easy. I think it is vital to understand why you need to make lifestyle changes in order to reduce your chances of getting diabetes.

Type 1 Diabetes

Type 1 is also called *juvenile* diabetes. It is not increasing, because it seems to be mostly congenital.

Type 1 diabetes is a condition in which the pancreas loses its ability to produce insulin, in part or totally. The common cause of type 1 diabetes is that the body's immune system attacks the pancreas with antibodies. Type 1 usually begins when the patient is young—hence the term juvenile—but can also be due to some kind of trauma to the pancreas. The frequency of type 1 diabetes has held steady, and it currently accounts for about 5 to 10 percent of all diabetes.

As noted, the role of insulin is to help sugar get into our body's cells after it has been digested and absorbed into the blood. Whenever we eat a meal, our pancreas releases insulin into the bloodstream so that the cells can use the sugar for energy. If this doesn't happen, the resulting electrolyte imbalances can lead to coma or death.

The signs that sugar levels are rising in the blood are increased thirst and urination, since the body is attempting to get rid of the excess sugar through the kidneys. Since the symptoms of type 1 diabetes are so dramatic and easily diagnosed, it is not normally recommended that people be screened for the disease. The most common treatment is lifelong insulin injections. Newer ways to administer insulin doses are currently being studied and implemented.

Type 2 Diabetes

Type 2 diabetes is a distinctly different disorder from type 1. It used to be referred to as adult-onset diabetes. This name no longer applies because, sadly, we are diagnosing type 2 diabetes in increasing numbers of children. The reason this disease was primarily one of adults is that it is caused by poor lifestyle behaviors, so it is truly alarming that it has become so common in children.

We used to think that type 2 diabetes was basically a delayed form of type 1, so treatment always involved stimulating the pancreas to make more insulin. Now we know the disease is more complicated than that. As I just explained, type 2 diabetes initially raises insulin levels, due to the cells being insulin resistant; insulin production begins to wane later on. We owe much of our understanding of this to the research of Gerald M. Reaven and his colleagues.[762]

Type 2 diabetes is rising dramatically around the world, and it is related to our lifestyle. Its early symptoms can be much subtler than those of type 1. Since there are so many people who don't realize they have the disease (about 5 million in the United States alone), it is important to be checked by your doctor.

So how do you know if you have it? According to the American Diabetes Association, a diagnosis of type 2 diabetes can be made based on any of the following criteria:

1. Plasma glucose while fasting 126 mg/dl or greater.
2. Showing symptoms of diabetes with casual plasma glucose of 200mg/dl or greater.
3. Having plasma glucose of 200 mg/dl during an oral glucose tolerance test.

If your doctor has not checked you for diabetes recently (or if you aren't sure), please make an appointment soon. You could have type 2 diabetes for a long time, and suffer a great deal of permanent damage, without knowing it.

The American Diabetes Association recommends that all individuals forty-five and older be tested for diabetes, especially those who have a BMI over 25. If one's blood sugar tests normal, tests should be repeated every three years. However, *you should be tested more frequently and from an earlier age* if you have the following risk factors:

1. You are overweight—BMI over 25.
2. You have a first-degree relative with diabetes.
3. You are a member of a high-risk ethnic population.

(Examples of such populations in the U.S. are Africans, Hispanics, Native Americans, Asians, and Pacific Islanders.)
4. You have delivered a baby weighing more than nine pounds or have a history of gestational diabetes.
5. Your HDL cholesterol level is 35 mg/dl or less and your triglyceride level is over 250.
6. You have high blood pressure.
7. A test has indicated that you have impaired glucose tolerance.

If you currently have type 2 diabetes, then please carefully follow your doctor's care. But don't stop at that. Even if you already have type 2 diabetes, many of the recommendations listed later in this chapter can still help either to reduce the amount of medication you need or to stop the progression of the disease. In rare cases, people who have been diagnosed with type 2 diabetes have been able to stop medication entirely, but that should only be done under the direction of a doctor. While I hope this book helps some people reduce their need for diabetes medication, my purpose is to work, as it were, *with* your doctor; the last thing I want to do is disrupt your relationship with him or her. Please never stop taking medication without the counsel and guidance of your physician. All I am saying here is that it's not too late to improve your health, even once you're given the diagnosis of type 2 diabetes.

A variety of medications are used to treat type 2 diabetics today.

Metformin reduces glucose output by the liver. Thiazolidinediones (TZDs) are insulin sensitizers, which improve glucose uptake in fat and muscle cells. We still use medications to stimulate the pancreas to make more insulin, but they are no longer the main treatment. Other medications are available, but my goal is to keep you from being put on medication altogether by turning your health around before you've been given the diagnosis of type 2 diabetes. We can accomplish that if we can diagnose metabolic syndrome or insulin resistance early enough and begin making serious lifestyle changes.

Metabolic Syndrome, or Insulin Resistance

There is a pattern of signs and symptoms that most patients show before they progress to full-blown type 2 diabetes. This grouping of symptoms, as first noted in the 1960s and 1970s, included several cardiovascular risk factors: hypertension, diabetes, lipid abnormalities, and obesity.[763] Reaven suggested that insulin resistance might be the cause. He referred to the grouping as syndrome X, but today it is most commonly called metabolic syndrome.

(There is some debate concerning the concept of metabolic syndrome. Reaven believes that all the qualities associated with the diagnosis are simply due to the normal progression of insulin resistance and that it is not necessarily a separate syndrome.[764] The American Diabetes Association prefers that the term "metabolic syndrome" be replaced by "cardiometabolic risk" to stress the association between diabetes, heart disease, and stroke.[765] I will use "metabolic syndrome," since it is widely recognized and accepted.)

There is currently a great deal of research being done with the goal of understanding the cause of metabolic syndrome. Some studies seem to indicate that insulin resistance is the cause of metabolic syndrome. However, at least two studies[766, 767] suggest that insulin resistance may not be the underlying cause of quite all the cardiovascular risk factors that make up metabolic syndrome. I will describe later in this chapter why I believe that metabolic syndrome has a second cause in addition to insulin resistance. In fact, this factor may be the cause of insulin resistance itself. And the cause matters. Knowing it tells us how to live in order to help reduce the incidence of type 2 diabetes and other chronic disease.

What's more, metabolic syndrome and insulin resistance are associated with very serious health consequences, even if one never develops type 2 diabetes. They significantly increase the risk of developing heart disease. And they are associated with an increased risk of cancer of the prostate,[768, 769] liver,[770] uterus,[771] colon,[772] breast,[773] pancreas,[774] and other health conditions. It is no coincidence that some of these cancers have been increasing globally right along with the epidemic of insulin resistance.

So what does all this mean to you?

You need to know *now* whether or not you already have metabolic syndrome. If you do, you'll need to get very serious about aggressively changing your lifestyle. In order to reverse or delay the progression of metabolic syndrome, you'll need to change more than one or two factors. If you know someone well who has type 2 diabetes, you realize that it is not to be taken lightly. Also, if you have had a great deal of difficulty losing weight, it may be on account of metabolic syndrome. That is, your inability to lose weight may have to do with health disorders you don't yet understand.

This is one reason why I'm spending so much time describing insulin resistance and metabolic syndrome. It has to be addressed if we want to lose weight and, more importantly, achieve optimal health.

ANOTHER THING THAT'S NOT ON YOUR DIET

Most diet-for-sale programs have not dealt with metabolic syndrome, or have taken wrong approaches. Some even make recommendations that worsen metabolic syndrome, which in turn makes it harder lose weight. It's easy to see why these weight-loss programs are generally unsuccessful, and why many people are so frustrated—especially when many of these diet plans have been written or promoted by scientists. I've had a unique, global practice in preventive medicine for twenty years, and the growing body of scientific literature and research, much of it cited here, only adds support to my position.

Certainly new studies will provide new insights, but enough is now known that I can show you the right path, in confidence that you won't have to change course significantly in the future.

Diagnosing Metabolic Syndrome

There are four well-known ways to diagnose metabolic syndrome.

1. Perhaps the most common set of criteria for diagnosis comes from the National Cholesterol Education Program's Adult Treatment Panel (NCEP ATP-III).[775] According to this program, metabolic syndrome can

be diagnosed if three or more of the following risk factors are present:

- Abdominal obesity as defined by waist circumference
  Men > 102 cm or 40 in.
  Women > 88 cm or 35 in.
- Triglycerides 150 mg/dl or greater
- HDL cholesterol
  Men < 40 mg/dl
  Women < 50 mg/dl
- Blood pressure of 130/85 mm Hg or higher, or under treatment for hypertension
- Fasting glucose of 110 to 125 mg/dl

2. Another method of diagnosing metabolic syndrome comes from the World Health Organization.[776] This report defines metabolic syndrome as insulin resistance or impaired glucose tolerance, together with at least two of the components listed below:

- Hypertension, defined as > 140/90 mm Hg, or if the patient is currently using antihypertensive medicine
- Dyslipidemia, defined as plasma triglyceride of > 150 mg/dl, or a low HDL cholesterol (< 35 mg/dl in men, < 40 mg/dl in women)
- Central or general obesity—waist to hip ratio > 0.9 in men, > 0.85 in women and/or body mass index > 30
- Microalbuminuria—urinary albumin excretion rate of > 20 mcg/minute or albumin : creatinine ratio > 30 mg/g

This definition is also accurate and predictive of cardiovascular disease, but clinically more difficult to work with, because of the glucose tolerance testing and microalbuminuria testing that are required.

3. The American Heart Association and National Heart, Lung, and Blood Institute[777] consider a patient to have metabolic syndrome if he or she meets three of the following criteria:

- Waist circumference of greater than 102 cm (40 in.) in men or 88 cm (35 in.) in women (Asian Americans should probably have cutoffs of 90 cm [35 in.] for men and 80 cm [31 in.] for women)
- Triglycerides greater than 150 mg/dl or under treatment for hypertriglyceridemia
- HDL-C of less than 40 mg/dl for men or less than 50 mg/dl for women, or under treatment for low HDL
- Blood pressure greater than 135/85 mm HG or under treatment for hypertension
- Fasting glucose of greater than 100 mg/dl or under treatment for elevated glucose

4. The fourth set of criteria is from the International Diabetes Foundation.[778] A person is given the diagnosis of metabolic syndrome if he or she has central obesity and meets two other criteria:

- Ethnically specific increased waist circumference:
  Europids—men > 94 cm, women > 80 cm
  South Asians—men > 90 cm, women > 80 cm
  Chinese—men > 90 cm, women > 80 cm
  Japanese—men > 85 cm, women > 80 cm
  South and Central Americans—men > 90 cm, women > 80 cm
  Sub-Saharan Africans—men > 94 cm, women > 80 cm
  Eastern Mediterranean and Middle East (Arab)—men > 94 cm, women > 80 cm
- Triglycerides > 150 mg/dl or under treatment for hypertriglyceridemia
- HDL-C < 40 mg/dl for men and < 50 mg/dl for women or under treatment for it
- Blood pressure > 135/85 or under treatment for hypertension
- Fasting glucose of > 100 mg/dl or diagnosed with diabetes

Some researchers now include inflammation as part of the definition of metabolic syndrome, too.[779]

Whichever method your doctor uses to diagnose metabolic syndrome, it is important for you to be tested very soon.

You also need to know if you are insulin resistant. There are many ways to determine insulin sensitivity. The method called hyperinsulinemic clamp is considered to be the gold standard but, unfortunately, requires prolonged insulin infusion and repeated blood sampling. We have used a method of measuring the insulin sensitivity that is similar to the Homeostasis Model Assessment (HOMA) and Quantitative Insulin Sensitivity Check Index (QUICKI) tests. These tests use *a single measurement* of fasting insulin and glucose. A simple measurement of a fasting insulin level above 5 is evidence that the syndrome may be beginning. We have been using this method for at least ten years, personally counseling over 15,000 people, and have found the method to be quite reliable and an accurate predictor of the progression of type 2 diabetes.

These tests have been shown in the studies to correlate well with direct gold standard measurements[780] and are useful in defining the metabolic syndrome and predicting the development of cardiovascular disease and type 2 diabetes.[781, 782] Through this method and personal contact with the patients in our program, we have gained special insights into metabolic syndrome and the way lifestyle contributes to it. Most researchers lack this insight, because they don't look at metabolic syndrome from an individualized perspective.

Our institute has added yet another method of diagnosing insulin resistance by using the specialized cholesterol test described in chapter 9. By looking at a combination of high triglyceride, low HDL2, and small, dense LDL cholesterol particles, we can often detect insulin resistance earlier than by testing for fasting insulin and glucose elevations. Reaven's team at Stanford University has confirmed the accuracy of using these tests.[783]

The Third National Health and Nutrition Examination Survey (NHANES) reported that the prevalence of metabolic syndrome in adults over the age of twenty years was 24 percent, but the age-specific rate increased rapidly. The prevalence in fifty-year-olds was more than 30 percent, and over 40 percent in people over sixty.[784] While those numbers apply to Americans, similar rates already apply to every industrialized nation in the world—or soon will if people don't make rapid, dramatic lifestyle changes.

The Cause of Insulin Resistance and Metabolic Syndrome

While the conventional wisdom is that elevated insulin is the cause of metabolic syndrome, my reading and experience point to a different—or at least additional—contributing factor.

Even for the best trained scientists, it is sometimes difficult to differentiate between causes and effects of diseases and health problems. That's a reason why so many studies use the word "associated" when two factors seem to be linked. It isn't always clear which one causes the other, or whether they have a common cause. But it is important to get the cause-and-effect relationships right with regard to metabolic syndrome. Only when we know the cause can we make the lifestyle changes necessary to reduce our chances of getting it, and the chronic diseases that it engenders.

And—surprise!—here's the list of factors that increase insulin resistance. As Captain Renault would say, "Round up the usual suspects."

- Diet high in saturated fats, dark meat, and trans fats[785, 786, 787]
- Lack of exercise[788]
- Abdominal obesity[789]
- Smoking[790]
- Inadequate fruit and vegetable intake[791]
- Elevated C-reactive protein[792, 793, 794, 795, 796, 797]
- Soft drinks (even diet sodas)[798]

Apparently all these factors harm the function of insulin receptors, thereby increasing insulin levels in the blood to some degree. Increased insulin in the blood may then lead to many of the health problems associated with metabolic syndrome. The underlying component that is consistent with all of these risk factors is inflammation, as demonstrated by certain blood markers such as C-reactive protein, tumor necrosis factor-alpha, and interleukin-6. In fact, these markers even seem to be the mediators that lead to health problems such as atherosclerosis.[799]

There's a lot more information about the nature and results of inflammation in chapters 2 and 3, so feel free to go back and re-read them if you'd like. Here I'll just list steps to reduce it, along with the insulin resistance it causes.

DR. DUKE'S GAME PLAN

How to Reduce Insulin Resistance

Here is a long list of things you can do to help reduce insulin resistance. You may not understand why some of these lifestyle changes work. Please review what was discussed in previous chapters. But I want to list them now so you can get started. Most of these steps are easy, and some of them are pleasant, like eating salmon and whole grains. Feel free to refer back to these pages after you've finished this book and gained a better understanding of why they work.

Here are twenty-two ways to reduce insulin resistance through lifestyle change:

1. Reduce saturated fats, trans fats, and omega-6 fats in your diet.[800, 801] The primary sources of these fats are red dark meat,[802, 803] palm oil, coconut oil, high-fat dairy products, and cheap oils such as corn oil or other partially hydrogenated oils.
2. Reduce high-fructose corn syrup.[804] Sports drinks and processed foods contain massive amounts of it.[805, 806] Read labels, please!
3. Eat fewer foods with high glycemic index, such as simple sugars.[807] (See Appendix C.)
4. Exercise—get your doctor's permission, and then just do it.[808, 809]
5. If you're obese, get down to a healthier weight range.[810, 811] Fat cells produce substances that increase insulin resistance. This is especially true of abdominal (visceral) fat. When the number or size of fat cells diminishes, the production of harmful substances also decreases.
6. Stop smoking *now*. Or else cut back as much as you possibly can.[812] The chemicals in smoke increase insulin resistance.
7. Get more omega-3 fat in your diet through food or by supplementation.[813, 814] Food sources include salmon, flax and flax oil, walnuts, olive oil and canola oil.

8. Get enough chromium.[815] This essential mineral stabilizes glucose metabolism.

9. Eat more whole grains.[816] Some diet doctors want you to cut back on whole grains because they are fairly high in carbohydrates. However, these are *complex* carbs—their consumption is associated with *decreased* insulin resistance.

10. Lower your C-reactive protein.[817] (Learn how in chapters 2 and 3.)

11. Increase your intake of dietary fiber.[818, 819] One of fiber's many benefits is that it stabilizes glucose metabolism. You get it mostly from fruits and vegetables. Yum!

12. Eat more monounsaturated fats.[820] That means olive oil, *paisan*.

13. Become a vegetarian.[821] In general, vegetarians have less insulin resistance. A vegetarian diet incorporates many of the qualities provided on this list. Even if you don't give up flesh, please eat at least five to seven servings of fruits and vegetables daily.

14. Get enough calcium.[822] This also stabilizes glucose metabolism. Eat it. Take supplements. (See #20 below.)

15. Buy low-fat, organic dairy products.[823, 824] The benefit here may be from a protein in the dairy product or from the calcium. (You might be surprised that I would recommend dairy products, since it has been argued that a protein in dairy milk promotes cancer. And in fact, a careful search of the scientific literature reveals that perhaps there is a slight increased risk of prostate cancer or its recurrence with milk consumption.[825, 826] Some researchers didn't find it to be a strong risk,[827] and many studies suggest that diary products offer protection from colon[828] and breast[829] cancer, and perhaps others.[830] Most likely, the bad components in milk related to prostate cancer are the fat and hormones given to cows. This is why I recommend low-fat milk from organically raised cows.)

16. Get enough magnesium.[831, 832]

17. Drink coffee.[833] There have been many studies involving coffee consumption and insulin resistance. Though some studies indicated that the reduced insulin resistance was mostly the caffeine, other studies have shown benefit from decaffeinated coffee, and greater benefit from regular coffee than would be expected from caffeine alone.[834] The phytonutrients within coffee obviously are at least par-

tially responsible for reducing insulin resistance. Interestingly, studies involving tea (which contains caffeine) have not commonly shown decreased insulin resistance. Some benefit from coffee has been seen with just one or two cups a day.

18. Push the protein component of your diet as high as 27 percent, but avoid proteins heavy in saturated or trans fats.[835]

19. Add ground cinnamon to cereals or other foods—a half to a full teaspoon a day—with the clearance of your doctor. In one study,[836] one to six grams were shown in forty days to lower fasting serum glucose 18 to 29 percent, triglycerides 23 to 30 percent, LDL cholesterol 7 to 27 percent, and total cholesterol 12 to 26 percent.

20. Take adequate amounts of vitamin D. People with higher vitamin D levels in their blood had the lowest risk of type 2 diabetes.[837] Vitamin D supplementation (> 800 IU daily) was associated with a reduced risk of development of type 2 diabetes.[838] In fact, combining a daily intake of > 1200 mg calcium and > 800 IU vitamin D was associated with a 33 percent lower risk of type2 diabetes. Vitamin D and calcium together have also been shown to reduce insulin resistance.[839]

21. Get adequate sleep, preferably seven to eight hours a night.[840]

22. Avoid soft drinks.[841, 842]

Of course, seek advice from your doctor before making any significant changes with regard to these steps. I know what works generally. You doctor knows you individually. ❖

Knowledge Is Your Best Defense

It's critically important to have your physician determine whether or not you have type 2 diabetes or insulin resistance. If you do have one of these disorders, please work closely with your physician and do your best to manage it. Both diseases are progressive, and they can cause significant damage even before you show symptoms. Following the twenty-two recommendations above will help reduce insulin resistance, and may help reduce or eliminate your need for medications.

Also, please remember that reducing insulin resistance is critical to helping you lose weight. Obesity increases the risk of insulin resistance, and insulin resistance contributes to obesity. It's a vicious cycle that has to be broken.

The next chapter brings together everything in this book. It's the master plan of the Optimum Health Revolution—twenty-five action steps you can take right away. Like any good plan, it isn't difficult to understand or manage. You're about to see how easy this revolution for optimal health really is.

PART V:

Twenty-Five Easy Steps
and Conclusions

CHAPTER 13

The Twenty-Five Easy
and Manageable Steps to
Optimal Health

I hope this book has been a profound educational experience for you so far. I hope I have shattered some misconceptions and brought you new insight and a new, wider, clearer view of what it takes to attain optimal health.

As with any formal education, the time comes to put what you've learned into action. That's where we are now. Or, to put it another way, our revolutionary plan is complete—now it's time to join the revolution and beat chronic disease. Are you ready to permanently be a part of the revolution?

The plan I've given you is an easy, practical guide for optimal health. It isn't complicated. You don't have to think about it before every move you make. Neither is it a miracle cure that promises you health via a single activity, food, supplement, medication, contraption or product.

Put these twenty-five steps into action and you'll be living a new, healthier life—not through some simple-minded "miracle," but by treating your body the way it is supposed to be treated. You'll feel better. You will significantly increase your chances of avoiding chronic disease. And you will be more likely to live longer and in better health.

But first, a word to people who want to take short cuts....

STOP! DO NOT READ FURTHER!

If it was your intent to skip the first twelve chapters of this book and go straight to the action steps, I applaud your eagerness. But I passionately want you to succeed in changing your lifestyle for the better. To make real, lasting change in the way we live, we have to believe deeply in what we're doing. And that kind of belief is the product of learning and knowing. To start here, at the end, is not much better than diving into another health fad, and you'll be more likely to give up. Start at the beginning, and you'll have the understanding and the grasp of details necessary to carry out our revolutionary plan wisely, safely, effectively, and for the rest of life.

These twenty-five action steps are a summary of everything you've learned from this book. The details, the research references, and the reasoning behind them can't be included here. That's why I wrote an entire book, instead of filming a thirty-minute infomercial. That and the fact that I'm not trying to sell you anything.

You wouldn't place your family's health in the hands of a "doctor" who somehow skipped medical school. This book exists to help you take greater charge of your own health. You need a little training to do that well and safely.

So please, *please* start at the beginning. I'll see you back here in a few days, and you'll be off and running toward a new, healthier lifestyle—with the confidence and motivation of someone who knows what he's doing and why he's doing it.

Finding the Time to Make These Twenty-Five Steps Work

If you are a typical citizen of the twenty-first century, you may be thinking: "Twenty-five steps? Twenty-*five*?! If they take one minute each I might be able to work them all in over the course of a week. Or maybe a month. Don't hold your breath."

Most of us are so overwhelmed by our busy lifestyles that we want to believe we can improve our health, lose weight, be more attractive, boost our energy, and reduce the risk of cancer and heart disease all on the fly. We want something that comes in a pill or a bottle or a jar. We want to have it all, but we don't want to spend any time in pursuit of "it all," because we have no more time to give.

So listen up, team: For the vast majority of you, winning optimal health won't require any more time than you currently have to give. The most time-consuming part is reading this book, and you're almost finished.

You'll need to spend a few days discussing this stuff with your spouse or significant other and your family. But beyond that, you're going to ease into a healthier lifestyle one step at a time, at a pace you can handle. *Most of the new behaviors you'll adopt will replace old behaviors*, so you won't need to find extra time.

I *will* suggest that if you have many of the risk factors that were discussed earlier in this book, then you should speed up the pace of change. But the big thing is to start now—make *some* of these changes, do whatever you can today.

Probably the hardest part of changing to an optimally healthy lifestyle is intellectual. We get stuck in our old ways of thinking. This is why a revolution is necessary. Everybody says that being overweight is unhealthy, and we're taught that the only way to become healthy is to focus on losing weight. Then we're taught that the only ways to lose weight are (1) to eat exactly the percentages of proteins, fats, and carbohydrates that are being touted by this week's diet guru, or (2) or to exercise until we drop. This has been the paradigm of popular health "science" all your life.

But where has this paradigm gotten us? We're getting fatter, there's still way too much heart disease, and the rates of diabetes and cancer are rising fast. See anything wrong with this picture?

However, a few ordinary people have found the right way to live to attain optimal health. We see a great many of them at our institute—people we've taught and from whom we've learned much.

So let's get started. The science behind these recommendations has been documented throughout this book. It's time to start walking the walk.

How to Work These Steps

These twenty-five steps will lead you toward optimal health. You are almost certainly taking some of them already. I've included spaces for you check off the ones that you are already taking and those you still need to start on.

These steps are *not* listed in order of importance. *They are all important!* They all reduce inflammation! The order in which you should make these changes depends on your family medical history, your current health problems or symptoms, and so on. In short, your greatest risk factors. Many of you may need to focus urgently on just a few of these steps. Others might do better to make small, gradual changes in all the steps. We're talking about *your* health risks and lifestyle, not mine.

Above all, you need to adopt your new lifestyle at a pace you can handle. I don't want you dropping out because you couldn't achieve unrealistic objectives. Any change in this direction is good. Your goal is simply to make progress. Every bit of progress you make is an achievement you can be proud of, and which has its own rewards. You approach optimal health by making positive lifestyle changes that you will be able to live with for the rest of your life.

You're not out to set records here. Whatever changes you make now, keep living those changes for several weeks before taking on another load of changes. Let these steps settle in so that they become habits in your daily life.

Twenty-Five Easy Steps to Optimal Health

NEED
TO   ALREADY
CHANGE   DOING

_____ _____ 1. **Eat more fruits and vegetables.** You need at least seven servings per day, and preferably nine. This is far easier than you think. "Servings" are commonly only half a cup in size. A big helping of green beans, broccoli or grapes might count as two servings or more. However, don't eat the same fruits and vegetables all the time. Include a variety of color in your choices. (See Appendix B.4.) The best way to eat fruits and vegetables is either raw or by steaming fresh or frozen ones. To review the benefits of eating a variety of fruits and vegetables, see chapters 9–12.

_____ _____ **2. Quit or decrease smoking.** Quitting is by far the best, but any reduction is helpful to your health. Avoid secondhand smoke as well. If you need help, see your doctor. If you can't stop, then please protect your family by not smoking near them.

_____ _____ **3. Eat more whole grains.** They contain fiber, minerals, and many other beneficial nutrients, as described throughout this book.

_____ _____ **4. Get help for depression or stress.** Contact a professional or your religious leader for assistance. It isn't a sign of weakness to get help—it's a sign of strength and hope. Generally, do your best to maintain a positive outlook on life. (See chapters 7, 9, and 10.)

_____ _____ **5. Calculate your BMI, waist-to-hip ratio, and percent body fat.** If it is elevated, as described in chapter 11, then you have a health risk that you need to reduce by following all of these twenty-five steps. The way to reduce obesity is to reduce all your risks for chronic disease as described throughout this book. Losing weight isn't a strategy for attaining optimal health, it's a result.

_____ _____ **6. Calculate how many calories you need.** See chapter 11 and Appendix A.7 for methods to determine the calories you need to take in daily. If you are overweight, obese, or have an elevated percent body fat, you should reduce your intake to 300 to 500 calories below the level determined in chapter 11. Obtain a nutritional assessment. Doing that—and following the rest of teachings in this book—will enable you to lose weight while you reduce your risk of chronic disease.

_____ _____ **7. Learn how to estimate your calorie intake.** Most people couldn't begin to guess how many calories they take in daily. But people who are really successful at losing weight generally have a reasonably accurate notion of their caloric consumption. In fact, you can quickly and easily train yourself so that accurately estimating calories is second nature. All you need is a small kitchen scale, measuring cups, and a chart showing the calories in different foods by weight (easy to find on the Internet). Then spend a day playing with your food. Do this for a day every week or two, and soon accurately estimating calories in your meals will be second nature. You don't have to be accurate to the last calorie. Hitting it within a couple hundred a day, on average, will do fine.

This information is priceless. It will blow your mind to see the mass of vegetables you can eat to take on just 300 calories. Here's an example: Half a cup of chopped raw broccoli has only twelve calories. So 300 calories' worth of broccoli equals 12½ cups. That's about ¾ of a gallon. This demonstrates the power and importance of plants. They're loaded with antioxidants that help reduce the risk of chronic disease, and they contain so much fiber and total mass that you can eat to your heart's content without taking on large amounts of calories.

_____ _____ **8. Wear sunscreen.** Preferably one rated SPF 30 or above. Also, avoid excessive exposure to the sun, and don't even go near a tanning bed.

_____ _____ **9. Eat carbohydrates with low glycemic index.** This factor is explained in chapters 6 and 9–12. Appendix C provides a reference for where you can find the glycemic index of many foods. You don't have to eat exclusively those carbohydrates with the very lowest glycemic index, but you should generally favor low over high. Don't follow the low glycemic index or load menus, instead use the charts just to find the low glycemic index and load carbohydrates (see Appendix C for further explanation). Among other benefits, you will feel full on less food and fewer calories, and go longer before you feel hungry again.

_____ _____ **10. Take basic supplements.** See chapter 8 for details, and get your doctor's clearance before starting.

_____ _____ **11. Kick the fad habit.** Stop obsessing about grams and ratios of fat, protein, and carbohydrates. Just eat the *good* fats, carbohydrates, and proteins as described throughout this book. And please don't jump on the next fad that comes out. If the "latest thing" doesn't correspond with the science presented here, just ignore it. The science provided here should stand the test of time. Remember—new isn't necessarily better.

_____ _____ **12. Exercise your religious faith.** Whatever you believe, believe it intensely. (See chapter 9.)

NEED
TO   ALREADY
CHANGE DOING

_____ _____ 13. **Avoid high-fructose corn syrup.** This is found in many foods, especially in sweetened drinks. It is so ubiquitous, we can't avoid it altogether, but we can cut way back. For starters, replace sweetened drinks with green tea, water, coffee, low-fat organic dairy products, and drinks artificially sweetened with Splenda®. (The latter are less than ideal, but they're not killing us nearly as fast as diabetes and obesity.) See chapter 11 and Appendices B.1 and B.2 for more.

_____ _____ 14. **Get enough rest.** For most of us, that's seven to eight hours a night. (See chapter 6.)

_____ _____ 15.**Use only canola and extra-virgin olive oil.** Replace all other oils, especially partially hydrogenated oils, with these two. This will reduce omega-6 and trans fats drastically. (See chapters 2–4, 6, and 9–12.)

_____ _____ 16.**Eat organic foods** as much as possible. Meats, dairy, fruits, vegetables, and grains. (See chapters 3, 4, and 6.)

_____ _____ 17.**Decrease alcohol use**, preferably to zero. Its contributions to health problems are greater than any benefits. If you drink a lot of alcohol and cutting back seems unthinkable to you, then you probably *really* need to think about it.

_____ _____ 18.**Get more omega-3** in your diet and (if cleared by your doctor) through supplementation. (See chapters 3, 4, 8, and 9.)

_____ _____ 19.**Reduce exposure to contagious diseases**, especially sexually transmitted diseases like venereal warts, hepatitis B, hepatitis C, HIV, et al. (See chapters 3, 6, and 10.)

NEED
TO   ALREADY
CHANGE DOING

_____ _____ **20. See your doctor.** You should be checked for the following at the minimum: cholesterol levels, homocys-
teine, blood pressure, thyroid stimulating hormone
(TSH), ferritin,* hs-C-reactive protein, PSA (in men, to
screen for the possibility of prostate cancer), fasting glucose, and fasting insulin. Better yet, follow the recommendations in Appendix A.

_____ _____ **21. Cut back on processed foods, including fast food
and snacks.** These are loaded with omega-6, trans fats,
chemicals, high-fructose corn syrup, and other horrible
stuff. You can find healthy food at some fast food restaurants, but it it's rare. Replace bad, processed snacks with
fruit, vegetables, and well-balanced food-bars.

_____ _____ **22. Move your body more.** That's how we burn calories
and build muscle. Increase the "exercise of daily living,"
as explained in chapters 3, 4, 6, and 9-12. Get clearance
from a doctor before switching from couch potato-ness
to intense exercise. If you're wondering where you might
find time for exercise, start by trading TV time for time
spent in motion.

_____ _____ **23. Reduce your exposure to chemicals.** This is
explained in chapters 3, 4, 6, 10, and 11, as well as in
Appendices B.1 and B.2. Besides reducing chemical
exposure via food, consider an air or water purification
system.

---

*Testing for ferritin measures total body iron. The levels I prefer are between 50 and 100. When levels are
higher, excess iron tends to destroy the tissues in which it is stored by oxidation. (To reduce excess iron,
donate blood, then have your ferritin rechecked.) If your ferritin is too low—below 20—talk to your doctor
about how you might be losing blood and about perhaps taking a short course of iron supplementation.)

NEED
TO   ALREADY
CHANGE DOING

_____ _____ **24. Reduce consumption of dark meats**, especially beef, pork, and processed meats (if bacteria don't even want it, it's probably not good for *you*, either), because of their omega-6 and chemical content (e.g., pesticides and herbicides.) Replace with lean, skinless, organic chicken, turkey, or fish. Try veggie burgers, and even try eating vegetarian a few days a week.

_____ _____ **25. Get genetic testing.** Ask your doctor about genetic tests as they become commercially available, in order to determine your inherited risk of chronic disease.

Persistence and Progress, Not Perfection

Now that you have your list, you can begin working on it. As you can see, it involves your total lifestyle. Take whatever steps you can now.

A key to a successful revolution of optimal health is to realize that nobody's perfect, not even you. Perfectionism ensures failure, because it sets a goal no one can attain. Perfectionism is a kind of obsession, which means it adds stress to your life, which is a risk factor for chronic disease. We're trying to get rid of those, not add new ones.

I'm certainly not perfect in my own lifestyle. For instance, I'm addicted to chocolate chip cookies. There's no way I could completely eliminate chocolate chip cookies from my life. The reason chocolate chip cookies have not killed me is that I do the vast majority of what I teach daily, so I can occasionally eat chocolate chip cookies without guilt or regret.

Aside from my cookie habit, I changed my lifestyle *gradually*, so that new ways of living became normal, habitual, and nearly effortless.

When you make gradual changes in your total lifestyle, you cannot fail. You make the changes that you want to make when you want to make them. It's not an all-or-nothing game. Do a little bit now and add a little bit more later. Every change you make is a success, a win.

How Do I Know This Will Work?

I know this game plan for optimal health works because I've seen thousands of people improve their health by making lifestyle changes—and I've documented the results for many of them. I know that it works because of the vast body of medical and scientific literature that supports the concepts I have taught you. If you control your caloric intake, eat more fruits, vegetables, whole grains, and lean meat, and increase your exercise of daily living, you *will* reduce your risk of chronic disease *and* lose weight.

Weight loss is only one of the many changes that will occur in your life, and you don't have to reach an "ideal" weight before you reduce your risk of chronic disease. Again, this is about progress.

And progress means reducing your risk factors. Follow these steps as you become ready. Be consistent. As you follow these Twenty-Five Easy and Manageable Steps to Optimal Health, you will lose weight, your percent body fat will drop, your muscle mass will increase, your waist-to-hip ratio will improve, you'll have more energy, and you will reduce your risk of chronic disease. You will enjoy a better quality of life and increase your chances of living longer.

Work these steps long enough and well, and you will see a day when you have reduced your risk factors as much as possible—and when your new lifestyle seems effortless, comfortable, and normal. **That's the day you'll know the revolution was successful and you won your optimal health.**

You'll wonder why it ever seemed hard.

There is one last chapter. It is about two people who are great examples of optimal health. One has gotten there recently, while the other, my father, has lived an optimal lifestyle his whole life.

I add these stories in the hopes that seeing these ideas at work in the lives of real people will be an inspiration to you.

Thank you for giving me the opportunity to share this knowledge with you and your family. I have great hope for you all.

CHAPTER 14

Two People Who Have
Achieved Optimal Health

Throughout recorded history, in virtually every culture, a few singu-
lar individuals have always risen to become champions. Champions
are widely recognized and praised for their accomplishments. They
become exemplars of virtue—of valor, skill, or intelligence. Sometimes
one is elevated to the status of champion on account of a single act at a
crucial moment. We memorialize our champions with statues, paintings,
legend, poetry, and song.

And yet most real champions don't get the recognition they deserve.
Many shy away from it.

This final chapter is devoted to the first two entrants into the Optimal
Health Hall of Fame. You would likely never hear of them in any other
way, because they are humble people whose accomplishments are not
the kind that make national headlines. But these two men have accomplished much and serve as role models for thousands.

The first is a middle-aged high school teacher who made lifestyle
changes over a very short time that have dramatically reduced his risk of
chronic disease. The second is Wayne Johnson, my father, a man who is
reaping the results of a lifelong devotion to optimal health. These two

men are great examples of the practical application of the principles taught in this book. I offer them to you as sources of great hope and inspiration.

The first of these stories shows that you can dramatically improve your risk of chronic disease in just a few months, and the second is proof that all your efforts are worth it.

Larry

Larry is a warm, engaging teacher at a public high school in the United States. At this writing he is forty-eight years old, has been married for twenty-four years, and has two children, Luke, thirteen, and Maren, seven. He's a guy with a great smile and sparkling blue eyes that express a sincere interest in every word you speak—not just curiosity but genuine caring. Larry is a big guy, but that doesn't stop you from wanting to give him a hug. He's a gentle giant. The quality that stands out most when you meet him is his biblically defined meekness, which is to say power under control. You can sense how the love that comes from a committed relationship with his Creator flows out and masters his strength. You can't help liking Larry and his equally admirable wife Cheri. They are great people by any definition.

Larry did not come to me in the best of health. In addition to his teaching job, his activities include coaching football and track, service to his church and his community, and a busy social life. There is a history of heart disease and cancer in Larry's family, and he was deeply concerned about how this might affect his own future. But his time commitments had gradually undermined his attempts to live a healthy lifestyle. Upon arrival at our center, Larry had metabolic syndrome and weighed 284 pounds. He had a waist-to-hip ratio of 0.99, blood pressure of 158/100, triglycerides of 647, and fasting insulin of 20.2 (I prefer a level of < 5). He was obese, with 32 percent body fat, meaning he was carrying ninety-one pounds of fat. He was following only two pillars of optimal health (Environment and Hygiene, and Mind and Spirit.) He had nine risk factors for heart disease, eight for cancer, and four for diabetes.

Larry is a coach and a former athlete. He had professional knowledge about how to "get in shape," but he lacked the ability to change his whole lifestyle. He wanted to be in better health, but he felt stuck. The cascade of conflicting information from popular media, diet marketers, and fad promoters had only deepened his frustration and subsequent stasis. Larry could have given up and accepted an early demise due to chronic disease, using "lack of time" as an excuse for his poor health, but he didn't. He refused to quit. Larry had the character and integrity to be honest about his lifestyle and confront deadly chronic disease with courage. As an educator, he knows the value of being teachable and has been a wonderful student of optimal health. He's motivated by a desire to be with his loving wife and family as long as possible, and to stand as an example for others.

After just four months of following the guidelines presented in the last chapter, Larry dramatically improved his health and reduced his risk of chronic disease. His weight dropped to 243 pounds and his body fat to 16.6 percent. He lost fifty-one pounds of fat and gained ten pounds of muscle. (Remember, even though the optimal health lifestyle is not promoted as a weight-loss program, if you are overweight and follow this lifestyle, you *will* lose excess weight.) He now follows all eight pillars of optimal health. His risk factors for both heart disease and cancer are reduced to the one he can't ever change—family history. He now has no risk factors for type 2 diabetes. His C-reactive protein is normal. With a blood pressure of 126/76, triglycerides of 81, HDL cholesterol of 52, waist-to-hip ratio of 0.92, and fasting insulin of 4.2, he no longer has metabolic syndrome.

In just four months, Larry is a new person.

This could happen to you, too.

How did Larry do it? He followed the teachings presented in this book.

How did he manage so much change with such a busy life? He eats smarter, which doesn't necessarily take more time. He exchanged some TV time for formal exercise and gets even more exercise through the activities of daily living. He reexamined his life's priorities and placed his health higher on the list. He learned how supplements can contribute to optimal health and takes them regularly. He learned how to calculate calories and now controls his caloric intake largely by eating more vegetables. He learned to control his stress through lifestyle changes, and has reduced all the risk factors he can.

How do we know that these are permanent changes in Larry—that it won't turn out to be just another fad? Though Larry made lifestyle changes faster than most people, he demonstrates the hallmark characteristic among people who are truly winning the fight for optimal health—he quickly got to the point at which the lifestyle is no longer work. Change always takes some initial effort, but soon these changes become both habit and belief, ingrained in your lifestyle. They become normal to you, requiring little or no effort. You're a new person.

Larry proves that it is possible to change one's life quickly and drastically. But even if the changes necessary to reduce your risk factors take years to complete, don't give up. It isn't how fast you change. It's how much you change and how permanent those changes become. Start down the right path and keep moving steadily and persistently until you attain the best lifestyle you're capable of living.

Larry feels great. He has far more energy and zest for life. For the first time in years, he is optimistic about his future, knowing that his risk for chronic disease is dramatically reduced. He is better off physically, medically, emotionally, mentally, and spiritually.

Today this man touches many lives. He is a living example of victory in the Optimal Health Revolution. He works to help others to find new hope, people who feel helpless and trapped in their bodies—just like he did.

The lifestyle Larry adopted doesn't involve gimmicks, fads, miracle products, or quick fixes. It combines the best of Eastern and Western medicine with a strong emphasis on prevention. It will stand the test of time, because it is based on the best of science. It changed Larry's life, and it can change yours.

Wayne

I'd like to conclude my book with the story of a great man whose journey toward optimal health began in boyhood. He is, at this writing, an unbelievably healthy eighty-seven-year-old man. He skis down intermediate slopes, cares for a one-acre yard, and shovels snow. His health is as much a reflection of his character as of his lifestyle. It is commonly taught that good health involves body, mind, and spirit, but character is a fourth element that isn't understood well enough in modern societies.

Admiration for good character has nearly been lost—many of us would have a hard time even defining it. But I have seen firsthand how integrity and character have impacted my father's health. I'll try to explain that, knowing that any written description of my dad will be inadequate. Few of us understand how character affects our health over time.

Dad was born in 1921 to a humble couple whose recent ancestors had immigrated to America in hope of finding a better life. Instead of looking to the United States to care for them or using their native languages as excuse for failure, his ancestors learned English and tried to make America better. During the Depression, Wayne's father Walter held several jobs. Even after the discouraging experience of having money stolen from him, he persisted in reaching out through hard work and industriousness to aid scores of neighbors who were suffering. This trait of reaching out to others became my father's hallmark characteristic. His love for others isn't the kind of superficial emotion we often see, but flows from his innermost being.

My father is very athletic. Prior to an injury in spring football practice during his sophomore year at UCLA, he played in the same backfield as the great Jackie Robinson and Bob Waterfield, who is now in the National Football League Hall of Fame. Robinson, the Major League Baseball Hall-of-Famer and the first African American to play major league baseball, sent our family Christmas cards for years afterward. In the innocence of childhood I thought nothing of this. I figured everyone got Christmas cards from Jackie Robinson. But in a time when it was very unusual for Americans of different skin colors to have close friendships, my father's love was not limited by foolish prejudices. He was and has always been concerned with the heart and character of a person.

During World War Two, Dad entered the Naval Air Corps and began training as a pilot in preparation for aircraft carrier service. One fateful day he was with a group of trainee pilots being flown to a new airfield when the transport plane made what pilots casually refer to as a "hard landing." You and I would call it a crash landing. The impact caused one of the trainees to hurtle forward through the plane's cabin. My dad reached out and caught the man, probably saving him from serious injury. However, Dad's own legs were injured so badly that he received an honorable discharge. This reflexive act of love may have saved my father's life, because half the pilots trained in his group were killed during the war.

In the city where I was raised, my dad is greatly admired for his compassion and integrity. He managed a branch of a small bank, and though the bank's vault—which often contained hundreds of thousands of dollars—lacked a time lock, the bank never lost a penny. He was such a keen judge of people that in over twenty years as a loan officer—during which time he made thousands of loans totaling many millions of dollars—losses on his loans totaled only about $300.

Dad was a loan officer before credit cards were widely available, so along with the large corporate loans, he averaged several small loans per day. My father was so loved and respected that people never wanted to let him down. He received checks from all over the country, as debtors who were forced by hard times to take seasonal jobs worked hard to repay him. When he left the bank, scores of people came in to wish him well, many of them crying, because of what he meant to their families. (When was the last time you had such emotions for your banker?) To this day, whenever I meet people who know my father, they always ask about him.

He was elected president of the city council after a group of council members with questionable integrity were voted off because the city was chronically in debt. The city was out of debt soon after he took office. Some former councilmen made threats of violence and even death against my dad *and* his family, but Dad refused to be intimidated. He remained steadfast in doing what was right, while taking action to protect our family. His integrity and character won.

We had a large yard, a basketball court, and a nearby lake. When I was in high school, as many as fifty of my friends would come to our house to play. Usually ten or so of my crowd would never make it to the court or the lake, but would end up sitting in the living room chatting with Dad. Many of my friends wished my father were theirs.

I could write a book about my dad and what it was like to be raised by him. Maybe I should. For now, though, I hope this brief glimpse gives you an idea of his character.

The point I want to make concerns the many ways in which his character affected his health.

First, he has given out so much love over the years that he is bathed in love in return. Most of us know how good it feels to be truly loved by a few special people, but can you imagine having the genuine love of hundreds?

My dad has always followed almost all of the steps outlined in this book. It came naturally to him. He never smoked, drank alcohol, or was gluttonous, and he has never been overweight. He has always participated in the activities of daily living and still does all his own yard work on a lot of nearly an acre. He has exercised by running or walking almost every day of his adult life. He is under the care of a doctor for his few health problems and takes his medications faithfully. He is an eternal optimist and attends church regularly. His faith is profound. He eats a very well-balanced, nutritious diet loaded with fruits and vegetables, and he takes supplements daily.

His priorities have always been in order. He didn't pursue wealth or fame. He made a career of lending money to businesses and individuals, and sometimes lent his own money to others, to help them get ahead or overcome hardship. He was accepted into the UCLA School of Medicine's first class but declined so that he could devote more time to our family. (This resulted in two of his children graduating from the UCLA School of Medicine.) My dad preferred spending time with his family to hanging around with adult friends. He would take us fishing, swimming, canoeing, or hiking almost every day of the summer. Now in his late eighties, he still beats me at golf and goes fishing and camping with my family. My children adore him. He babysits our preschooler and has helped me in the last year with yard work that would wear out the average thirty-year-old.

His honesty allows him to sleep well at night. He has an inner peace that few know, which comes from living a pure life. He doesn't make a show of his religious faith, but is always quietly reaching out to people in need. Some people show their religious devotion in odd, destructive ways. People of character resolve differences rationally and through dialogue. They help innocent people in need.

The values of many people in modern society are out of whack in ways that harm their health. Material wealth is fine as far as it goes. But for too many, the greedy pursuit of wealth and fame causes stress that results in heart disease or cancer. My father has always had the humility to avoid that kind of behavior and the ravages of illness that often come with it. Nearly all my father's contemporaries who took the striving, money-obsessed path are dead, but my father lives a healthy, happy, vigorous life.

Our society recognizes its champions in terms of symbols: wealth, fame, Nobel Prizes, gold records, Academy Awards, headlines, tribute shows on television, stars on the Hollywood Walk of Fame. My dad never got that kind of recognition, but there is no finer human being or better example of optimal health. Most of the people modern societies hold up as heroes pale in comparison.

I am privileged to have been raised by this unsung hero, the greatest earthly personification of love that I know. His lifestyle is optimal. He is the complete man—physically, mentally, spiritually, and in character. He lives a happy, loving, peaceful, hopeful, active, healthy life that I'm sure will culminate with his heavenly Father saying, "Well done, thou good and faithful servant."

APPENDICES

Appendix A

A.1 Health Checkup Recommendations

Males

Under eighteen years old
    1. Yearly exams by doctor
    2. BMI checked yearly
    3. Monthly testicular exams beginning at age fifteen

Ages eighteen to forty
    1. Complete physical exam every three years, including urinalysis and blood work
    2. Cholesterol check every three years
    3. Blood pressure check every two years
    4. Vision check by your doctor every three years
    5. Dental: yearly dentist exam and cleaning every six months
    6. Skin cancer: self exam and during yearly physical exam
    7. Tetanus/diphtheria inoculation: every ten years
    8. Testicular self exams monthly and by physician during yearly exam
    9. Percent body fat yearly

Ages forty to fifty
    1. Complete physical exam yearly, including urinalysis and blood testing with CBC, chemistry panel, fasting glucose, hs-C-reactive protein, homocysteine, VAP cholesterol panel, liver panel, fasting insulin, and omega-3 levels
    2. Digital rectal exam yearly for prostate and rectal abnormalities
    3. Stool for occult blood yearly
    4. Complete eye exam by ophthalmologist
    5. Yearly prostate-specific antigen (PSA)
    6. Baseline exercise treadmill and every three years depending

on risk

7. Bone density every three years (more frequently if problems are already present)

Over fifty years old

1. Continue yearly physical exam, rectal exam, PSA, and yearly stool for occult blood
2. Sigmoidoscopy every three to five years or colonoscopy every ten years (more frequently for high-risk individuals or when problems are already present)
3. Pneumococcal shot: over age sixty-five, given once in lifetime (check with your doctor if you have high-risk condition or were vaccinated before age sixty-five)
4. Consider yearly influenza shots

Females

Under eighteen years old

1. Yearly exams by doctor
2. PAP and pelvic exam at least yearly once sexual activity begins
3. BMI checked yearly

Ages eighteen to thirty-five

1. Complete physical exam every three years, including urinalysis and blood work
2. Blood pressure check every two years
3. Clinical (i.e., by physician) breast exam yearly
4. PAP test and pelvic yearly
5. Self breast exam monthly (preferably one week after period begins)
6. VAP cholesterol check every three to five years
7. Vision check by your doctor at least every three years
8. Dental: yearly dentist exam and cleaning every six months
9. Skin cancer: self exam and during complete yearly physical exam

10. Tetanus/diphtheria inoculation: every ten years
11. Percent body fat yearly

Ages thirty-five to thirty-nine
1. Baseline mammogram
2. Continue recommendations for age eighteen to thirty-five

Ages forty to fifty
1. Complete physical exam yearly with urinalysis and blood work that includes CBC, chemistry panel, liver panel, VAP cholesterol panel, hs-C-reactive protein, homocysteine, fasting glucose, fasting insulin, and omega-3 levels
2. Mammogram yearly
3. Digital rectal exam yearly with stool for occult blood
4. Complete eye exam by ophthalmologist
5. Bone density every three years (more frequently if problems are already present)
6. Baseline exercise treadmill every three years depending on risk
7. Otherwise, continue recommendations for eighteen to thirty-five and thirty-five to thirty-nine

Over fifty years old
1. Continue yearly physical exam, rectal exams, and stool for occult blood
2. Continue yearly PAP, mammogram, breast, and pelvic exam until your doctor decides the rate may be reduced
3. Sigmoidoscopy every three to five years or colonoscopy every ten years (more frequently for high-risk individuals or when problems are already present)
4. Pneumococcal shot: over age sixty-five given once in lifetime (check with your doctor if you have high-risk condition or were vaccinated before age sixty-five)
5. Consider yearly influenza shots after age fifty

A.2 The Best Method for Determining Cholesterol Status

We use a special cholesterol test at our institute that measures actual levels of all kinds of cholesterol rather than estimating some of it. We evaluate a more detailed range of cholesterol values, the importance of which I will explain presently. We recommend treatments that are specific to these different cholesterol values as well. However, if your cholesterol is elevated, please discuss the information presented here with your doctor rather than "treating" your condition yourself. Partial knowledge can be as dangerous as no knowledge.

We obtain real (not calculated) LDL levels. These are referred to as R-LDL. In addition, we obtain lipoprotein (a), IDL, VLDL-3, HDL-2, HDL-3, LDL size and pattern, total cholesterol, and triglycerides.*

The accuracy of this method and the additional values it provides dramatically increase our ability to detect abnormalities and thereby provide for accurate treatment. The standard cholesterol therapy drugs don't treat some of these additional cholesterol values, as you will see below.

Lipoprotein (a) (Lp[a]). This is a molecule that looks very similar to R-LDL except that it has a special protein attached that inhibits the breakdown of clots. It is a risk factor for heart disease by itself and more than doubles the risk.[843] This value should be less than 10 mg/dl. If lipoprotein (a) is elevated and HDL is low, studies show that you would have 8.3 times the chance of developing heart disease.[844] There is also a very strong chance that this inherited trait is passed on to your children. Therefore, if your Lp(a) level is elevated, you should have your immediate family checked as well. Elevated Lp(a) may be lowered by taking omega-3. Current medicine recommendations are to treat with a combination of niacin and either statins or fenofibrates. Therefore, if your Lp(a) is elevated, you should discuss it with your doctor.

IDL cholesterol. IDL causes heart disease faster than R-LDL. This value should be less than 20 mg/dl. There is also a high chance that you will

---

*To decode the abbreviations in this sentence: LDL is low-density lipoprotein; IDL is intermediate-density lipoprotein; VLDL is very-low-density lipoprotein; HDL is high-density lipoprotein.

transfer this IDL trait to your children, so if your value is elevated you should have your immediate family checked for it as well. IDL is commonly lowered by reducing the amount of saturated fats in your diet and taking omega-3. If this isn't beneficial, you may need to talk to your doctor about taking medicines called statins in combination with niacin.

LDL size and pattern. LDL particles are primarily of two different sizes with corresponding patterns. They can either be small and dense (pattern B) or large and buoyant (pattern A). Small dense pattern B LDL increases the risk of heart attacks 6.9 times.[845] Without this knowledge, you could have a normal cholesterol level in the past, and still be at an increased risk for heart attack. You can change from a pattern B to A by taking omega-3. If this isn't helpful, you may need to talk to your doctor about taking niacin, glutathione or fenofibrates.

VLDL-3. This value is directly measured and it is best to be below 10. These small, dense particles increase the risk of heart disease.[846] Elevated levels can be reduced with omega-3 and by reducing other fats in your diet. If this isn't helpful, you may need to talk to your doctor about taking niacin or fenofibrates.

HDL-2. HDL is considered the good cholesterol. HDL-2 is large and buoyant and the more protective of the two HDLs. Low HDL-2 is a risk factor for heart disease, even if the rest of the cholesterol panel is normal.[847] It is best if this value is greater than 10 mg/dl in men and greater than 25 mg/dl if women. Low HDL-2 can be elevated by exercise (after you've gotten clearance from a doctor), omega-3, and niacin.

HDL-3. This HDL is smaller and denser than HDL-2 and not as protective. Its value should be greater than 30 mg/dl in men and 25 mg/dl in women.

A.3 BMI Chart

Body Weight (pounds)

Height (inches)	Normal						Overweight					Obese										Extreme Obesity														
BMI	19	20	21	22	23	24	25	26	27	28	29	30	31	32	33	34	35	36	37	38	39	40	41	42	43	44	45	46	47	48	49	50	51	52	53	54
58	91	96	100	105	110	115	119	124	129	134	138	143	148	153	158	162	167	172	177	181	186	191	196	201	205	210	215	220	224	229	234	239	244	248	253	258
59	94	99	104	109	114	119	124	128	133	138	143	148	153	158	163	168	173	178	183	188	193	198	203	208	212	217	222	227	232	237	242	247	252	257	262	267
60	97	102	107	112	118	123	128	133	138	143	148	153	158	163	168	174	179	184	189	194	199	204	209	215	220	225	230	235	240	245	250	255	261	266	271	276
61	100	106	111	116	122	127	132	137	143	148	153	158	164	169	174	180	185	190	195	201	206	211	217	222	227	232	238	243	248	254	259	264	269	275	280	285
62	104	109	115	120	126	131	136	142	147	153	158	164	169	175	180	186	191	196	202	207	213	218	224	229	235	240	246	251	256	262	267	273	278	284	289	295
63	107	113	118	124	130	135	141	146	152	158	163	169	175	180	186	191	197	203	208	214	220	225	231	237	242	248	254	259	265	270	278	282	287	293	299	304
64	110	116	122	128	134	140	145	151	157	163	169	174	180	186	192	197	204	209	215	221	227	232	238	244	250	256	262	267	273	279	285	291	296	302	308	314
65	114	120	126	132	138	144	150	156	162	168	174	180	186	192	198	204	210	216	222	228	234	240	246	252	258	264	270	276	282	288	294	300	306	312	318	324
66	118	124	130	136	142	148	155	161	167	173	179	186	192	198	204	210	216	223	229	235	241	247	253	260	266	272	278	284	291	297	303	309	315	322	328	334
67	121	127	134	140	146	153	159	166	172	178	185	191	198	204	211	217	223	230	236	242	249	255	261	268	274	280	287	293	299	306	312	319	325	331	338	344
68	125	131	138	144	151	158	164	171	177	184	190	197	203	210	216	223	230	236	243	249	256	262	269	276	282	289	295	302	308	315	322	328	335	341	348	354
69	128	135	142	149	155	162	169	176	182	189	196	203	209	216	223	230	236	243	250	257	263	270	277	284	291	297	304	311	318	324	331	338	345	351	358	365
70	132	139	146	153	160	167	174	181	188	195	202	209	216	222	229	236	243	250	257	264	271	278	285	292	299	306	313	320	327	334	341	348	355	362	369	376
71	136	143	150	157	165	172	179	186	193	200	208	215	222	229	236	243	250	257	265	272	279	286	293	301	308	315	322	329	338	343	351	358	365	372	379	386
72	140	147	154	162	169	177	184	191	199	206	213	221	228	235	242	250	258	265	272	279	287	294	302	309	316	324	331	338	346	353	361	368	375	383	390	397
73	144	151	159	166	174	182	189	197	204	212	219	227	235	242	250	257	265	272	280	288	295	302	310	318	325	333	340	348	355	363	371	378	386	393	401	408
74	148	155	163	171	179	186	194	202	210	218	225	233	241	249	256	264	272	280	287	295	303	311	319	326	334	342	350	358	365	373	381	389	396	404	412	420
75	152	160	168	176	184	192	200	208	216	224	232	240	248	256	264	272	279	287	295	303	311	319	327	335	343	351	359	367	375	383	391	399	407	415	423	431
76	156	164	172	180	189	197	205	213	221	230	238	246	254	263	271	279	287	295	304	312	320	328	336	344	353	361	369	377	385	394	402	410	418	426	435	443

A.4 BMI Chart for Boys

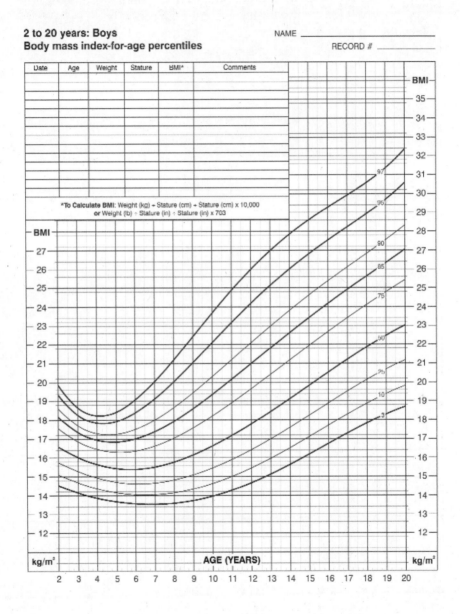

2 to 20 years: Boys
Body mass index-for-age percentiles

NAME _____

RECORD # _____

*To Calculate BMI: Weight (kg) ÷ Stature (cm) ÷ Stature (cm) x 10,000
or Weight (lb) ÷ Stature (in) ÷ Stature (in) x 703

AGE (YEARS)

SOURCE:http://www.cdc.gov/nchs/data/nhanes/growthcharts/set2clinical/cj41l073.pdf

A.5 BMI Chart for Girls

2 to 20 years: Girls
Body mass index-for-age percentiles

NAME _____

RECORD # _____

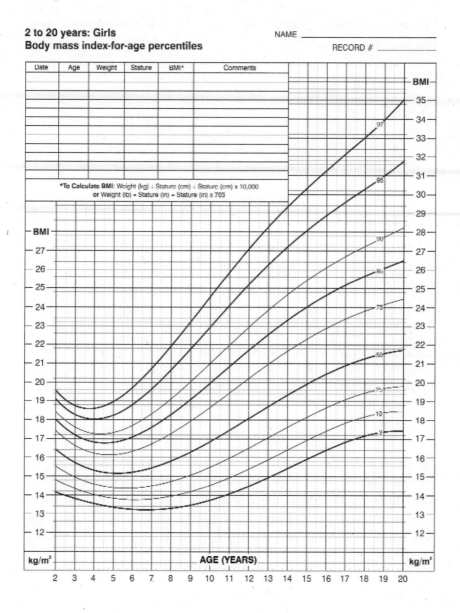

SOURCE:http://www.cdc.gov/nchs/data/nhanes/growthcharts/set2clinical/cj41l074.pdf

A.6 Cost of Obesity

Expected Lifetime Medical Care Costs of Selected Obesity-related Diseases, Discounted 3% by Sex, Age Group, and BMI

Sex and Age Group	Expected Liftime Costs, $, by BMI, kg/m²			
	22.5	27.5	32.5	37.5
Men				
35-44	16,200	20,200	25,300	31,700
45-54	19,600	24,000	29,600	36,500
55-64	22,000	26,100	31,200	37,400
Women				
35-44	15,200	18,900	23,800	29,700
45-54	18,800	23,200	28,700	35,300
55-64	21,900	26,500	32,200	39,000

The direct and indirect costs of health care associated with diabetes (a disease made worse by obesity) in the U.S. during 1997 were an estimated $98 billion.[848] Annual hospital days were 74 percent higher among the severely overweight and 34 percent higher among the moderately overweight.[849] Hospital costs associated with childhood obesity have more than tripled since 1981, soaring to $127 million per year.[850]

Obesity cost the United States $123 billion in 2001, including direct and indirect health-care costs like lost productivity.[851] The Centers for Disease Control states that the annual costs for an obese person are 37.7 percent more (or $732 higher) than the costs for a normal-weight person. Obese Medicare patients cost $1,486 more per year.[852] Nearly 40 million workdays are lost each year due to obesity-related causes, and over 65 million physician office visits annually are due to obesity-related problems.[853]

A.7 How to Calculate Daily Calorie Needs

	MALES				FEMALES		
Activity level	Sedentary*	Mod. Active*	Active*	Activity level	Sedentary*	Mod. Active*	Active*
AGE				AGE			
2	1000	1000	1000	2	1000	1000	1000
3	1000	1400	1400	3	1000	1200	1400
4	1200	1400	1600	4	1200	1400	1400
5	1200	1400	1600	5	1200	1400	1600
6	1400	1600	1800	6	1200	1400	1600
7	1400	1600	1800	7	1200	1600	1800
8	1400	1600	2000	8	1400	1600	1800
9	1600	1800	2000	9	1400	1600	1800
10	1600	1800	2200	10	1400	1800	2000
11	1800	2000	2200	11	1600	1800	2000
12	1800	2200	2400	12	1600	2000	2200
13	2000	2200	2600	13	1600	2000	2200
14	2000	2400	2800	14	1800	2000	2400
15	2200	2600	3000	15	1800	2000	2400
16	2400	2800	3200	16	1800	2000	2400
17	2400	2800	3200	17	1800	2000	2400
18	2400	2800	3200	18	1800	2000	2400
19-20	2600	2800	3000	19-20	2000	2200	2400
21-25	2400	2800	3000	21-25	2000	2200	2400
26-30	2400	2600	3000	26-30	1800	2000	2400
31-35	2400	2600	3000	31-35	1800	2000	2200
36-40	2400	2600	2800	36-40	1800	2000	2200
41-45	2200	2600	2800	41-45	1800	2000	2200
46-50	2200	2400	2800	46-50	1800	2000	2200
51-55	2200	2400	2800	51-55	1600	1800	2200
56-60	2200	2400	2600	56-60	1600	1800	2200
61-65	2000	2400	2600	61-65	1600	1800	2000
66-70	2000	2200	2600	66-70	1600	1800	2000
71-75	2000	2200	2600	71-75	1600	1800	2000
76 and up	2000	2200	2400	76 and up	1600	1800	2000

Source: USDA

Recommended calories per day based on sex, age, and activity level.

Sedentary: Engages in less than 30 minutes a day of moderate physical exercise
Mod. Active: Engages in 30 to 60 minutes a day of moderate physical exercise
Active: Engages in at least 60 minutes a day of moderate physical exercise

A.8 Macronutrition and Weight Loss

There are over a thousand diet books now on the market, and many of these provide recommendations that differ widely from solid science.[854] In fact, many authors even ridicule current scientific research while basing their program on either old science or unsubstantiated theories. But it is poor logic to throw out all of established medicine just because you have points of disagreement. Many of the originators of current popular diet and health programs, by discarding most established scientific guidelines, have thrown out the good information along with the bad. They are standing on very shaky ground as they go from one fad to another.

A very important question to ask yourself is this: "What makes a program successful?" Is it how much weight you lose in the shortest time period? Is it how much temporary energy you have? Is it how much weight you can lose after three months? Or is it something other than what the magazines and tabloids babble about, like how much weight you can lose *and keep off forever* while staying away from diseases that can harm you?

Most of the popular diet programs cause you to lose weight very rapidly, short-term. Sadly, these programs either cause you to lose water and muscle weight, or else put such demands on your body that they can be very risky. You should not define the success of a program in terms of how fast you lose weight or how many pounds you can shed in ninety days. Success should be defined by how much weight you can lose and keep off forever. An example of long-term success comes from the U.S. National Weight Control Registry,[855] which has followed thousands of people who have maintained an average weight loss of 13.6 kg (or thirty pounds) over an average of 5½ years. These people had a diet of approximately 24 percent of calories from fat, 19 percent of calories from protein and 56 percent of calories from carbohydrates. The National Weight Control Registry is not theoretical; it observes people who have had proven success. Their intake of food macronutrients fit within those recommendations of the Institute of Medicine and our guidelines—not those of the extreme low-fat or low-carb programs.

Essentially all other popular diets and lifestyle programs have weight loss or weight management as their main goal, and these have often made percentages of macronutrients (carbohydrate, fat, and protein) the key element of their instruction. Most diet and lifestyle programs can be divided up into three basic categories. The first category is extremely low-fat and low-calorie diets. The second category is extremely low-carbohydrate and lower-calorie diets that replace carbohydrates with either fat or protein. The third category utilizes more of a balanced macronutrient intake and lower calories. As we have seen from an article in JAMA,[856] all of the popular diets provide modestly reduced body weight after one year, but there is no selective advantage for one program over another as far as weight loss is concerned. All of the promises of miracle breakthroughs and claims of selective advantages of their particular diet have proven to be untrue.

This study from JAMA that I just quoted is very powerful for many reasons. First of all, participants were randomly selected for the weight loss programs. Previous research concerning certain diet programs involved individuals who already believed in the program and would therefore be biased. It's not surprising that these biased participants would lose weight over a short time period. Second, the JAMA study followed the programs for one year. Most all of the previous research followed participants in diet programs for only three months, which is too short a time. It is certainly possible to lose weight on almost any program in three months. I could market a pickle or celery diet and people who believed in it would lose weight in three months. Third, the researchers noted carefully the numbers of participants who did not complete the study. By the end of one year, half the people following the more extreme diets (low-fat and low-carb) had dropped out and resumed eating as they had before. Of those following the more moderate diets, only 35 percent stopped the program by the end of one year.

Also, there is significant confusion over the definition of a low-carbohydrate diet. The term "low-carb" has been horribly misused and misunderstood. I recently saw a cable TV program on which presenter praised low-carb diets and gave examples of how to prepare them. Then he proceeded to stir-fry some vegetables. Apparently he is very uninformed concerning carbohydrates! Many vegetables are mainly carbohydrates. I would agree that he had prepared a wonderful, healthy meal, but the people on his program who lost weight did it primarily with complex carbohydrates.

There are bad carbohydrates and good carbohydrates. (See Appendix C to learn about glycemic index and load, which will help you understand the difference between good and bad carbs.) The bad ones are simple sugars and carbohydrates with high glycemic index. In general, complex carbohydrates are the good ones. Complex carbohydrates include whole-grain breads, whole-grain cereals, fruits, and vegetables. Please don't let these uninformed fad authors chase you away from incredibly valuable food. Whole grains and complex carbohydrates protect you from heart disease, cancer, diabetes, and other chronic diseases. Please don't let their lack of knowledge cause you any more confusion. Just like the extremely low-fat diets of the past caused people to neglect omega-3, today's low-carb diets cause you to miss whole grains, fruits, and vegetables.

The low-carb fad can be downright dangerous when complex carbohydrates are replaced with harmful fats, like trans fatty acids. Adopt such a diet and you will lose the protection from chronic disease contained in whole grains and the phytonutrients of fruits and vegetables, replacing them with fats that increase inflammation and advance chronic diseases such as heart disease, type 2 diabetes, and cancer. The originator of much of this work created his diet program long before the understanding of inflammation's contribution to chronic disease was available, and his work is very outdated scientifically.

Other authors have replaced carbohydrates with high-protein foods. But it is important to realize that there are good and bad sources of protein. All of the essential amino acids that are required for normal growth and metabolism can be obtained from nonfat milk or soy products. They can also be obtained from beans if you're knowledgeable. Extremely high protein intake, even if it is from a safe source, is unsupported in scientific literature. With extreme protein intake, you will be missing much of the complex carbohydrate nutrient protection necessary to reduce the risk of chronic disease. According to the Institute of Medicine of the National Academies,[857] Acceptable Macronutrient Distribution Range (AMDR) for protein is 10 to 35 percent for adults. The AMDR for young children is 5 to 20 percent, and for older children it's 10 to 30 percent.

If the diet program you've been following recommends a protein intake out of this range, its authors do not have the scientific background to prove their stance. In addition, the AMDR for fat is 20 to 35 percent and for carbohydrate is 45 to 65 percent of calories for adults.

The majority of popular diet programs have given only lip service to total bodily health. Their authors have proposed narrowly focused and sometimes dangerous methods for reducing weight, as though weight loss by any means were the key to improved health. In fact, most of these authors promote their ideas as if all good health revolved around their diets. Tragically, though, most of the programs have not taken your total health into consideration; they have made recommendations that can even worsen it.

For those of you who have tried many weight-loss programs without long-term success, there is hope. You will need to approach this program not as a temporary change in diet, but a true and permanent change of your lifestyle. Begin slowly with a few changes now, then make a few more changes later. Be patient. Throw away your bathroom scale; you shouldn't focus on measuring your weight loss. Your focus should simply be on reducing your risk factors. Do that, and then watch what happens to your body. It will be exciting, and after a while you'll become used to all the changes you've made. You won't feel as if it's work or sacrifice. That is when you'll have reached optimal health.

If you have not been successful with weight loss and your health is getting worse, it is most likely because you're not living a lifestyle that will reduce inflammation. You can't live two contradictory lifestyles simultaneously and expect to be successful. The steps taken by the people in the U.S. National Weight Control Registry have led part of the way in the right direction. They have a good start that the rest of us need to follow, then go beyond. **Your main focus should be on the prevention of chronic disease, not weight reduction.** Reconstruct your thinking! I know that's not easy for some of us to do, but it is necessary if you want to be successful with weight management and achieving optimal health.

A.9 Cytokines and the Innate Immune System

Cytokines are a structurally diverse group of chemicals. These chemicals have elaborate, abstruse names, like tumor necrosis factor alpha (tnf-alpha), interleukin-1, interleukin-6, interleukin-8, and interleukin-12. All of these cytokines have important local and total-body effects. I'll explain some of those effects here, so you can have an idea of the kind of good they do—and how they can hurt you if they are produced in excess. I'll even use some symbols, so you can understand at a glance what some of these chemicals do:

| MOVES CELLS THROUGH WALLS | MAKES BLOOD VESSELS LEAK | STIMULATES ACTIVITY | ATTRACTS | INCREASES TEMPERATURE |

Interleukin-1 (IL-1)

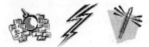

IL-1 turns on certain immune system cells (lymphocytes) that destroy certain kinds of tissue. It allows white blood cells to move through blood vessel walls so they can fight infections in adjacent tissue. It increases body temperature, which helps kill germs, triggers the adaptive immune response, stimulates the bone marrow to make more white blood cells and stimulates the release of CRP and other highly active proteins. Also, IL-1 produces IL-6.

Interleuken-6 (IL-6)

IL-6 increases body temperature, triggers the adaptive immune response, stimulates white blood cell production and activation, and stimulates releases of active proteins like CRP.

Interleuken-8 (IL-8)

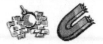

IL-8 attracts, gathers, and activates white blood cells and helps them transfer through blood vessel walls.

Interleuken-12 (IL-12)

IL-12 incites natural killer cells to kill at a rate between twenty and one hundred times higher than normal.

Tumor Necrosis Factor Alpha (TNF-alpha)

TNF-alpha increases the ability of blood vessels to leak (which is a good thing when it comes to normal immune system function), increases the ability of white blood cells to transfer across blood vessel walls and triggers local blood clotting in small vessels. The clotting action helps prevent infections from entering the bloodstream. (However, if too much TNF-alpha is released, this clotting can cause shock and the failure of vital organs.) It also raises body temperature, stimulates the adaptive immune system, increases white blood cell production, and causes active proteins like CRP to be released.

Cytokines also activate complement proteins that increase the activity of the immune system. Conversely, one pathway of complement activation (alternative) is part of the innate immunity and can stimulate cytokine release. So this is kind of a circular switch system, in which many switches control other switches.

A.10 Labeling and Definitions of Organic Food Products

If a product claims to be "100 % organic"
1. It *must* be 100 percent organic, not counting water or salt.
2. It *must* show an ingredient statement if it consists of more than one ingredient.
3. It *must* list the Certifying Agent that certified the product as organic.
4. It *may* use the term "100 percent organic."
5. It *may* use the "USDA organic" seal and/or that of the Certifying Agent that works with the USDA.

If a product claims to be "organic"
1. It *must* contain at least 95 percent organic ingredients, not counting water or salt.
2. It *must not* contain added sulfites.
3. It *may* contain up to 5 percent non-organically produced ingredients.
4. It *must* list the Certifying Agent that certified the product as organic.
5. It *may* use the term "organic" to modify the product name.
6. It *may* use the "USDA organic" seal and/or that of the certifying agent that works with the USDA.

If a product claims to be "made with organic ingredients"
1. It *must* contain at least 70 percent organic ingredients.
2. It *must not* contain added sulfites.
3. It *may* contain up to 30 percent non-organically produced ingredients.
4. It *must* list the organic ingredients as "organic" when other organic labeling is shown.
5. It *must* list the Certifying Agent that certified the product as organic.
6. It *may* use the phrase "made with organic _____."
7. It *may* use the Certifying Agent seal but must not use the "USDA organic" seal.

If the product claims to have *some* organic ingredients
1. It *may* contain less than 70 percent organic ingredients.
2. It *may* contain over 30 percent non-organically produced ingredients.
3. It *must* list the organic ingredients as "organic" when other organic labeling is shown.
4. It *must not* have the "USDA organic" seal, the Certifying Agent seal or any other reference to organic contents.

Source: www.ams.usda.gov/nop/ProdHandlers/labelTable.htm

Appendix B

B.1 Food Contents to Avoid

There are many ingredients listed on food packages that you should reduce or avoid. **This does not mean that you can't have any food containing these ingredients, but that reduction or control is wise.** You can eat anything on this list as long as you monitor its amount and eat it sparingly.

Avoid or eat sparingly: ingredients and foods that are high in saturated fat, artificial trans fats, and preservatives

1. Hydrogenated Fats/Partially Hydrogenated Oils—the number-one source of artificial trans fat
2. Palm oil
3. Coconut oil
4. Lard
5. Shortening
6. The phrase "One or more of the following oils" (chances are the company put a drop of canola oil into a vat of lard.)
7. Whole milk (go for low-fat or nonfat and look for organic to avoid added chemicals and hormones)
8. Cream
9. Milk fat
10. Buttermilk
11. Butter
12. Stick margarine (look for margarine in a tub and make sure it has no trans fats)
13. Cheese (look for low-fat versions)
14. Egg yolks (especially if not free-range organic)
15. Beef and other dark meats (Occasional intake is OK, especially if they are free range.)
16. Pork (Pigs are cute, but they are the garbage disposals of the barnyard. They will literally eat garbage, animal waste,

and things that other animals have rejected. They can accu
mulate higher levels of chemicals, hormones, etc., in their
meat. Be careful of any animal that is the garbage disposal of
its environment, for example, certain shellfish and catfish.)

17. Bacon (There are about fifteen reasons for not eating bacon.
Try a veggie substitute.)
18. Hot dogs (This is how meat packing plants get rid of their
garbage.)
19. Hamburgers
20. Pepperoni, salami, baloney, and any other preserved meats
(If bacteria aren't even interested, then it's probably not
good for you.)
21. Sausage (another word for preservatives)

Avoid or eat sparingly: pre-prepared/packaged foods that are often
sources of saturated and/or trans fats, too much salt, and lots of preservatives (Try to eat fresh whenever possible!)

1. Biscuit and cake mixes
2. Cinnamon rolls
3. Corn/potato/tortilla chips (look for baked varieties)
4. Doughnuts
5. Flavored popcorn
6. Pastries
7. Cookies

Consume only moderately: ingredients that are high in omega-6 fatty
acids (Instead, emphasize sources of monounsaturated and omega-3
polyunsaturated fatty acids such as olive oil and canola oil.)

1. Corn oil
2. Cottonseed oil
3. Sunflower oil
4. Safflower oil
5. Peanut oil
6. Sesame oil

7. Grapeseed oil

8. Soybean oil (Soybeans are OK, though.)

Cooking methods that can signal bad things:

1. "Deep fried"
2. "Fried"
3. "Smoked"
4. "Alfredo"

Other ingredients to watch out for:

1. High-fructose corn syrup (HFCS) (Lots of reasons to not use this. It has been associated with increased risk of obesity, increased risk of diabetes, accelerating the aging process,[858] increasing inflammation,[859] increasing triglycerides, and increasing harmful LDL cholesterol,[860, 861] among other suspected problems.)

2. Salt

3. Sugar

4. Enriched wheat (This means all natural, beneficial ingredients have been removed and it needs enrichment to have any significant value.)

5. "Multigrain" (Often manufacturers have taken the beneficial ingredients out of several grains, leaving only enriched grains. They use the word "multigrain" as advertising, but there is still very little natural vitamin and mineral content left in the product. The term "whole grain" usually indicates much better nutritional value.)

6. Non-diet soft drinks, as they contain way too much sugar

7. Alcohol (Everyone in the world has heard about the benefits of red wine but the greatest benefit most likely is resveratrol, which is in the grape skin and can be obtained by drinking grape juice.)

8. Artificial sweeteners (Avoid overuse and try to emphasize Splenda®, which is also referred to as "sucralose," when you do need one since it has the strongest support for safety.

Aspartame's safety should be rechecked, especially for children of early age. For Stevia®, the U.S. FDA and European Community Scientific panel declared it unsafe for food. It comes from the stevia plant and has two main chemicals: stevioside and rebaudioside A. Stevioside didn't appear to be an increased risk of cancer. Rebaudioside A has apparently never been tested for cancer risk, and some soft drink companies plan to use this as their form of Stevia®. So use it sparingly until adequate testing has been done.)[862]

9. Chemicals in general (Generally good to not consume products with many chemicals because some increase inflammation.)

    a. Butylated Hydroxyanisole (BHA) (The Department of Health and Human Services considers BHA to be "reasonably anticipated to be a human carcinogen.")

    b. Cyclomate (May increase the potency of other carcinogens.)

    c. Sodium benzoate (When used with ascorbic acid— which is safe by itself— the sodium benzoate can form small amounts of harmful a chemical, benzene. It may be safe without the ascorbic acid.)

    d. Sodium nitrite, sodium nitrate (Preserves red color in meat. They can break down to nitrosamines, which are harmful chemicals.)

For additional information about product safety, you may want to check www.cspinet.org/reports/chemcuisine.htm. This list is not exhaustive, but it should provide enough guidelines to protect you from many harmful foods.

When you first look at food labels, it will seem like every food item you use has at least one of the above products in it. Don't panic. It takes some time and patience to find them, but there are many manufacturers who produce common, ordinary products or meals that are prepared in a healthy way. The health-food section of large grocery stores is a good place to start. Be careful, though; just because it's in the health-food section doesn't mean it's healthy. You still need to be careful to avoid the contents listed above. It may seem frustrating at first, but hang in there. Your health is worth it. You can spend a little time now to find good quality foods, or you can spend time and money later to treat the diseases the bad foods tend to increase.

Don't be afraid to try non-meat products, like vegetarian burgers or bacon. Many people have even found they like the taste of the vegetable substitute better!

B.2 Plastic Food Container Safety

The containers our food and drinks come in are also very important. Some plastics have a warning on them cautioning us against using the container in the microwave oven or in dishwashers. Some of you may have ignored these warnings, thinking that if the cheap piece of plastic melted, you'd just throw it away. But it turns out that those little warnings that you can just barely read may be incredibly important. One example is a chemical commonly added to plastics called Bisphenol A.

Bisphenol A (BPA) was originally developed as a synthetic estrogen in the 1930s. When a similar chemical was found to cause cancer, BPA was taken out of medical use. In the 1950s, it was found that BPA helped to harden plastics. The only problem is that when food is heated in the plastic container or put in a dishwasher, the BPA comes out of the plastic and can enter your food. BPA has been shown to increase the risk of breast cancer and prostate cancer in rats.[863]

Here's what we recommend:

1. Avoid plastic containers with recycling numbers 7, 6, and 3 on the bottom. (These are the numbers used in the U.S., but you should check your own government guidelines if you live elsewhere.)
2. Store or prepare food in glass, porcelain, or stainless steel.
3. Don't microwave plastic food containers or wash them in the dishwasher.
4. Use polyethylene terephthalate (PETE) instead of polycarbonate plastic. In the U.S., PETE has the recycling number 1 on it. Number 2 is OK as well.

B.3 Omega-3 Fish Consumption Guidelines

Many sources of seafood have been contaminated with mercury, which damages the nervous system and the brain. This is especially true for developing children. Pregnant or nursing women or children:

1) Shouldn't eat fish that have a high mercury content—swordfish, tilefish or king mackerel.
2) Shouldn't eat more than 12 oz a week of seafood that's low in mercury—salmon, catfish, shrimp, and canned light tuna.
3) Shouldn't eat more than 1½ oz per week of tuna steak or canned albacore for every 50 pounds (24 kg) of body weight.

Everyone else can eat more fish, but safety standards aren't known for sure.

B.4 Optimal Health Revolution Modification of the USDA "My Pyramid" 2,000-Calorie Menu

There are many health and weight-loss programs that provide very specific diets for their readers, but that is not my purpose here. In fact, I believe that the main reason many people quit diet programs is that the menus provided are too restrictive or complicated.

The purpose of Appendix B.4 is twofold. First, I want to provide general guidelines so that you can tailor your menu to fit your natural preferences. Second, I want to show how I would modify a very sound program ("My Pyramid" from the U.S. Department of Agriculture[864]) to make it fit the teachings I've provided throughout this book. I will list the 2,000-calorie "My Pyramid" menu in the left column below, with the corresponding changes that I would make in the right column. These guiding principles will demonstrate how you might approach your menu planning.

One caveat: 2,000 calories may not be the intake you personally need to maintain or lose weight, so please determine your caloric intake as shown in chapter 11, then make appropriate adjustments.

If your current eating habits are not as good as the "My Pyramid" diet, I suggest that you begin your new lifestyle by following the principles of that diet. Remember, you don't have to be perfect to improve your health, and following most of the "My Pyramid" diet would be a great step toward optimal health. Any dietary changes will at first seem awkward. Just keep going, because these changes will soon seem normal to you.

If you already have taken some solid steps toward eating a good diet, then focus on the Optimal Health Revolution modifications. These recommendations will take you to a new level of healthy eating, and will significantly reduce the inflammation associated with chronic disease.

If these changes are too hard for you, relax. Any step you take is helpful. Feel proud of the changes that you have made, and take more steps when you are able. Please don't obsess over the foods and menus. Eating should be fun, not stressful. Remember, good eating habits are only one of the pillars of optimal health. Don't put all your efforts here. Keep your eyes on the larger picture of optimal health.

Most people have found the following dietary guidelines surprisingly simple, tasty and easy to follow. I think you will be pleasantly surprised.

USDA "MY PYRAMID" SEVEN-DAY 2,000-CALORIE DIET	OPTIMAL HEALTH REVOLUTION MODIFICATIONS

Day 1

BREAKFAST	BREAKFAST
Breakfast Burrito:	**Breakfast Burrito:**
1 flour tortilla (7" diameter)	1 organic whole-grain tortilla
1 scrambled egg (in 1 tsp soft margarine)	1 organically raised free-range chicken egg high in omega-3 or organic egg whites (in olive oil)
1/3 cup black beans (low salt)	1/3 cup black beans (low salt)
2 tbsp salsa	diced green and red peppers
1 cup orange juice	1/4 cup diced olives
1 cup fat-free milk	1/4 cup diced tomato
	2 tbsp organic salsa
LUNCH	
Roast Beef Sandwich:	1 whole orange
1 whole-grain sandwich bun	1 cup organic fat-free milk
3 oz lean roast beef	
2 slices tomato	MIDMORNING SNACK
1/4 cup shredded romaine lettuce	1 cup organically grown carrots
1/8 cup sautéed mushrooms (in 1 tsp oil)	1 medium apple
1½ oz part-skim mozzarella cheese	
1 tsp yellow mustard	LUNCH
	Roast Beef Sandwich:
¾ cup baked potato wedges	1 whole-grain sandwich bun
1 tbsp ketchup	3 oz organically grown lean beef
1 unsweetened beverage	2 slices tomato
	1/4 cup mixed baby greens or spinach
DINNER	1/8 cup sautéed mushrooms (in 1 tsp olive or canola oil)
Stuffed Broiled Salmon:	1½ oz organic skim mozzarella cheese
5 oz salmon filet	1 tsp yellow mustard
1 oz bread stuffing mix	
1 tbsp chopped onions	
1 tbsp diced celery	1½ cups steamed frozen mixed veggies
2 tsp canola oil	1 plum
½ cup saffron (white) rice	2 cups green tea or coffee
1 oz slivered almonds	
½ cup steamed broccoli (with 1 tsp soft margarine)	
1 cup fat-free milk	

USDA "MY PYRAMID" SEVEN-DAY 2,000-CALORIE DIET	OPTIMAL HEALTH REVOLUTION MODIFICATIONS
Day 1 (con't)	

SNACKS	**AFTERNOON SNACK**
1 cup cantaloupe	1 banana
	DINNER
	Broiled Pacific Salmon:
	5 oz Pacific or Norwegian salmon filet sautéed in 2 tsp canola or olive oil
	½ cup wild rice
	1 cup steamed broccoli
	1 tsp vegetable oil spread with no trans fats (non-hydrogenated)
	1 cup fat-free organic milk
	SNACKS
	1 cup cantaloupe

Day 2	

BREAKFAST	**BREAKFAST**
Hot Cereal:	Hot Cereal:
½ cup cooked oatmeal	1 cup cooked oatmeal
2 tbsp raisins	¼ cup dried figs
1 tsp soft margarine	1 tsp vegetable oil spread
	1 tsp flaxseeds
½ cup fat-free milk	
1 cup orange juice	½ cup fat-free organic milk
	1 whole orange
	1 cup green tea or coffee
	MIDMORNING SNACK
	1 cup celery sticks with 1 tbsp canola oil–based dressing/dip

USDA "MY PYRAMID" SEVEN-DAY 2,000-CALORIE DIET	OPTIMAL HEALTH REVOLUTION MODIFICATIONS

Day 2 (con't)

LUNCH	**LUNCH**
Taco Salad:	**Taco Salad:**
2 oz tortilla chips	2 oz organic whole-grain tortilla
2 oz ground turkey sautéed in 2 tsp	chips made with canola oil or whole-
sunflower oil	grain pita bread
½ cup black beans (low salt)	2 oz ground turkey sautéed in 2 tsp
½ cup iceberg lettuce	canola or olive oil
2 slices tomato	½ cup black beans (low salt)
1 oz low-fat cheddar cheese	½ cup mixed baby greens
2 tbsp salsa	2 slices tomato
½ cup avocado	1 oz low-fat soy cheddar cheese
1 tsp lime juice	2 tbsp organic salsa
	½ cup avocado
1 unsweetened beverage	1 tsp lime juice
	1 unsweetened beverage
DINNER	½ cup grapes
Spinach Lasagna:	
1 cup lasagna noodles, cooked (2 oz	**AFTERNOON SNACK**
dry)	1 cup snap peas
⅔ cup spinach	
½ cup ricotta cheese	**DINNER**
½ cup tomato sauce with tomato bits	**Spinach Lasagna:**
1 oz part-skim mozzarella cheese	1 cup whole-grain lasagna noodles,
	cooked (2 oz dry)
1 whole-wheat dinner roll	⅔ cup spinach
1 cup fat-free milk	½ cup low-fat organic cottage cheese
	½ cup organic tomato sauce
	1 oz soy mozzarella cheese
SNACKS	
½ oz dry-roasted almonds	½ cup steamed green beans
¼ cup pineapple	1 whole-wheat dinner roll
2 tbsp raisins	1 cup fat-free milk
	SNACKS
	½ oz walnuts
	¼ cup pineapple
	1 cup blackberries

USDA "MY PYRAMID" SEVEN-DAY 2,000-CALORIE DIET	OPTIMAL HEALTH REVOLUTION MODIFICATIONS
Day 3	

BREAKFAST	**BREAKFAST**
Cold Cereal:	**Cold Cereal:**
1 cup bran flakes	1 cup organic whole-grain cereal
1 cup fat-free milk	1 cup fat-free organic milk
1 small banana	1 small banana or peach
	1 tsp flaxseeds
1 slice whole-wheat toast	
1 tsp soft margarine	1 slice whole-wheat toast
	1 tsp vegetable oil spread
1 cup prune juice	
	3 prunes
	1 cup green tea
LUNCH	
Tuna Sandwich:	**MIDMORNING SNACK**
2 slices rye bread	1 cup broccoli with 1 tbsp canola
3 oz tuna (packed in water, drained)	oil–based dressing/dip
2 tsp mayonnaise	
1 tbsp diced celery	**LUNCH**
¼ cup shredded romaine lettuce	**Tuna Sandwich:**
2 slices tomato	2 slices rye bread
	3 oz tuna (packed in water, drained)
1 medium pear	2 tsp canola-based mayonnaise
1 cup fat-free milk	1 tbsp diced celery
	¼ cup shredded mixed baby greens
DINNER	2 slices tomato
Roasted Chicken Breast:	
3 oz boneless, skinless chicken breast	1 medium pear
	1 cup fat-free milk
1 large baked sweet potato	
	AFTERNOON SNACK
½ cup peas and onions	1 cup fresh cherries
1 whole-wheat dinner roll	
1 tsp soft margarine	
1 cup leafy greens salad	
3 tsp sunflower oil and vinegar dressing	

USDA "My Pyramid" Seven-Day 2,000-Calorie Diet	Optimal Health Revolution Modifications
Day 3 (con't)	
Snacks	**Dinner**
¼ cup dried apricots	**Roasted Chicken Breast:**
1 cup low-fat fruited yogurt	3 oz boneless, skinless, organically grown chicken breast
	1 large baked sweet potato
	½ cup peas and onions
	1 whole-wheat dinner roll
	1 tsp vegetable spread
	1 cup mixed baby green salad
	3 tsp canola oil and vinegar dressing
	1 cup coffee
	Snacks
	¼ cup dried apricots
	²/₃ medium papaya
Day 4	
Breakfast	**Breakfast**
1 whole-wheat English muffin	1 whole-wheat English muffin
2 tsp soft margarine	1 tsp vegetable spread
1 tbsp jam or preserves	2 tsp jam or preserves
1 medium grapefruit	1 medium grapefruit
1 hard-cooked egg	1 hard-cooked egg from free-range,
1 unsweetened beverage	organically grown chicken
	1 cup tomato juice (low salt)
Lunch	
White Bean Vegetable Soup:	**Midmorning snack**
1¼ cup chunky vegetable soup	½ of 5" diameter cantaloupe
½ cup white beans	
2 oz breadsticks	
8 baby carrots	
1 cup fat-free milk	

USDA "MY PYRAMID" SEVEN-DAY 2,000-CALORIE DIET	OPTIMAL HEALTH REVOLUTION MODIFICATIONS

DINNER	**LUNCH**
Rigatoni with Meat Sauce:	**White or Pinto Bean Vegetable Soup:**
1 cup rigatoni pasta (2 oz dry)	1¼ cup chunky vegetable soup
½ cup tomato sauce with tomato bits	½ cup white or pinto beans
2 oz extra lean cooked ground beef	
(sautéed in 2 tsp vegetable oil)	2 oz whole-grain bread or bread-
3 tbsp grated Parmesan cheese	sticks
	8 baby carrots
	1 cup fat-free organic milk
Spinach Salad:	
1 cup baby spinach leaves	**AFTERNOON SNACK**
½ cup tangerine slices	1 large pear
½ oz chopped walnuts	
3 tsp sunflower oil and vinegar	**DINNER**
dressing	**Rigatoni with Meatless Veggie Sauce:**
	1 cup whole-grain rigatoni pasta (2
1 cup fat-free milk	oz dry)
	½ cup organic tomato sauce
	2 oz meatless veggie substitute
SNACKS	3 tbsp fresh Parmesan cheese
1 cup low-fat fruit yogurt	
	Spinach Salad:
	1 cup baby spinach leaves
	½ cup tangerine slices
	½ oz chopped walnuts
	3 tsp canola oil and vinegar dressing
	1 cup steamed kale
	1 cup fat-free organic milk
	SNACKS
	½ cup soy vanilla frozen dessert (ice-cream substitute)
	½ cup blueberries

USDA "MY PYRAMID" SEVEN-DAY 2,000-CALORIE DIET	OPTIMAL HEALTH REVOLUTION MODIFICATIONS

Day 5

BREAKFAST

Cold Cereal:
1 cup puffed wheat cereal
1 tbsp raisins
1 cup fat-free milk
1 small banana

1 slice whole wheat toast
1 tsp soft margarine
1 tsp jelly

LUNCH

Smoked Turkey Sandwich:
2 oz whole-wheat pita bread
¼ cup romaine lettuce
2 slices tomato
3 oz sliced smoked turkey breast
1 tbsp mayo-type salad dressing
1 tsp yellow mustard

½ cup apple slices
1 cup tomato juice (low salt)

DINNER

Grilled Top Loin Steak:
5 oz grilled top loin steak

¾ cup mashed potatoes
2 tsp soft margarine

½ cup steamed carrots
1 tbsp honey

2 oz whole-wheat dinner roll
1 tsp soft margarine

1 cup fat-free milk

BREAKFAST

Cold Cereal:
1 cup organic whole-grain cereal
½ cup red grapes
1 cup fat-free organic milk
1 tsp flaxseeds
1 small banana

1 slice whole grain toast
1 tsp vegetable spread
1 tsp jelly

MIDMORNING SNACK

1 cup broccoli with 1 tbsp canola-based dressing/dip

LUNCH

Turkey Sandwich:
2 oz whole-grain pita bread
¼ cup mixed baby greens
2 slices tomato
3 oz sliced organically grown, oven-roasted turkey breast
1 tsp canola oil–based mayo spread
1 tsp yellow mustard

½ cup apple slices
1 cup tomato juice (low salt)

AFTERNOON SNACK

1 cup fresh carrots

USDA "MY PYRAMID" SEVEN-DAY 2,000-CALORIE DIET	OPTIMAL HEALTH REVOLUTION MODIFICATIONS
Day 5 (con't)	

SNACKS
1 cup low-fat fruited yogurt
	DINNER
	Waldorf Salad:
	    2 cups mixed baby greens
	    ¼ sliced apple
	    4 sliced strawberries
	    8 sliced red grapes
	    2 tbsp chopped walnuts
	    2 tbsp canola or olive oil–based dressing
	    4 oz sliced grilled organic skinless chicken
	
	    2 oz whole-wheat dinner roll
	    1 tsp vegetable spread
	
	    1 cup fat-free organic milk
	
	SNACKS
	4" wedge of honeydew melon

Day 6	

BREAKFAST
French Toast:
    2 slices whole-wheat French toast
    2 tsp soft margarine
    2 tbsp maple syrup
 	
    ½ medium grapefruit
    1 cup fat-free milk
	BREAKFAST
	French Toast:
	    2 slices whole-grain bread dipped in
	    1 egg (from free range, organic chicken)
	    2 tsp vegetable spread
	    1 tbsp pure maple syrup
	
	    1 orange
	    1 cup fat-free organic milk
	
	MIDMORNING SNACK
	1 large pear

USDA "My Pyramid" Seven-Day 2,000-Calorie Diet	Optimal Health Revolution Modifications
Day 6 (con't)	

LUNCH
Vegetarian Chili on Baked Potato:

1 cup kidney beans (low salt)
½ cup tomato sauce with tomato bits
3 tbsp chopped onions
1 oz low-fat cheddar cheese
1 tbsp vegetable oil
1 medium baked potato

½ cup cantaloupe
¾ cup lemonade

DINNER
Hawaiian Pizza:

2 slices cheese pizza
1 oz Canadian bacon
¼ cup pineapple
2 tbsp mushrooms
2 tbsp chopped onions

Green Salad:

1 cup leafy greens
3 tsp sunflower oil and dressing

1 cup fat-free milk

SNACKS
5 whole wheat crackers (low salt)
⅛ cup hummus
½ cup fruit cocktail (in water or juice)

LUNCH
Vegetarian Chili on Baked Potato:

1 cup kidney beans (low salt)
½ cup organic tomato sauce
3 tbsp chopped onions
1 oz soy cheddar cheese
1 tbsp canola or olive oil
1 medium baked potato

½ cup steamed lima beans
½ cup cantaloupe
¾ cup fresh-squeezed lemonade

AFTERNOON SNACK
1⅔ cup fresh raspberries

DINNER
Vegetarian Burger:

1 whole-grain hamburger bun
1 cup mixed baby greens
1 vegetarian meatless patty
2 tbsp mushrooms cooked in olive or canola oil
2 slices tomatoes
1 tbsp catsup
2 tsp yellow mustard

Green Salad:

1 cup mixed baby greens
3 tsp canola oil and vinegar dressing

1 cup fat-free organic milk

SNACKS
5 whole wheat crackers (low salt)
⅛ cup organic hummus
1 peach

USDA "MY PYRAMID" SEVEN-DAY 2,000-CALORIE DIET	OPTIMAL HEALTH REVOLUTION MODIFICATIONS
Day 7	

### BREAKFAST	### BREAKFAST
Pancakes:	**Pancakes:**
3 buckwheat pancakes	3 pancakes (made from whole-grain
2 tsp soft margarine	pancake mix, 1 free-range organic
3 tbsp maple syrup	egg, 2 tsp canola oil, and ½ cup fat-free organic milk)
½ cup strawberries	2 tsp vegetable spread
¾ cup honeydew melon	2 tbsp pure maple syrup
½ cup fat-free milk	
	½ cup strawberries
	¾ cup honeydew melon
### LUNCH	½ cup fat-free milk
Manhattan Clam Chowder:	
3 oz canned clams (drained)	### MIDMORNING SNACK
¾ cup mixed vegetables	1 cup celery
1 cup canned tomatoes (low salt)	
10 whole wheat crackers	### LUNCH
	Manhattan Clam Chowder:
1 medium orange	3 oz canned clams (drained)
1 cup fat-free milk	¾ cup mixed vegetables
	1 cup canned tomatoes (low salt)
### DINNER	1 slice whole-grain bread
Vegetable Stir-Fry:	1 medium orange
4 oz tofu (firm)	1 cup fat-free milk
¼ cup green and red bell peppers	
½ cup bok choy	### AFTERNOON SNACK
2 tbsp vegetable oil	1 cup snap peas
1 cup brown rice	
	### DINNER
1 cup lemon-flavored iced tea	**Vegetable Stir-Fry:**
	4 oz organic tofu (firm)
	¼ cup green and red bell peppers
	½ cup bok choy
	2 tbsp olive or canola oil
	1 cup wild rice
	1 cup green tea

USDA "MY PYRAMID" SEVEN-DAY 2,000-CALORIE DIET	OPTIMAL HEALTH REVOLUTION MODIFICATIONS
Day 7 (con't)	
SNACKS	SNACKS
1 oz sunflower seeds	4 whole walnuts
1 large banana	1 large banana
1 cup low-fat fruited yogurt	½ cup soy frozen dessert with 1 cup blueberries

Please remember, you don't have to follow this menu perfectly. Just take the steps you can now and advance at your own pace. Another hundred pages could be written to provide exact details of nutrient intake of different caloric levels, but that is beyond the scope of this book. Enough is being provided here to give you a good foundation on which to be victorious in the revolution for optimal health.

Appendix C—Glycemic Index and Glycemic Load

Glycemic index is the relative ability of a gram of carbohydrate in food to increase the level of sugar in the blood during the first two hours after it's consumed. The first list of foods and their corresponding glycemic indexes was published over twenty years ago.[865] Foods with a high glycemic index produce higher levels of sugar in the blood than foods with low glycemic indexes. Initially there was controversy as to the significance of the concept, but it is now widely recognized as a reliable, physiologically based classification of food. The Food and Agriculture Organization of the United Nations and the World Health Organization recommends that to promote good health we need to consume a high-carbohydrate diet (> 55 percent of total calories), with the great majority of carbohydrates having a low glycemic index.[866] Generally, a glycemic index of less than 55 is considered low and more than 70 is considered high.

As noted in this book, carbohydrates with high glycemic index are associated with increased risk of heart disease[867] and diabetes.[868] Foods with low glycemic index are associated with protection from developing obesity,[869] colon cancer,[870] breast cancer,[871] ovarian cancer,[872] and stomach cancer.[873]

Glycemic load differs from glycemic index in that it is a measure of the total effect that a food has on raising the sugar level in the blood. It takes into account both the type and quantity of a sugar within a food. For example, a given fruit may have a high glycemic index because of the type of sugar it contains, yet have a relatively low glycemic load because it contains a small amount of that sugar and therefore won't raise the blood level of sugar very much. You need to know both the quality and quantity of sugar in a food to determine its total effect on the body. Generally, a glycemic load of less than 10 is low and more than 20 is high.

The glycemic index of a given food can vary depending on how it is prepared, how it is tested, and the country or region where it was grown. Breads from different manufacturers have different components and therefore different effects on the body. Fruit from different parts of the world have different sugar content based on different soils, climates, farming methods, and harvesting practices. When you use the glycemic index, first search for the country in which you live or the foods that match your normal diet. Second, look for the brand names of the products you normally purchase. If your brand has a high glycemic load, seek to replace it with a brand that has low glycemic load, or choose something else to eat.

Why I Don't Recommend a Completely Low Glycemic Load Menu

Sydney University and the Glycemic Research Service staff have done outstanding research on glycemic index. With the scientific knowledge available to them twenty years ago, they advanced this field tremendously. But the concept of chronic inflammation's role in causing chronic disease was largely unknown when they began their work. Subsequently, there are some people who have concluded that high glycemic index and load foods cause disease, but in light of the most recent research, this is where I differ.

Actually, the most recent scientific literature reveals a deeper cause of chronic disease—inflammation—which is discussed extensively throughout this book. The reason that low glycemic load diets have shown disease reduction is because they reduce inflammation, not just because they reduce the glycemic load in and of itself. It is my contention that the greatest benefit of low glycemic load diets is their reduction of inflammation. High glycemic load diets have been shown to be associated with increased inflammation.[874]

Unfortunately, I don't recommend the low glycemic load menus. They were designed with only one purpose in mind—to reduce glycemic load—but they don't necessarily reduce inflammation. For example, some menus I've seen recommend that you eat inflammatory protein like dark meat and fats because they have a low glycemic load. These menus are reasonable, but they certainly weren't designed with reduction of inflammation in mind. Therefore, please use the tables only to find low glycemic index and load carbohydrates, not for any other reason.

Now that you understand this critical point, the glycemic index tables can help you significantly reduce your risk of chronic disease. They can help you choose carbohydrates that you enjoy and that will protect you. Please use them carefully and wisely. (The tables can be found in number 76 of the *American Journal of Clinical Nutrition*, in Foster-Powell's "International table of glycemic index and glycemic load values: 2002."[875])

References

1   World Health Organization. Obesity: Preventing and Managing the Global Epidemic, Report of a WHO Consultation. Geneva: World Health Organization. WHO Technical Report Series 894; 2000.

2   King H, et al. Global burden of diabetes, 1995–2025. Diabetes Care 198; 21: 1414–1431.

3   Jemal A, et al. Trends in the leading causes of death in the United States, 1970–2002. JAMA 2005; 294: 1255–1259.

4   He J, et al. Major causes of death among men and women in China. NEJM Sept 15, 2005; 353(11): 1124–1134.

5   Braunwald E, et al. Cardiovascular medicine at the turn of the millennium: triumphs, concerns and opportunities. NEJM 1997; 337: 1360–1369.

6   Magadle R, et al. C-reactive protein levels and arterial abnormalities in the offspring of patients with premature myocardial infarction. Cardiol 2003; 100(1): 1–6.

7   Kang ES, et al. Relationship of serum high sensitivity C-reactive protein to metabolic syndrome and the microvascular complications in type 2 diabetes. Diabetes Res Clin Pract 2005 Aug; 69(2): 151–159.

8   Rohde LE, et al. Survey of C-reactive protein and cardiovascular risk factors in apparently healthy men. Am J Cardiol 1999 Nov 1; 84(9): 1018–1022.

9   Blake GJ, et al. Blood pressure, C-reactive protein, and the risk of future cardiovascular events. Circulation 2003 Dec 16; 108(24): 2993–2999.

10 Savoia C, et al. Reduction of C-reactive protein and the use of hypertensives. Vasc Health Risk Manag 2007; 3(6): 975–983.

11 Vongpatanasin W, et al. C-reactive protein causes down regulation of vascular angiotensin subtype 2 receptors and systolic hypertension in mice. Circulation 2007; 115: 1020–1028.

12 Esposito K, et al. Effect of weight loss and lifestyle changes on vascular inflammatory markers in obese women: a randomized trial. JAMA 2003 Apr 9; 289(14): 1799–1804.

13 Douglas KM, et al. Relationship between depression and C-reactive protein in a screening population. Psychosom Med 2004 Sept–Oct; 66(5): 679–683.

14 Christ-Crain M, et al. Elevated C-reactive protein and homocysteine values: Cardiovascular risk factors in hypothyroidism? A cross-sectional and a double-blind, placebo controlled trial. Atherosclerosis 2003 Feb; 166(2): 379–386.

15 Park HS, et al. Relationship of obesity and visceral adiposity with serum concentrations of CRP, TNF-alpha and IL-6. Diabetes Res Clin Pract 2005 Jul; 69(1): 29–35.

16 Black PH. The inflammatory response is an integral part of the stress response: Implications for atherosclerosis, insulin resistance, type II diabetes and metabolic syndrome. Brain Behav Immun 2003 Oct; 17(5): 350–364.

17 Mohrschladt MF, et al. C-reactive protein in patients with familial hypercholesterolemia: No effect of symvastatin therapy. Atheroscl 2001 Aug; 157(2): 491–494.

18 Tannock LR, et al. Cholesterol feeding increases C-reactive protein and serum amyloid A levels in lean insulin-sensitive subjects. Circulation 2005; 111: 3058–3062.

19 Plasma homocysteine predicts progression of atherosclerosis. Atherosclerosis 2005 Jul; 181(1): 159–165.

20 King DE, et al. The relationship between attendance at religious services and cardiovascular inflammatory markers. Int J Psychiatry Med 2001; 31(4): 415–425.

21 King DE, et al. C-reactive protein, diabetes, and attendance at religious services. Diabetes care 2002; 25(7): 1172–1176.

22 Gao X, et al. Plasma C-reactive protein and homocysteine concentrations are related to frequent fruit and vegetable intake in Hispanic and non-Hispanic white elders. J Nutr 2004 Apr; 134(4): 913–918.

23 Lopez-Garcia E, et al. Consumption of (n-3) fatty acids is related to plasma biomarker of inflammation and endothelial activation in women. J Nutr 2004; 134(7): 1806–1811.

24 Folsum AR, et al. C-reactive protein and incident coronary heart disease in Atherosclerosis

Risk In Communities (ARIC) study. Am Heart J 2002 Aug; 144(2): 233–238.

25   Erlinger TP, et al. C-reactive protein and the risk of incidence colorectal cancer. JAMA 2004; 291(5): 585–590.

26   Rohde LE, et al. Survey of C-reactive protein and cardiovascular risk factors in apparently healthy men. Am J Cardiol 1999 Nov 1; 84(9): 1018–1022.

27   Esposito K, et al. Effect of weight loss and lifestyle changes on vascular inflammatory markers in obese women: a randomized trial. JAMA 2003 Apr 9; 289(14): 1799–1804.

28   Park HS, et al. Relationship of obesity and visceral adiposity with serum concentrations of CRP, TNF-alpha and IL-6. Diabetes Res Clin Pract 2005 Jul; 69(1): 29–35.

29   Black PH. The inflammatory response is an integral part of the stress response: Implications for atherosclerosis, insulin resistance, type II diabetes and metabolic syndrome. Brain Behav Immun 2003 Oct; 17(5): 350–364.

30   King DE, et al. Relation of dietary fat and fiber to elevation of c-reactive protein. Am J Cardiol 2003 Dec 1; 92(11): 1335–1339.

31   Gao X, et al. Plasma C-reactive protein and homocysteine concentrations are related to frequent fruit and vegetable intake in Hispanic and non-Hispanic white elders. J Nutr 2004 Apr; 134(4): 913–918.

32   Volpato S, et al. Relationship of alcohol intake with inflammatory markers and plasminogen activator inhibitor-1 in well-functioning older adults: Health, Aging, and Body composition Study. Circ 2004 Feb 10; 109(5): 607–612.

33   Nettleton JA, et al. Dietary patterns are associated with biochemical markers of inflammation and endothelial activation in the Multi-Ethnic Study of Atherosclerosis (MESA). Am J Clin Nutr 2006 Jun; 83(6): 1369–1379.

34   Larrousse M, et al. Increased levels of atherosclerosis markers in salt-sensitive hypertension. Am J Hypertens. 2006 Jan; 19(1): 87–93.

35   Leung WK, et al. Transgenic cyclooxygenase expression and high salt enhanced susceptibility to chemical-induced gastric cancer development in mice. Carcinogenesis 2008 Aug; 29(8): 1648–1654.

36   Pope CA 3rd, et al. Ambient particulate air pollution, heart rate variability, and blood markers of inflammation in a panel of elderly subjects. Environ Health Perspect 2004 Mar; 112(3): 339–345.

37   Stolzenberg-Solomon RZ, et al. Meat and meat mutagen intake and pancreatic cancer risk in NHI-AARP cohort. Cancer Epidemiol Biomarkers Prev 2007 Dec; 16(12): 2664.

38   Martinez ME, et al. Meat intake, preparation methods, mutagens, and colorectal adenomas recurrences. Carcinogenesis 2007 Sep; 28(9): 2019–2027.

39   Harris RE. Cyclooxygenase-2 (Cox-2) and the inflammogenesis of cancer. Subcell Biochem 2007; 42: 93–126.

40   Urbanski A, et al. Ultraviolent light induces increased circulating interleukin-6 in humans. J Invest Dermatol 1990 Jun; 94(6): 808–811.

41   Shima M, et al. Comparative study of C-reactive protein in chronic hepatitis B and chronic hepatitis C. Tohoku J Exp Med 1996 Mar; 178(3): 287–297.

42   Timms PM, et al. Circulating MMP9, vitamin D and variation in the TIMP-1 response with VDR genotype: Mechanisms for inflammatory damage in chronic disorders? QJM 2002 Dec; 95(12): 787–796.

43   Erlinger TP, et al. C-reactive protein and the risk of incidence colorectal cancer. JAMA 2004; 291(5): 585–590.

44   Kang ES, et al. Relationship of serum high-sensitivity C-reactive protein to metabolic syndrome and microvascular complications in type 2 diabetes. Diab Res Clin Prac 2005 Aug; 69(2): 151–159.

45   Park HS, et al. Relationship of obesity and visceral adiposity with serum concentrations of CRP, TNF-alpha and IL-6. Diabetes Res Clin Pract 2005 Jul; 69(1): 29–35.

46 Gao X, et al. Plasma C-reactive protein and homocysteine concentrations are related to frequent fruit and vegetable intake in Hispanic and non-Hispanic white elders. J Nutr 2004 Apr; 134(4): 913–198.

47 Esposito K, et al. Effect of weight loss and lifestyle changes on vascular inflammatory markers in obese women: A randomized trial. JAMA 2003 Apr 9; 289(14): 1799–1804.

48 Robertson AK, et al. T cells in atherogenesis: For better or for worse? Arterioscler Thromb Vasc Biol 2006; 26: 2421–2432.

49 Frostegard J, et al. Cytokine expression in advanced human atherosclerotic plaques: dominance of pro-inflammatory (Th 1) and macrophage-stimulating cytokines. Atherosclerosis 1999; 145: 33–43.

50 Libby P. Inflammation and cardiovascular disease mechanisms. Am J Clin Nutr 2006; 83(suppl): 456–460.

51 Libby P, et al. Inflammation and atherosclerosis. Circulation 2002; 105: 1135–1143.

52 Pradhan AD, et al. C-reactive protein, interleukin-6, and the risk of developing type 2 diabetes mellitus. JAMA 2001; 286: 327–334.

53 Festa A, et al. Elevated levels of acute-phase proteins and plasminogen activator inhibitor-1 predict the development of type 2 diabetes: The insulin resistance atherosclerosis study. Diabetes 2002; 51: 1131–1137.

54 Festa A, et al. Progression of plasminogen activator inhibitor-1 and fibrinogen levels in relation to incident type 2 diabetes. Circulation 2006; 113: 1753–1759.

55 Shoelson SE, et al. Inflammation and insulin resistance. J Clin Invest 2006; 116: 1793–1801.

56 Pradhan AD, et al. C-reactive protein is independently associated with fasting insulin in non-diabetic women. Atheroscler Thromb Vasc Biol 2003; 23: 650–655.

57 Murray CJ, et al. Alternative projections of mortality and disability by cause 1990–2020: Global Burden of Disease Study. Lancet 1997; 349: 1498–1504.

58 Gunter MJ, et al. A prospective study of serum C-reactive protein and colorectal cancer risk in men. Cancer Res 2006; 66: 2483–2487.

59 Pradhan A. Obesity, metabolic syndrome and type 2 diabetes: Inflammatory basis of glucose metabolic disorder. Nutr Rev. 2007 Dec 11; 65(12): S152–S156.

60 Seddon JM, et al. Association between C-reactive protein and age-related macular degeneration. JAMA 2004 Feb 11; 291(6): 704–710.

61 Yasojima K, et al. Human neurons generate C-reactive protein and amyloid P: Upregulation in Alzheimer's disease. Brain Res 2000 Dec 22; 887(1): 80–89.

62 Vermeire S, et al. C-reactive protein as a marker for inflammatory bowel disease. Inflamm Bowel Dis 2004 Sep; 10(5): 661–665.

63 Hunot S, et al. Neuroinflammatory processes in Parkinson's disease. Ann Neurol 2003; 53 Suppl 3: S49–S58, Disc S58–S60.

64 Olafsdottir IS, et al. C-reactive protein levels are increased in non-allergic but not allergic asthma: A multicentre epidemiologic study. Thorax 2005 Jun; 60(6): 451–454.

65 Otterness IG, et al. An analysis of 14 molecular markers for monitoring osteoarthritis. Relationship of the markers to clinical endpoints. Osteoarthritis Cartilage 2001 Apr; 9(3): 224–231.

66 Van Dijk EJ, et al. C-reactive protein and cerebral small-vessel disease. Circulation 2005; 112: 900–905.

67 Itzkowitz SH, et al. Inflammation and cancer IV. Colorectal cancer in inflammatory bowel disease: The role of inflammation. Am J Physiol Gastrointest Liver Physiol 2004; 287: G7–G17.

68 Catassi C, et al. Association of celiac disease and intestinal lymphomas and other cancers. Gastroenterology 2005; 128 (Suppl): 79–86.

69 Nardone G, et al. Review article: Heliobacter pyloric and molecular events in precancerous gastric lesions. Aliment Pharmacol Ther 2004; 20: 261–270.

70   Payette H, et al. Insulin-like growth factor-1 and interleukin-6 predict sarcopenia in very old community-living men and women. The Framingham Heart Study. J Am Geriatr Soc 2003; 51: 1237–1243.

71   Sebastian C, et al. MacrophAging: A cellular and molecular review. Immunobiology 2005; 210: 121–126.

72   Linnane AW, et al. Mitochondrial DNA mutations as an important contributor to aging and degenerative diseases. Lancet 1989; 1: 642–645.

73   Wallace DC. A mitochondrial paradigm of metabolic and degenerative diseases, aging, and cancer: A dawn of evolutionary medicine. Annu Rev Genet 2005; 39: 359–407.

74   Santoro A, et al. Mitochondrial DNA involvement in human longevity. Biochem Biophys Acta 2006; 1757: 1388–1399.

75   Verma S, et al. A self-fulfilling prophecy: C-reactive protein attenuates nitric oxide production and inhibits angiogenesis. Circulation 2002; 106: 913–919.

76   Pasceri V, et al. Direct proinflammatory effects of C-reactive protein on human endothelial cells. Circulation; 102: 2165–2168.

77   Danenberg HD, et al. Increased thrombosis after arterial injury in human C-reactive protein-transgenic mice. Circulation 2003; 108: 512–515.

78   Verma, et al. C-reactive protein and atherothrombosis—Beyond a biomarker: An actual partaker of lesion formation. Am J Physiol Regul Integr Comp Physiol 2003; 285: R1253–R1256.

79   Scannapieco FA, et al. Association of periodontal infections with atherosclerotic and pulmonary diseases. J Periodontal Res 1999 Oct; 34(7): 340–345.

80   Poynter JN, et al. Statins and the risk of colorectal cancer. NEJM May 26, 2005; 352(21): 2184–2192.

81   Ridker PM, et al. Rosuvastatin to prevent vascular events in men and women with elevated C-reactive protein. N Engl J Med 2008 Nov 9;359:2195-2207.

82   Ridker PM, et al. Measurement of C-reactive protein for the targeting of statin therapy in the primary prevention of acute coronary events. N Eng J Med 2001;344:1959-1965.

83   Berger JS, et al. Aspirin for the primary prevention of cardiovascular events in women and men. JAMA 2006; 295: 306–313.

84   Jacobs EJ, et al. A large cohort study of aspirin and other nonsteroidal anti-inflammatory drugs and prostate cancer incidence. J Natl Cancer Inst July 2005; 97(13): 975–980.

85   Sansbury LB, et al. Use of nonsteroidal anti-inflammatory drugs and risk of colon cancer in a population-based, case-controlled study of African Americans and whites. Am J Epidemiol 2005 Sep 15; 162(6): 548–558.

86   The Omega Diet. 1999. HarperCollins Publishers Inc., 10 East Third St., New York, NY.

87   Chung CP, et al. High prevalence of the metabolic syndrome in patients with systemic lupus erythematosus: Association with disease characteristics and cardiovascular risk factors. Ann Rheum Dis 2007 Feb; 66(2): 208–214.

88   Pacifici R, et al. Effect of surgical menopause and estrogen replacement on cytokine release from human blood mononuclear cells. Proc Natl Acad Sci USA 1991; 88: 5134–5138.

89   Kimble RB, et al. Simultaneous block of interleukin-1 and tumor necrosis factor is required to completely prevent bone loss in the early post-ovarectomy period. Endocrinology 1995; 136: 3054–3061.

90   Ishimi Y, et al. IL-6 is produced by osteoblasts and induces bone absorption. J Immunol 1990; 145: 3297–3303.

91   Hill PA, et al. The cellular actions of interleukin-11 on bone resorption in vitro. Endocrinology 1998; 139: 1564–1572.

92   Ross R. Atherosclerosis—An inflammatory disease. N Engl J Med 1999; 340: 115–126.

93   Libby P. Inflammatory mechanisms: The molecular basis of inflammation and disease. Nutr Rev Dec 2007; (11) 65(12): S140–S146.

94   Kelley GL, et al. High dietary fructose induces a hepatic stress response resulting in choles-terol and lipid dysregulation. Endocrinology 2004; 145(2): 548–555.

95   Lopez-Garcia E, et al. Consumption of trans fatty acids is related to plasma biomarkers of inflammation and endothelial dysfunction. J Nutr 2005; 135(3): 562–566.

96   Tannock LR, et al. Cholesterol feeding increases C-reactive protein and serum amyloid A lev-els in lean insulin-sensitive subjects. Circulation 2005; 111: 3058–3062.

97   Ghosh S, et al. Elevation of C-reactive protein in serum of Channa punctatus as an indicator of water pollution. Indian J Exp. Biol. 1992 Aug; 30(8): 736–737.

98   Ford ES. Does exercise reduce inflammation? Physical activity and C-reactive protein among US adults. Epidemiology 2002; 13: 561–568.

99   Taaffe DR, et al. Cross-sectional and prospective relationships of interleukin-6 and C-reactive protein with physical performance in elderly persons: MacArthur studies of successful aging. J Gerontol A Biol Sci Med Sci 2000; 55: M709–M715.

100   Colbert LH, et al. Physical activity, exercise, and inflammatory markers in older adults: find-ings from the Health, Aging and Body Composition Study. J Am Geriatr Soc. 2004; 52: 1098–1104.

101   Church TS, et al. Reduction of C-reactive protein levels through use of a multivitamin. Am J Med 2003; 115(9): 702–707.

102   Fuller B, et al. Anti-inflammatory effects of Co Q10 and colorless carotinoids. J Cosmet Dermatol 2006 Mar; 5(1): 30–38.

103   Kritchevsky SB, et al. Serum carotenoids and markers of inflammation among nonsmokers. Am J Epidemiol. 2000 Dec 1; 152(11): 1065–1071.

104   Rayssiguier Y, et al. High fructose consumption combined with low dietary magnesium intake may increase the incidence of the metabolic syndrome by inducing inflammation. Magnes Res 2006 Dec; 19(4): 237–243.

105   Largo R, et al. Glucosamine inhibits IL-1 beta-induced NFKappa activation in human osteoarthritic chondrocytes. Osteoarthritis Cartilage 2003 Apr; 11(4): 290–298.

106   Bischoff SC. Quercetin: Potentials in the prevention and therapy of disease. Curr Opin Clin Nutr Metab Care 2008 Nov; 11(6): 733–740.

107   Gao X, et al. Plasma C-reactive protein and homocysteine concentrations are related to fre-quent fruit and vegetable intake in Hispanic and non-Hispanic white elders. J Nutr 2004 Apr; 134(4): 913–918.

108   Chen Y, et al. Are there age-related changes in flavonoids bioavailability? Phytochemicals, Aging and Health. 2008. CRC Press, Boca Raton, FL Edited by Meskin MS, et al. pgs. 19–38.

109   Rayssiguier Y, et al. High fructose consumption combined with low dietary magnesium intake may increase the incidence of the metabolic syndrome by inducing inflammation. Magnes Res 2006 Dec; 19(4): 237–243.

110   Aljada A, et al. Increase in intranuclear nuclear factor kappaB and decrease in inhibitor kappaB in mononuclear cells after a mixed meal: Evidence for a proinflammatory effect. Am J Clin Nutr 2004; 79: 682–690.

111   Ludwig DS. Glycemic load has come of age. J Nutr 2003; 133: 2695–2696.

112   Liu S, et al. Relation between a diet with a high glycemic load and plasma concentrations of high-sensitivity C-reactive protein in middle-aged women. Am J Clin Nutr 2002 Mar; 75(3): 492–498.

113   McCarty MF. Low-insulin-response diets may decrease plasma C-reactive protein by influenc-ing adipocyte function. Med Hypotheses 2005; 64: 385–387.

114   Giles JT, et al. Serious infections associated with anticytokine therapies in the rheumatic dis-eases. J Intensive Care Med 2004; 19: 320–334.

115   Sohn HY, et al. Cyclooxygenase inhibition and atherothrombosis. Curr Drug Targets 2006; 7: 1275–1284.

References

116 Juni P, et al. COX2 inhibitors, traditional NSAIDS and the heart. Brit Med J 2005; 330: 1342.

117 Gauldie J, et al. Smad3 signaling involved in pulmonary fibrosis and emphysema. Proc Am Thorac Soc 2006; 3: 696–702.

118 Langman MJS. Ulcer complications and NSAIDS. Am J Med 1998; 84(2A): 15.

119 Pathak SK, et al. Oxidative stress and cyclooxygenase activity in prostate carcinogenesis, targets for chemoprotective strategies. Eur J Cancer 2005; 41(1): 61.

120 Patel S, et al. Association between serum vitamin D metabolite levels and disease activity in patients with early inflammatory polyarthritis. Arthritis Rheum 2007 Jul; 56(7): 2143–2149.

121 Targher G, et al. Serum 25-hydroxyvitamin D3 concentrations and carotid artery intima-media thickness among type 2 diabetic patients. Clin Endocrinol (Oxf) 2006 Nov; 65(5): 593–597.

122 Pittas AG, et al. The effects of calcium and vitamin D supplementation on blood glucose and markers of inflammation in nondiabetic adults. Diabetes Care 2007 Jul; 30(7): e81.

123 Motivala SJ, et al. Sleep and immunity: Cytokine pathways linking sleep with health outcomes. Curr Dir Psychol Sci 2007; 16: 21–26.

124 Vgontzas AN, et al. Adverse effects of modest sleep restriction on sleepiness, performance and inflammatory cytokines. J Clin Endocrinol Metab 2004; 89: 2119–2126.

125 Irvin MR, et al. Sleep deprivation and activation of morning levels of cellular and genomic markers of inflammation. Arch Intern Med 2006; 166: 1756–1762.

126 Meier-Ewert HK, et al. Effect of sleep loss on C-reactive protein, an inflammatory marker of cardiovascular risk. J Am Coll Cardiol 2004; 43: 678–683.

127 Lenny WK, et al. Transgenic cyclooxygenase-2 expression and high salt enhanced susceptibility to chemical-induced gastric cancer development in mice. Carcinogenesis 2008 Aug; 29(8): 1648–1654.

128 Sabatine MS, et al. Prognostic significance of the Centers for Disease Control/American Heart Association high sensitive C-reactive protein cut points for cardiovascular and other outcomes in patients with stable coronary artery disease. Circulation 2007; 115: 1528–1536.

129 Blaine JM. Using C-reactive protein to predict cardiovascular risk in older patients. Clin Geriatrics 2007 Aug; 15(8): 20–25.

130 Weinberg RB. Apolipoprotein A-IV polymorphisms and diet-gene interactions. Curr Opin Lipidol 2002; 13(2): 125–134.

131 Jeunemaitre X, et al. Molecular basis of human hypertension. Role of angiotensinogen. Cell 1992; 71: 169–180.

132 John SWM, et al. Genetic decreases in atrial natriuretic peptide and salt sensitive hypertension. Science 1995; 267: 679–681.

133 Robinson DR, et al. Dietary marine lipids suppress the continuous expression of interleukin-1B gene transcription. Lipids 1996; 31 (Suppl): S23–S31.

134 Urakaze M, et al. Dietary marine lipids suppress IL-1B mRNA levels in lipopolysaccharide stimulated monocytes. Clin Res 1991; 23.

135 Corton JC, et al. Peroxisome proliferators—Activated receptor gamma coactivator-1 in caloric restriction and other models of longevity. J Gerontol A Biol Sci Med Sci 2005; 60: 1494–1509.

136 Forman BM, et al. Hypolipidemic drugs, polyunsaturated fatty acids, and eicosanoids are ligands for peroxisome proliferators-activated receptors alpha and delta. Proc Natl Acad Sci USA 1997; 94: 4312–4317.

137 Ulricke B, et al. Fatty acids and gene expression. In: Zempleni J, Daniel H, eds. *Molecular Nutrition*. Cambridge MA:CABl Publishing; 2003: 121–134.

138 Hayes CE, et al. The immunological functions of the vitamin D endocrine system. Cell Mol Biol 2003; 49(2): 277–300.

139 Ames BN, et al. High-dose vitamin therapy stimulates variant enzymes with decreased coen-

zyme binding affinity (increased K[m]): Relevance to genetic disease and polymorphisms. Am J Clin Nutr 2002; 75(4): 616–658.

140 Hatakeyama D, et al. Zinc suppresses IL-6 synthesis by prostaglandin F2alpha in osteoblasts: Inhibition of phospholipase C and phospholipase D. J Cell Biochem 2002; 85(3): 621–628.

141 Li Y, et al. Vitamin E suppression of microglial activation is neuroprotective. J Neurosci Res 2001; 66(2): 163–170.

142 Booth FW, et al. Exercise and gene expression: Physiological regulation of the human genome through physical activity. J of Physiology 2002; 543: 399–411.

143 Booth FW, et al. Exercise controls gene expression. American Scientist 2005; 93: 28–35.

144 Lampe JW, et al. Brassica, biotransformation and cancer risk: genetic polymorphisms alter the preventive effects of cruciferous vegetables. J Nutr 2002; 132(10): 2991–2994.

145 Komatsu K, et al. Inhibitory action of (-)-epigallocatechin gallate on a radiation induced mouse oncogenic transformation. Cancer Lett 1997; 112(2): 135–139.

146 Shen F, et al. Suppression of IL-8 gene transcription by resveratrol in phorbol ester treated human monocytic cells. J Asian Nat Prod Res 2003; 5(2): 151–157.

147 Chen C, et al. Induction of detoxifying enzymes by garlic organosulfur compounds through transcription factor Nrf2: Effect of chemical structure and stress signals. Free Radic Biol Med 2004; 37(10): 1578–1590.

148 Aneja R, et al. Theaflavin, a black tea extract, is a novel anti-inflammatory compound. Crit Care Med 2004; 32(10): 2097–2103.

149 Kelley GL, et al. High dietary fructose induces a hepatic stress response resulting in cholesterol and lipid dysregulation. Endocrinology 2004; 145(2): 548–555.

150 Lai CQ, et al. Dietary intake of n-6 fatty acids modulates effects of apolipoprotein A5 gene on plasma fasting triglycerides, remnant lipoprotein concentrations, and the lipoprotein particle size. The Framingham Heart Study. Circulation 2006; 113: 2062–2070.

151 Estruch R, et al. Effects of a Mediterranean-style diet on cardiovascular risk factors: A randomized trial. Ann Int Med 2006; 145: 1–11.

152 Gibney M. Lipogene: An integrated project of the EU Sixth Framework Programme for Research and Technology Development (2004–2009). Available at www.ucd.ie/lipogene.

153 Nutrigenetics and Nutrigenomics. Simopoulis AP, et al (eds). 2004 Vol. 93. Karger, Basel, Switzerland.

154 Chodorowski Z, et al. Longevity of physicians and medical students born from 1880 to 1904 Przegl Lek 2003; 60(4): 249–250.

155 Sri Kantha S. Centenarian scientists: an unusual cluster newly formed in the 20th century. Med Hypothesis 2001; 57(6): 750–753.

156 Nishi M, et al. Lifespan of Japanese male medical doctors. J Epidemiol 1999; 9(5): 315–319.

157 Tai YT, et al. Adverse effects from traditional Chinese medicine: A critical reappraisal. J Hong Kong Med Assoc. 1993 pt; 45(3): 197–201.

158 Keen RW, et al. Indian herbal remedies for diabetes as cause of lead poisoning. Postgrad Med J 1994; 70: 113–114.

159 Nortier JL, et al. Urothelial carcinoma associated with the use of Chinese herb (Aristolochia Fangchi). NEJM 2000 Jun; 342(23): 1686–1892.

160 Ospina MB, et al. Meditation practices for health: State of the research. Evid Rep Technol Assess (Full Rep). 2007 Jun; (155): 1–263.

161 Wild S, et al. Global prevalence of diabetes. Diabetes May 2004; 27(5): 1047–1053.

162 www.who.int/chp/chronic_disease_report/en.

163 USA Today 1/9/07 Page 1.

164 Palinski W, et al. Developmental programming: Maternal hypercholesterolemia and immunity influence susceptibility to atherosclerosis. Nutr Rev Dec 2007(11); 65(12): S182–S187.

165 Romero R, et al. Inflammation in pregnancy: Its roles in reproductive physiology, obstetrical complications and fetal injury. Nutr Rev Dec 2007 (11); 65(12): S194–S202.

166 Insall W Jr,, et al. The fatty acids of human milk from mothers on diets taken ad libitum. Biochem J 1959; 72: 27–33.

167 Innis SM. Polyunsaturated fatty acids in human milk: An essential role in infant development. Adv Exp Med Biol 2004; 554: 27–43.

168 Innis SM. Human milk and formula fatty acids. J Pediatr 1992; 120(42): 56–61.

169 Kennedy ET, et al. Popular diets: Correlation to health, nutrition and obesity. J Am diet Assoc. 2001; 101: 411–420.

170 Andersen RE, et al. Effects of lifestyle activity versus structured aerobic exercise in obese women. JAMA 1999; 281: 335–340.

171 Hu FB, et al. Television watching and other sedentary behavior in relation to risk of obesity and type 2 diabetes mellitus in women. JAMA 2003 Apr 9; 289(14): 1785-91.

172 Howard RA, et al. Physical activity, sedentary behavior, and the risk of colon and rectal cancer in the NIH-AARP Diet and Health Study. Cancer Causes Control 2008 Nov;19(9):939-53.

173 Podewils LJ, et al. Physical activity, APOE genotype, and dementia risk; findings from the Cardiovascular Health Cognition Study. Am J Epidemiol. 2005 April; 161(7): 639-51.

174 Lee IM, et al. Physical activity and coronary heart disease in women: is "no pain, no gain" passé? JAMA 2001 Mar 21; 285(11): 1447-54.

175 Lee CD, et al. Physical activity and stroke risk: a meta-analysis. Stroke 2003 Oct;34(10): 2475-81.

176 Hooker SP, et al. Cardiorespiratory fitness as a predictor of fatal and nonfatal stroke in asymptomatic women and men. Stroke 2008 Aug [Epub ahead of print].

177 Nelson ME, et al. Effects of high-intensity strength training on multiple risk factors for osteoporotic fractures. A randomized controlled trial. JAMA 1994 Dec 28; 272(24): 1909-14.

178 Manini T, et al. Daily activity energy expenditure and mortality among older adults. JAMA 2006; 296: 171–179.

179 Shephard RJ, et al. Maximal oxygen uptake and independence in old age. Br J Sports Med 2008 April [Epub ahead of print].

180 Ford ES. Does exercise reduce inflammation? Physical activity and C-reactive protein among US adults. Epidemiology 2002; 13: 561–568.

181 Taaffe DR, et al. Cross-sectional and prospective relationships of interleukin-6 and C-reactive protein with physical performance in elderly persons: MacArthur studies of successful aging. J Gerontol A Biol Sci Med Sci 2000; 55: M709–M715.

182 Colbert LH, et al. Physical activity, exercise, and inflammatory markers in older adults: Findings from the Health, Aging and Body Composition Study. J Am Geriatr Soc 2004; 52: 1098–1104.

183 Benbrook C, et al. New evidence confirms the nutritional superiority of plant-based organic foods. 2008 Mar; www.organic-center.org.

184 Seo M, et al. Enhancing effect of chlorinated organic solvents on histamine release and inflammatory mediator production. Toxicology 2008 Jan 14; 243(1–2): 75–83.

185 Gao X, et al. Plasma C-reactive protein and homocysteine concentrations are related to frequent fruit and vegetable intake in Hispanic and non-Hispanic white elders. J Nutr 2004 Apr; 134(4): 913–918.

186 Osganian SK, et al. Vitamin C and the risk of coronary heart disease in women. J Am Coll Ccardiol 2003; 42(2): 246–252.

187 Spiegel K, et al. Brief communication: Sleep curtailment in healthy young men is associated with decreased leptin levels, elevated ghrelin levels, and increased hunger and appetite. Ann Intern Med. 2004 Dec 7; 141(11): 846–850.

188 Hublin C, et al. Sleep and mortality: A population-based 22-year follow-up study. Sleep 2007; 30: 1245–1253.

189 Belenky G, et al. Patterns of performance degradation and restoration during sleep restriction

and subsequent recovery: A sleep dose-response study. J Sleep Res 2003; 12: 1–12.

190 Van Dongen HP, et al. The cumulative cost of additional wakefulness: Dose-response effects on neurobehavioral functions and sleep physiology from chronic sleep restriction and total sleep deprivation. Sleep 2003; 26: 117–126.

191 Van Cauter E, et al. Roles of circadian rhythmicity and sleep in human glucose regulation. Endocrinology Reviews 1997; 18: 716–738.

192 Schibler U. Circadian time keeping: The daily ups and downs of genes, cells and organisms. Prog Brain Res 2006; 153: 271–282.

193 Motivala SJ, et al. Sleep and immunity: cytokine pathways linking sleep and health outcomes. Curr Dir Psychol Sci 2007; 16: 21–26.

194 Vgontzas AN, et al. Adverse effects of modest sleep restriction on sleepiness, performance and inflammatory cytokines. J Clin Endocrinol Metab 2004; 89: 2119–2126.

195 Irvin MR, et al. Sleep deprivation and activation of morning levels of cellular and genomic markers of inflammation. Arch Intern Med 2006; 166: 1756–1762.

196 Meier-Ewert HK, et al. Effect of sleep loss on C-reactive protein, an inflammatory marker of cardiovascular risk. J Am Coll Cardiol 2004; 43: 678–683.

197 Shamsuzzaman AS, et al. Elevated C-reactive protein in patients with obstructive sleep apnea. Circulation 2002; 105: 2462–2464.

198 Gangwisch JE, et al. Inadequate sleep as a risk factor for obesity: Analysis of NHANES 1. Sleep 2005; 28: 1289–1296.

199 Tamakoshi A, et al. Self-reported sleep duration as a predictor of all-cause mortality: Results from the JACC study, Japan. Sleep 2004; 27: 51–54.

200 Dominici F, et al. Fine particulate air pollution and hospital admission for cardiovascular and respiratory diseases. JAMA 2006; 295: 1127–1134.

201 Lynch DJ. Pollution poisons China's progress. USA Today, July 4, 2005.

202 www.cbsnews.com/stories/2008/03/10/health/main3920454.shtml.

203 USA Today, April 22, 2008.

204 Perez-de-Albeniz. Int J Psychotherapy March 2000; 5(1): 49–59.

205 Ospina MB, et al. Meditation Practices for Health: State of the Research Evidence Report/Technological Assessment No. 155. (Prepared by the University of Alberta Evidence-based Practice Center under Contract No. 290-02-0023.) AHRQ Publication No. 07-E010. Rockville, MD: Agency for Healthcare Research and Quality. June 2007.

206 Diaz JR, et al. Micronutrient deficiencies in developing and affluent countries. Eur J Clin Nutr 2003; 57 Suppl 1: S70–S72.

207 Mandelbaum-Schmid J. Vitamin and mineral deficiencies harm one-third of the world's population, says new report. Bull World Health Organ 2004; 82(3): 230–231.

208 Black R. Micronutrient deficiency—An underlying cause of morbidity and mortality. Bull World Health Organ 2003; 81(2): 79.

209 Macfarlane GD, et al. Hypovitaminosis D in a normal, apparently healthy urban European population. J Steroid Biochem Mol Biol 2004; 89–90(1–5): 621–622.

210 Fraser DR. Vitamin D deficiency in Asia. J Steroid Biochem Mol Biol 2004; 89–90(1–5): 491–495.

211 Nesby-O'Dell S, et al. Hypovitaminosis D prevalence and determinants among African-American and white women of reproductive age: Third National Health and Nutrition Examination Survey, 1988 to 1994. Am J Clin Nutr 2002; 76(1): 187–192.

212 Diaz JR, et al. Micronutrient deficiencies in developing and affluent countries. Eur J Clin Nutr 2003; 57 Suppl 1: S70–S72.

213 Stephenson LS, et al. Global malnutrition. Parisitology 2000; 121 Suppl: S5–S22.

214 Ge KY, et al. Dietary intake of some essential micronutrients in China. Biomed Environ Sci 2001; 14(4): 318–324.

215 Ramakrishnan U. Prevalence of micronutrient malnutrition worldwide. Nutr Rev 2002;60(5

Pt 2): S46-52.

216 Lewis SM, et al. Assessment of antioxidant nutrient intake of a population of southern US African-American and Caucasian women of various ages when compared to dietary reference intakes. J Nutr Health Aging 2003; 7(2): 121–128.

217 Ervin RB, et al. Mineral intakes of elderly adult supplement and non-supplement users in the third national health and nutrition examination survey. J Nutr 2002; 132(11): 3422–3427.

218 Matsumura Y. Nutrition trends in Japan. Asia Pac J Clin Nutr 2001; 10 Suppl: S40–S47.

219 Bates CJ, et al. Micronutrients: highlights and research challenges from the 1994–5 National Diet and Nutrition Survey of people aged 65 years and over. Br J Nutr 1999; 82(1): 7–15.

220 Ames BN, et al. Are vitamin and mineral deficiencies a major cancer risk? Nat Rev Cancer 2002; 2(9): 694–704.

221 Hampl JS, et al. Vitamins C deficiency and depletion in the United States: The Third National Health and Nutrition Examination Survey, 1988–1994. Am J Public Health 2004; 94(5): 870–875.

222 Fletcher RH, et al. Vitamins for chronic disease prevention in adults. JAMA 2002; 287: 3127–3129.

223 Radimer K, et al. Dietary supplement use by US adults: Data from the National Health and Nutrition Examination Survey, 1999–2000. Am J Epiemiol 2004; 160(4): 339–349.

224 Ervin RB, et al. Prevalence of leading types of dietary supplements used in the Third National Health and Nutrition Examination Survey, 1988–94. Adv Data 2004; (349): 1–7.

225 Hensrud, D, et al. Underreporting the use of dietary supplements and nonprescription medications among patients undergoing a periodic health examination. Mayo Clin Proc 1999; 74: 443–447.

226 Beitz R, et al. Use of vitamin and mineral supplements in Germany. Bundesgesundheitsblatt Gesundheitsforschung Gesundheitsschutz 2004; 47(11): 1057–1065.

227 Kim SH, et al. Use of vitamins, minerals, and other dietary supplements by 17- and 18-year-old students in Korea. J Med Food 2003; 6(1): 27–42.

228 Knudsen VK, et al. Use of dietary supplements in Denmark is associated with health and former smoking. Public Health Nutr. 2002; 5(3): 463–468.

229 Troppmann L, et al. Natural health product use in Canada. Can J Public Health 2002; 93(6): 426–430.

230 Horwath CC, et al. Dietary supplement use in a randomly selected group of elderly Australians. Results from a large nutrition and health survey. J Am Geriatr Soc 1989; 37(8): 689–696.

231 Chan K. Some aspects of toxic contamination in herbal medicines. Chemosphere 2003; 52(9): 1361.

232 Antioxidant supplements for prevention of gastrointestinal cancers: A systematic review and meta-analysis. Lancet 2004; 364: 1219–1228.

233 The HOPE and HOPE-TOO Trial Investigators. Effects of long-term vitamin E supplementation on cardiovascular events and cancer. JAMA 2005; 293: 1338–1347.

234 Bonaa KH, et al. Norvit Trial Investigators. Homocysteine lowering and cardiovascular events after myocardial infarction. NEJM April 13, 2006; 354(15): 1578–1588.

235 Loscalzo J. Homocysteine trials: Clear outcomes for complex reasons. NEJM April 13, 2006; 354(15): 1629–1632.

236 Chambers JC, et al. Plasma homocysteine concentrations and the risk of coronary heart disease in UK Indian Asian and European men. Lancet 200; 355: 523–527.

237 Ferguson LR. Dissecting the nutrigenomics, diabetes, and gastrointestinal disease interface: From risk assessment to health intervention. OMICS 2008 Aug 19 [Epub ahead of print.]

238 Winichagoon P. Limitations and resolutions for dietary assessments of micronutrient intake. Asia Pac J Clin Nutr 2008; 17 Suppl 1: 296–298.

239 Ames, BN. DNA damage from micronutrient deficiencies is likely to be a major cause of can-

cer. Mutat Res 2001 Apr 18; 475(1–2): 7–20.

240 Giovannucci E. Tomatoes, tomato-based products, lycopene and cancer: Review of the epidemiological literature. J Natl Cancer Inst 1999 Feb 17: 91(4): 317–331.

241 Aalinkeel R, et al. The dietary bioflavenoid quercetin selectively induces apoptosis in prostate cancer cells by down-regulating the expression of heat shock protein 90. Prostate 2008 Aug 25 [Epub ahead of print].

242 Rossebo AB, et al. N Engl J Med 2008 Sept 25; 359(13): 1343–1356.

243 Dietary Supplements Cause 600 'Adverse Events'. USA Today Sept 23 2008.

244 Newman DJ, et al. Natural products as sources of new drugs over the period of 1981–2002. J Nat Prod 2003; 66: 1022.

245 Newman DJ, et al. Natural products as sources of new drugs over the last 25 years. J Nat Prod 2007; 70: 461.

246 Dove A. Drug screening–Beyond the bottleneck. Nat Biotechnol 1999; 17(9): 859.

247 Saper, RB, et al. Heavy metal content of Ayurvedic herbal medicine products. JAMA 2004 Dec 15; 292(23): 2868–2873.

248 Yoong JKC. Heavy-metal meals of mercury. NEJM Jan 19, 2006; 354: e3.

249 Khandpur S, et al. Chronic arsenic toxicity from Ayurvedic medicines. Int J Dermatol 2008 Jun; 47(6): 618–621.

250 Church TS, et al. Reduction of C-reactive protein levels through use of a multivitamin. Am J Med 2003; 115(9): 702–707.

251 French AE, et al. Folic acid fortification is associated with a decline in neuroblastoma. Clin Pharmacol Ther 2003 Sep; 74(3): 288–294.

252 Koren G. Fam Prac News. July 1, 2006:39.

253 Ames BN. DNA damage from micronutrient deficiencies is likely to be a major cause of cancer. Mutat Res 2001 Apr 18; 475(1–2): 7–20.

254 Prisco D, et al. Effect of medium-term supplementation with a moderate dose of n-3 polyunsaturated fatty acids on blood pressure in mild hypertensive patients. Thromb Res 1998; 1(3): 105–112.

255 Storlien LH, et al. Fatty acids, triglycerides and syndromes of insulin resistance. Prostaglandins Leukot Essen Fatty Acids 1997 Oct; 57(4–5): 379–385.

256 Lopez-Garcia E, et al. Consumption of (n-3) fatty acids is related to plasma biomarker of inflammation and endothelial activation in women. J Nutr 2004; 134(7): 1806–1811.

257 Bucher HC, et al. N-3 polyunsaturated fatty acids in coronary heart disease: A meta-analysis of randomized controlled trials. Am J Med 2002; 112: 298–304.

258 Morris MC, et al. Consumption of fish and n-3 fatty acids and risk of incident Alzheimer disease. Arch Neurol 2003 Jul; 60(7): 940–946.

259 Sampath H, et al. Polyunsaturated fatty acid regulation of gene expression. Nutr Rev 2004 Sep; 62(9): 333–339.

260 Corton JC, et al. Peroxisome proliferator-activated receptor gamma coactivator 1 in caloric restriction and other models of longevity. J Gerontol A Biol Sci Med Sci 2005; 60: 1494–1509.

261 Forman BM, et al. Hypolipidemic drugs, polyunsaturated fatty acids, and eicosanoids are ligands for peroxisome proliferators-activated receptors alpha and delta. Proc Natl Acad Sci USA 1997; 94: 4312–4317.

262 Ulrike B, et al. Fatty acids and gene expression. In: Zempleni J, Daniel H, eds. Molecular Nutrition. Cambridge MA: CABl Publishing; 2003: 121–134.

263 Anderson P, et al. Endogenous anti-inflammatory neuropeptides and proresolving lipid mediators: A new therapeutic approach for immune disorders. J Cell Mol Med 2008 June 12 [Epub ahead of print].

264 Hall MN, et al. A 22-year prospective study of fish, N-3 fatty acid intake, and colorectal cancer risk in men. Cancer Epidemiol Biomarkers Prev 2008 May; 17(5): 1136–1143.

References

265 Edwards IJ, et al. Omega-3 fatty acids and PPAP gamma in cancer. PPAR Res 2008; 2008: 358052.

266 *The Omega Diet*. 1999. HarperCollins Publishers Inc., 10 East Third St, New York, NY.

267 Teegarden D. Calcium intake and reduction in weight or fat mass. J Nutr 2003 Jan; 133(1): 249S–251S.

268 http://ods.od.nih.gov/factssheets/calcium.asp. Accessed August 7, 2005.

269 Slattery M, et al. Lifestyle and colon cancer: An assessment of factors associated with risk. Am J Epidemiol 1999; 150: 869–877.

270 Kampman E, et al. Calcium, vitamin D, sunshine exposure, dairy products and colon cancer risk. Cancer Causes Control 2000; 11: 459–466.

271 Biasco G, et al. European trials on dietary supplementation for cancer prevention. Ann N Y Acad Sci 1999; 8889: 152–156.

272 Cunnane SC, et al. High alpha-linolenic aacid flaxseed (Linum usitastissimum): Some nutritional properties in humans. Br J Nutr 1993; 69: 443–453.

273 Homocysteine Lowering Trialists' Collaboration. Lowering blood homocysteine with folic acid based supplements: Meta-analysis of randomized trials. BMJ 1998; 316: 894–898.

274 Giovannucci E, et al. Multivitamin use, folate, and colon cancer in women in the Nurse's Health Study. Ann Intern Med 1998; 129(7): 517–524.

275 Shirodaria C, et al. Global improvement of vascular function and redox state with low dose folic acid. Circulation 2007; 115: 2262–2270.

276 de Bree A, et al. Folic acid improves vascular reactivity in humans: A meta-analysis of randomized controlled trials. Am J Clin Nutr 2007 Sept; 83(3): 610–617.

277 Martins D, et al. Prevalence of cardiovascular risk factors and the serum levels of 25-hydroxyvitamin D in the United States–Data from the Third National Health and nutrition Examination Survey. Arch Int Med 2007; 167: 1159–1165.

278 Schauber J, et al. The vitamin D pathway: A new target for the control of the skin's immune response? Exp Dermatol 2008 Jun 18 [Epub ahead of print].

279 Ingraham BA, et al. Curr Med Res Opin 2008 Jan; 24(1): 139–149.

280 Krishnan AV, et al. Calcitrol as a chemoprotective and therapeutic agent in prostate cancer: Role of anti-inflammatory activity. J Miner Res 2007 Dec 22 Suppl 2: v74–80.

281 Dobnig H, et al. Independent association of low serum 25-hydroxyvitamin D and 1,25 dihydroxyvitamin D levels with all-cause and cardiovascular mortality. Arch Intern Med 2008 Jun 23; 168(12): 1340–1349.

282 Melamed ML, et al. 25-hydroxyvitamin D levels and the risk of mortality in the general population. Arch Intern Med 2008 Aug 11; 168(15): 1629–1637.

283 Rabinovitz H, et al. Blood glucose and lipid levels following chromium supplementation in diabetic elderly patients on rehabilitation program. Program Abstracts, 53rd Annual Scientific Meeting. Gerontological Society of America. Gerontologist 2000; 40: 38.

284 Anderson RA, et al. Elevated intakes of supplemental chromium improve glucose and insulin variables in individuals with Type II diabetes. Diabetes 1997; 46: 1786–1791.

285 Ludwig DS, et al. Dietary fiber, weight gain, and cardiovascular disease risk in young adults. JAMA 1999 Oct 27; 282(16): 1539–1546.

286 Jensen MK, et al. Intakes of whole grains, bran, and germ and the risk of coronary heart disease in men. Am J Clin Nutr 2004 Dec; 80(6): 1492–1499.

287 Lopez-Ridaura R, et al. Magnesium intake and risk of type 2 diabetes in men and women. Diabetes Care 2004 Jan; 27(1): 134–140.

288 Rayssigquier Y, et al. High fructose consumption combined with low dietary magnesium intake may increase the incidence of the metabolic syndrome by inducing inflammation. Magnes Res 2006 Dec; 19(4): 237–243.

289 Soja AM, et al. Treatment of congestive heart failure with coenzyme Q10 illuminated by meta-analysis of clinical trials. Mol Aspects Med 1997; 18: S159–S168.

290 Singh RB, et al. Effect of hydrosoluble coenzyme Q10 on blood pressures and insulin resistance in hypertensive patients with coronary artery disease. J Hum Hypertens 1999; 13: 203–208.

291 Burke BE, et al. Randomized, double-blind, placebo-controlled trial of coenzyme Q10 in isolated systolic hypertension. South Med J 2001; 94: 1112–1117.

292 Shults CW, et al. Effects of coenzyme Q10 in early Parkinson's disease: Evidence of slowing the functional decline. Arch Neurol 2002; 59: 1541–1550.

293 Fuller B, et al. Anti-inflammatory effects of CoQ10 and colorless carotenoids. J Cosmet Dermatol 2006 Mar; 5(1): 30–38.

294 Lonn E, et al. Effects of long-term vitamin E supplementation on cardiovascular events and cancer: A randomized controlled trial. JAMA Mar 16, 2005; 293(11): 1338–1347.

295 Schutte AE, et al. Cardiovascular effects of oral supplementation of vitamin C, E and folic acid in young healthy males. Int J Vitam Nutr Res 2004 Jul;74(4):285-95

296 Singh U, et al. Vitamin E, oxidative stress, and inflammation. Annu Rev Nutr 2005; 25: 151–174.

297 Wu D, et al. Age-associated increase in PGE2 synthesis and COX activity in murine macrophages is reversed by vitamin E. Am J Physiol 1998; 275(3pt1): c661–c668.

298 Chan JM, et al. Supplemental vitamin E intake and prostate cancer risk in a large cohort of men in the United States. Cancer Epidemiol Biomarkers Prev 1999; 8: 893–899.

299 Pelucchi C, et al. Dietary intake of selected micronutrients and gastric cancer risk: An Italian case-controlled study. Ann Oncol Jul 31, 2008 [Epub ahead of print].

300 Masaki KH, et al. Association of vitamin E and C supplement use with cognitive function and dementia in elderly men. Neurology 2000; 54: 1265–1272.

301 Ravaglia G, et al. Effect of micronutrient status on natural killer cell immune function in healthy free-living subjects aged >/= 90y. Am J Clin Nutr 2000; 71: 590–598.

302 Lu QY, et al. Inverse associations between plasma lycopene and prostate cancer. Cancer Epidemiol Biomarkers Prev 2001; 10: 749–756.

303 Michaud DS, et al. Intake of specific carotenoids and risk of lung cancer in 2 prospective US cohorts. Am J Clin Nutr 2000; 72: 990–997.

304 Giovannucci E. Tomatoes, tomato-based products, lycopene and cancer: Review of the epidemiological literature. J Natl Cancer Inst Feb 17, 1999; 91(4): 317–331.

305 Kritchevsky SB, et al. Serum carotenoids and markers of inflammation among non-smokers. Am J Epidemiol Dec 1, 2000; 152(11): 1065–1071.

306 Imai K, et al. Cross-sectional study of effects of drinking green tea on cardiovascular and liver diseases. BMJ 1995; 310: 693–696.

307 Inoue M, et al. Regular consumption of green tea and the risk of breast cancer recurrence: Follow-up study from the Hospital-based Epidemiologic Research Program at Aichi Cancer Center (HERPACC), Japan Cancer Lett 2001; 167: 175–182.

308 Bushman JL. Green tea and cancer in humans: A review of the literature. Nutr Cancer 1998; 31(3): 151–159.

309 Nemecz G. Green tea. US Pharmacist, May 2000: 67–70.

310 Ross GW, et al. Association of coffee and caffeine intake with the risk of Parkinson's disease. JAMA 2000; 238: 2674–2679.

311 Pan T, et al. Potential therapeutic properties of green tea polyphenols in Parkinson's disease. Drugs Aging 2003; 20(10): 711–721.

312 Dai Q, et al. Fruit and vegetable juices and Alzheimer's disease. The Kame Project Am J Med Sep 2006; 119(9): 751–759.

313 Commenges D, et al. Intake of flavonoids and risk of dementia. Eur J Epidemiol Apr 2000; 16(4): 357–363.

314 Bastianetto S, et al. Neuroprotective effects of green and black teas and their catechin gallate esters against beta-amyloid-induced toxicity. Eur J Neurosci Jan 2006; 23(1): 55–64.

315 Choi YT, et al. The green tea polyphenols (-)-epigallocatechin gallate attenuates beta-amyloid-induced neurotoxicity in cultured hippocampal neurons. Life Sci Dec 21, 2001; 70(5): 603–614.

316 Ono K, et al. Potent anti-amyloidogenic and fibril-destabilizing effects of polyphenols in vitro. Implications for the prevention and therapeutics of Alzheimer's disease. J Neurochem Oct 2003; 87(1): 172–181.

317 Riviere C, et al. Inhibitory activity of stilbenes on Alzheimer's beta-amyloid fibrils in vitro. Bioorg Med Chem Jan 15, 2007; 15(2): 1160–1167.

318 Hsu S, et al. Chemoprotective effects of green tea polyphenols correlate with reversible induction of p57 expression. Anticancer Res 2001; 21: 3743.

319 Hsu S, et al. Green tea polyphenol targets the mitochondria in tumor cells inducing caspase 3-dependant aptosis. Anticancer Res 2003; 23: 1533.

320 Ahmed S, et al. Green tea polyphenol epigallocatechin-3-gallate (EGCG) differentially inhibits interleukin-1 beta-induced expression of matrix metalloproteinase-1 and -13 in human chondrocytes. J Pharmacol Exp Ther 2004; 308: 767.

321 Tedeschi E, et al. Green tea inhibits human inducible nitric-oxide synthase expression by down-regulating signal transducer and activator of transcription-1 alpha activator. Mol Pharmacol 2004; 61: 111.

322 Ackermann RT, et al. Garlic shows promise for improving some cardiovascular risk factors. Arch Intern Med 2001; 161: 813–824.

323 Ibid.

324 Key TJ, et al. A case-control study of diet and prostate cancer. Br J Cancer 1997; 76: 678–687.

325 Clark LC, et al. Decreased incidence of prostate cancer with selenium supplementation: Results of a double-blind cancer prevention trial. Br J Urol 1998; 81: 730–734.

326 Rayman MP. The importance of selenium to human health. Lancet 2000; 356: 233–241.

327 Correa P, et al. Chemoprevention of gastric dysplasia: Randomized trial of antioxidant supplements and anti-Heliobacter pylori therapy. J Natl Cancer Inst 2000; 92: 1881–1888.

328 Yokoyama T, et al. Serum vitamin C concentration was inversely associated with subsequent 20-year incidence of stroke in a Japanese rural community: The shibata study. Stroke 2000; 31: 2287–2294.

329 Solonen JT, et al. Antioxidant Supplementation in Atherosclerosis Prevention (ASAP) study: A randomized trial of the effect of vitamin E and vitamin C on the 3-year progression of carotid atherosclerosis. J Intern Med 2000; 248: 377–386.

330 Knekt P, et al. Antioxidant vitamins and coronary heart disease risk: A pooled analysis of 9 cohorts. Am J Clin Nutr 2004 Dec; 80(6): 1508–1520.

331 Pavelka K, et al. Glucosamine sulfate use and delay of progression of knee osteoarthritis: A 3-year, randomized, placebo-controlled, double-blind study. Arch Int Med 2002; 162: 2113–2123.

332 Largo R, et al. Glucosamine inhibits IL-1beta-induced NFKappaB activation in human osteoarthritic chondrocytes. Osteoarthritis Cartilage Apr 2003; 11(4): 290–298.

333 Faith SA, et al. Resveratrol suppresses nuclear factor-kappa B in herpes simplex virus infected cells. Antiviral Res 2006; 72: 242–251.

334 Aviram M, et al. Pomegranate phenolic antioxidant activities protect against cardiovascular disease. In: Phytochemicals, Aging and Health. 2008. CRC Press. Meskin MS, Bidlack WR, and Randolph RV. Boca Raton, FL. 135–154.

335 Aviram M, et al. Pomegranate juice consumption for 3 years by patients with carotid artery stenosis reduces common carotid intima-media thickness, blood pressure and LDL oxidation. Clin Nutr 2004: 24, 423.

336 Cole GM, et al. Neuroprotective effects of curcumin. Adv Exp Med Biol. 2007; 595: 197.

337 Al-Omar FA, et al. Immediate and delayed treatments with curcumin prevent fore-brain ischemia-induced neuronal damage and oxidative insult in rat hippocampus. Neurochem

Res 2006; 31: 611.

338 Xu Y, et al. Curcumin reverses impaired hippocampal neurogenesis and increases serotonin receptor 1A mRNA and brain-derived neurotrophic expressor in chronically stressed rats. Brain Res 2007; 116: 9.

339 Panchal H, et al. The antiproliferative and antioxidant curcumin influences gene expression of C6 rat glioma in vitro. Exp Gerontol 2007; 42: 1.

340 Mainster MA. Violet and blue light blocking interocular lenses: Photoprotection versus photoreception. Br J Ophthalmol 2006; 90(6): 784–792.

341 Kim SR, et al. Photooxidation of A2-PE a photoreceptor outer segment fluorophore and protection by lutein and zeaxanthin. Exp Eye Res 2006; 82(5): 828–839.

342 Bastianetto S, et al. The ginkgo biloba extract (EGb 761) protects hippocampal neurons against cell death induced by B-amyloid. Eur J Neurosci Jun 2000; 12(6): 1882–1890.

343 Yao Z, et al. The ginkgo biloba extract EGb 761 rescues the Pc12 neuronal cells from beta-amyloid induced cell death by inhibiting the formation of beta-amyloid-derived diffusible neurotoxic ligands. Brain Res Jan 19, 2001; 889(1–2): 181–190.

344 Stackman RW, et al. Prevention of age-related spatial memory deficits in a transgenic mouse model of Alzheimer's disease by chronic ginkgo biloba treatment. Exp Neurol Nov 2003; 184(1): 510–520.

345 Bischoff SC. Quercetin: Potentials in the prevention and therapy of disease. Curr Opin Clin Nutr Metab Care 2008 Nov; 11(6): 733–740.

346 Aalinkeel R, et al. The dietary bioflavonoid quercetin selectively induces apoptosis in prostate cancer cells by down-regulating the expression of the heat shock protein 90. Prostate Aug 25, 2008 [Epub ahead of print].

347 Acta Ophthalmol Scan 1998; 76: 224–229.

348 Leeuwen R, et al. Dietary intake of antioxidants and risk of age-related macular degeneration JAMA 2005; 294: 3101–3107.

349 Kirsh VA, et al. Supplemental and dietary Vitamin E, beta-carotene and Vitamin C intakes and prostate cancer risk. J Natl Cancer Inst Feb 15, 2006; 98(4): 245–254.

350 Wei EK, et al. Plasma Vitamin B6 and the risk of colorectal cancer and adenoma in women. J Natl Cancer Inst May 4, 2005; 97(9): 684–692.

351 Albert CM, et al. Dietary alpha-linolenic acid intake and the risk of sudden cardiac death and coronary heart disease. Circulation 2005; 112: 3232–3238.

352 Cochrane Database Syst. Rev 2004; 1: CD004526: Cochrane Database Syst. Tev 2001; 1: CD000227.

353 Bischoff-Ferrari HA, et al. Fracture prevention with Vitamin D supplementation: A meta-analysis of randomized controlled trials. JAMA May 11, 2005; 293: 2257–2264.

354 Forman JD. 2006 American Society for Hypertension. Family Practice News, July 1, 2006; 14.

355 Pittas AG, et al. The effects of calcium and vitamin D supplementation on blood glucose and markers of inflammation in nondiabetic adults. Diabetes Care Jul 2007; 30(7): e81.

356 Altman RD, et al. Commentary: Osteoarthritis of the knee and glucosamine. Osteoarthritis cartilage Jul 17, 2006: Epub.

357 Largo R, et al. Glucosamine inhibits IL-1beta-induced NFkappaB activation in human osteoarthritic chondrocytes. Osteoarthritis Cartilage Apr 2003; 11(4): 290–298.

358 Shults CW, et al. Effects of coenzyme Q10 in early Parkinson's disease: Evidence of slowing the functional decline. Arch Neurol 2002; 59: 1541–1550.

359 Patter GR, et al. Chromium picolinate positively influences the glucose transporter system via affecting cholesterol homeostasis in adipocytes cultured under hyperglycemic diabetic conditions. Mutat Res Jul 24, 2006; Epub.

360 Braunwald E, et al. Cardiovascular medicine at the turn of the millennium: Triumphs, concerns and opportunities. NEJM 1997; 337: 1360–1369.

361 Acton RT, et al. Genetics and cardiovascular disease. Ethn Dis 2004 Autumn; 14(4): S2-8-16.

362 Panagiotakos DB, et al. An integrated assessment of family history on the risk of developing acute coronary syndromes (CARDIO 2000 Study) Acta Cardiol Aug 2004; 59(4): 383–390.

363 Michos ED, et al. Relation of family history of premature coronary heart disease and metabolic risk factors to risk of coronary arterial calcium in asymptomatic subjects. Am J Cardiol Mar 1, 2005; 95(5): 655–657.

364 Murabito J, et al. Sibling cardiovascular disease as a risk factor for cardiovascular disease in middle-aged adults. JAMA 2005; 294: 3117–3123.

365 Kornman KS, et al. Candidate genes as potential links between periodontal and cardiovascular diseases. Ann Periodontol 2001; 648–657.

366 Resnick HE, et al. Prevalence and clinical implications of American Diabetes Association-defined diabetes and other categories of glucose dysregulation in older adults. J Clin Epidemiol 2001; 54: 869–876.

367 Beckman JA, et al. Diabetes and Atherosclerosis-Epidemiology, Pathophysiology, and Management. JAMA 2002; 287(19): 2570–2581.

368 US Office on Smoking and Health. The Health Consequences of Smoking: Cardiovascular Diseases: A Report of the Surgeon General. Washington DC: US Government Printing Office; 1989: 179–203.

369 Wald NJ, et al. Prospective study of effect of switching from cigarettes to pipes or cigars on mortality from three smoking-related diseases. BMJ 1997; 314: 1860–1863.

370 Jacobs EJ, et al. American Cancer Society, Atlanta. Cigar smoking and death from coronary heart disease in a prospective study of US men. Arch Intern Med November 8, 1999; 159: 2413–2418.

371 Howard G, et al. Cigarette smoking and progression of atherosclerosis—The Atherosclerosis Risk in Communities (ARIC) Study. JAMA 1998; 279(2): 119–124.

372 Mittleman MA, et al. Triggering myocardial infarction by marijuana. Circulation 2001; 103: 2805–2809.

373 Otsuka R, et al. Acute effects of passive smoking on the coronary circulation in healthy young adults. JAMA 2001; 286(4): 436–441.

374 Ezzati M, et al. Role of smoking in global and regional cardiovascular mortality. Circ 2005; 112: 489–497.

375 www.who.int/tobacco/health_priority/en/index.html.

376 Wells AJ. Passive smoking as a cause of heart disease. J Am Coll Cardiol 1994; 24: 546–554.

377 DiFranza JR, et al. Effect of maternal cigarette smoking on pregnancy complications and sudden infant death syndrome. J Fam Pract 1995; 40: 385–394.

378 Bero LA, et al. Sponsored symposia on environmental tobacco smoke. JAMA 1994; 271: 612–617.

379 Barnes DE, et al. Why review articles on the health effects of passive smoking reach different conclusions. JAMA 1998; 279: 1566–1570.

380 US Environmental Protection Agency. Respiratory Health Effects of Passive Smoking: Lung Cancer and Other Disorders. Washington DC: US Environmental Protection Agency; 1992.

381 US Department of Health and Human Services. The Health Consequences of Involuntary Smoking: A Report of the Surgeon General. Rockville, Maryland: US Public Health Service; 1986.

382 National Academy of Sciences. Environmental Tobacco Smoke: Measuring Exposures and Assessing Health Effects. Washington DC: National Academy Press; 1986.

383 Barnoya J, et al. Cardiovascular effects of secondhand smoking. Circ 2005; 111: 2684–2698.

384 USA Today June 6, 2006.

385 Fichenberg CM, et al. Association of the California Tobacco Control Program with declines in cigarette consumption and mortality from heart disease. N Engl J Med 2000; 343(24): 1772–1777.

386 Chobanian AV, et al. The seventh report of the joint national committee on prevention, detec-

tion, evaluation, and treatment of high blood pressure. The JNC 7 report. JAMA 2003; 289(19): 2560–2572.

387 Eastern Stroke and Coronary Heart Disease Collaborative Research Group. Blood pressure, cholesterol, and stroke in eastern Asia. Lancet 1998; 352: 1801–1807.

388 Vongpatanasin W, et al. C-reactive protein causes down-regulation of vascular angiotensin subtype 2 receptors and systolic hypertension in mice. Circulation 2007; 115: 1020–1028.

389 Savoia C, et al. Reduction of C-reactive protein and the use of anti-hypertensives. Vasc Health Risk manag 2007; 3(6): 975–983.

390 Chobanian AV, et al. The seventh report of the joint national committee on prevention, detection, evaluation, and treatment of high blood pressure. The JNC 7 report. JAMA 2003; 289(19): 2560–2572.

391 Berlin JA, et al. A meta-analysis of physical activity in the prevention of coronary heart disease. Am J Epidemiol 1990; 132: 612–628.

392 Sesso HD, et al. Physical activity and coronary heart disease in man—The Harvard Alumni Health Study. Circulation 2000; 102: 975–980.

393 Lee I-M, et al. Physical activity and coronary heart disease in women. JAMA 2001; 285(11): 1447–1454.

394 Tanasescu M, et al. Exercise type and intensity in relation to coronary heart disease in men. JAMA 2002; 288: 1994–2000.

395 Manson JE, et al. Walking compared with vigorous exercise for the prevention of cardiovascular events in women. N Engl J Med 2002; 347: 716–725.

396 Andersen RE, et al. Effects of lifestyle activity versus structured aerobic exercise in obese women. JAMA 1999; 281: 335–340.

397 Dunn AL, et al. Comparison of lifestyle and structured interventions to increase physical activity and cardiorespiratory fitness. JAMA 1999; 281: 327–334.

398 Volk B, et al. Consultant May 2006. www.consultantlive.com.

399 Irwin ML, et al. Effects of exercise on total and intra-abdominal body fat in postmenopausal women. JAMA 2003; 289: 323–330.

400 Hu FB, et al. Walking compared with vigorous physical activity and risk of Type II diabetes in women. JAMA 1999; 282: 1433–1439.

401 Boule NG, et al. Effects of exercise on glycemic control and body mass in Type II diabetes mellitus. JAMA 2001; 286: 1218–1227.

402 Eur Heart J 2003; 24: 1473–1480.

403 Manson JE, et al. Body weight and mortality among women. N Engl J Med 1995; 333: 677–685

404 Rimm EB, et al. Body size and fat distribution as predictors of coronary heart disease among middle-aged and older US men. Am J Epidemiol 1995; 141: 1117–1127.

405 Al Suwaidi J, et al. Association between obesity and coronary atherosclerosis and vascular remodeling. Am J of Cardiol 2001; 88: 1300–1303.

406 Yan LL, et al. Midlife body mass index and hospitalization and mortality in older age. JAMA 2006; 295: 190–198.

407 Wei M, et al. Relationship between low cardiorespiratory fitness and mortality in normal-weight, overweight and obese men. JAMA 1999; 282(16): 1547–1553.

408 Levine GN, et al. Cholesterol reduction in cardiovascular disease. Clinical benefits and possible mechanisms. N Engl J Med 1995; 332: 512–521.

409 Scandinavian Simvastatin Survival Study Group. Randomized trial of cholesterol lowering the and 4444 patients with coronary heart disease: the Scandinavian Simvastatin Survival Study (4S). Lancet 1994; 344: 1383–1389.

410 Sheperd J, et al. Presentation of coronary heart disease with pravastatin in men with hypercholesterolemia. N Engl J Med 1995; 333: 1301–1307.

411 White CW, et al. Effect of an aggressive lipid-lowering strategy on progression of atherosclerosis in the left main coronary artery from patients in the post coronary artery bypass graft

trial. Circulation 2001; 104: 2660–2665.

412 Expert Panel on Detection, Evaluation, and Treatment of High Blood Cholesterol in Adults. The Executive Summary of the Third Report of the National Cholesterol Education Program (NCEP) Expert Panel on Detection, Evaluation, and Treatment of High Blood Cholesterol in Adults (Adult Treatment Panel III). JAMA 2001; 285: 2486–2497.

413 Pischon T, et al. Non-high-density lipoprotein cholesterol and apolipoprotein B in the prediction of coronary heart disease in men. Circulation 2005; 112: 3375–3383.

414 Genest J, et al. Lipoprotein cholesterol, apolipoprotein A-1 and B and lipoprotein (a) abnormalities in men with premature coronary artery disease. J Am Coll Cardiol 1992; 19: 792–802.

415 Estruch R, et al. Effects of the Mediterranean-style diet on cardiovascular risk factors: A randomized trial. Ann Intern Med 2006; 145: 1–11.

416 Mozaffarian D, et al. Medical progress: Trans fatty acids and cardiovascular disease. NEJM April 2006; 354(15): 1601–1613.

417 Sun Q, et al. A prospective study of trans fatty acids in erythrocytes and risk of coronary artery disease. Circulation 2007;115: 1858–1865.

418 Lai CQ, et al. Dietary intake of n-6 fatty acids modulates effect of apolipoprotein A5 gene on plasma fasting triglycerides, remnant lipoprotein concentrations, and lipoprotein particle size. The Framingham Heart Study. Circulation 2006; 113: 2062–2070.

419 Sachs FM, et al. Effects on blood pressure of reduced dietary sodium and the dietary approaches to stop hypertension (DASH) diet. NEJM 2001; 344: 3–10.

420 Appel L, et al. Effects of protein, monounsaturated fat, and carbohydrate intake on blood pressure and serum lipids. JAMA 2005; 294: 2455–2464.

421 Howard BV, et al. Low-fat dietary pattern and risk of cardiovascular disease. JAMA 2006; 295: 655–666.

422 Rissanen TH, et al. Low intake of fruits, berries and vegetables is associated with excess mortality in man: The Kuopio Ischemic Heart Disease Risk Factor (KIHD) study. J Nutr 2003; 133(1): 199–204.

423 Pereira MA, et al. Dietary fiber and risk of coronary heart disease: A pooled analysis of cohort studies. Arch Int Med 2004; 164(4): 370–376.

424 Tucker KL, et al. The combination of high fruit and vegetable and low saturated fat intakes is more protective against mortality in aging men than is either alone: The Baltimore Longitudinal Study of Aging J Nutr 2005; 135(3): 556–561.

425 Lock K, et al. The global burden of disease attributable to low consumption of fruits and vegetables: The implications for the global strategy on diet. Bull World Health Organ 2005; 83(2): 100–108.

426 Knekt P, et al. Antioxidant vitamins and coronary heart disease risk: A pooled analysis of 9 cohorts. Am J Clin Nutr 2004 Dec; 80(6): 1508–1520.

427 Rowan PJ, et al. Depressive symptoms have an independent, gradient risk for coronary heart disease incidence in a random, population-based sample. Ann Epidemiol 2005; 15(4): 316–320.

428 Marzari C, et al. Depressive symptoms and development of coronary heart disease events: The Italian longitudinal study. J Gerontol A Biol Sci Med Sci 2005; 60(1): 85–92.

429 Whooley M. Depression and cardiovascular disease. JAMA 2006; 295: 2874–2881.

430 Barth J, et al. Depression as a risk factor for mortality in patients with coronary heart disease: A meta-analysis. Psychosom Med 2004; 66(6): 802–813.

431 Nabkasorn C, et al. Effects of physical exercise on depression, neuroendocrine stress hormones and physiological fitness in adolescent females with depressive symptoms. Eur J Public Health Aug 26, 2005 [Epub ahead of print].

432 Hornstein C. Stress, anxiety and cardiovascular disease: An interdisciplinary approach. Vertex 2004; 15 Suppl 1: 21–31.

433 Critchley HD, et al. Mental stress and sudden cardiac death: Asymmetric midbrain activity as a linking mechanism. Brain 2005; 128(Pt 1): 75–85.

434 *Family Practice News.* May 15, 2006: 20.

435 Pignalberi C, et al. Psychological stress and sudden death. Ital Heart J Suppl. 2002; 3(10): 1011–1021.

436 Brunner EJ, et al. Adrenocortical, autonomic, and inflammatory causes of the metabolic syndrome. Circulation 2002; 106: 2659–2665.

437 Osler W. The faith that heals. British Med J 1910; 1470–1472.

438 NIH Consensus Conference. Methodological approaches to the study of religion, health, and aging. National Institute of Aging and Fetzer Institute, March 16–17, 1995.

439 Byrd RC. Positive therapeutic benefits of intercessory prayer in a coronary care unit population. South Med J 1998; 81(7): 826–829.

440 Harrris WS, et al. A randomized, controlled trial of the effects of remote, intercessory prayer on outcomes in patients admitted to the coronary care unit. Arch Intern Med 1999; 159: 2273–2278.

441 Larson DB, et al. The impact of religion on men's blood pressure. J Religion Health 1989; 28: 265–278.

442 Comstock GW, et al. Church attendance and health. J Chronic Dis 1972; 25: 665–672.

443 Oxman TE, et al. Lack of social participation or religious strength or comfort as risk factors for death after cardiac surgery in the elderly. Psychosomatic medicine 1995; 57: 5–15.

444 Koenig HG, et al. Use of hospital services, religious attendance, and religious affiliation. Southern Medical Journal 1998; 91(10): 925–932.

445 Koenig HG, et al. Attendance at religious services, interleukin-6, and other biological parameters of immune system in older adults. Int J Psych Med 1997; 27(3): 233–250.

446 Lutgendorf SK, et al. Religious participation, interleukin-6, and mortality in older adults. Health Psychol. Sep 2004; 23(5): 465–475.

447 King DE, et al. The relationship between attendance at religious services and cardiovascular inflammatory markers. Int J Psychiatry Med 2001; 31(4): 415–425.

448 Strawbridge WJ, et al. Frequent attendance at religious services and mortality over 28 years. Am J Public Health 1997; 87: 957–961.

449 Hummer RA, et al. Religious involvement and U.S. adult mortality. Demography May 1999; 36(2): 273–285.

450 Chambers JC, et al. Plasma homocysteine concentrations and risk of coronary heart disease in UK Indian Asians and European men. Lancet 2000; 355: 523–527.

451 Cappuccio FP, et al. Homocysteine levels in men and women of different ethnic and cultural background living in England. Atherosclerosis 2002; 164: 95–102.

452 Senaratne MP, et al. Possible ethnic differences in plasma homocysteine levels associated with coronary artery disease between South Asian and East Asian immigrants. Clin Cardiol 2001; 24: 730–734.

453 HOPE 2 Investigators. Homocysteine lowering with folic acid and B vitamins in vascular disease. NEJM April 13, 2006; 354(15): 1567–1577.

454 Bonaa, KH, et al. NORVIT trial investigators. Homocysteine lowering and cardiovascular events after acute myocardial infarction. NEJM April 13, 2006; 354(15): 1578–1588.

455 Nasir K, et al. Elevated homocysteine is associated with reduced regional left ventricular function. The Multi-Ethnic Study of Atherosclerosis. Circulation 2007; 115: 180–187.

456 Shirodana C, et al. Global improvement of vascular function and redox state with low dose folic acid. Circulation 2007; 115: 2262–2270.

457 Vermeulen EGJ, et al. Effect of homocysteine lowering treatment with folic acid plus vitamin B6 on progress in of subclinical atherosclerosis: A randomized, placebo-controlled trial. Lancet 2000; 355: 517–522.

458 Jublanc C, et al. Hypothyroidism and cardiovascular disease: Role of new risk factors and

coagulation parameters. Semin Vasc Med 2004; 4(2): 145–151.

459 Tuzcu A, et al. Subclinical hypothyroidism may be associated with elevated C-reactive protein (low-grade inflammation) and fasting hyperinsulinemia. Endocr J 2005; 52(1): 89–94.

460 Imaizumi M, et al. Risk for ischemic heart disease and all-cause mortality in subclinical hypothyroidism. J Clin Endocrinol Metab 2004; 89(7): 3365–3370.

461 Hu FB, et al. Fish and Omega-3 PUFA intake and risk of coronary heart disease in women. JAMA 2002; 287: 1815–1821.

462 Japan Public Health Center-Based (JPHC) Study Cohort I. Intake of fish and n3 fatty acids and risk of coronary heart disease among Japanese. Circulation 2006; 113: 195–202.

463 Waite N, et al. The impact of fish-oil supplements on insulin sensitivity. J Hum Nutr Diet 2008 Jul 15; 21(4): 402–403.

464 Albert CM, et al. Blood levels of long-chain n-3 PUFA and the risk of sudden death. N Eng J Med 2002; 346: 1113–1118.

465 Leaf A, et al. Prevention of fatal arrhythmias in high-risk subjects by fish oil in n-3 fatty acid intake. Circulation 2005; 112: 2762–2768.

466 Mozaffarian D, et al. Effect of fish oil on heart rate in humans. Circulation 2005; 112: 1945–1952.

467 Harris WS, et al. Effects of fish oil on the VLDL triglyceride kinetics in humans. J Lipid Res 1990; 31: 1549.

468 Morris MC, et al. Does fish oil lower blood pressure? A meta-analysis of controlled trials. Circulation 1993; 88: 523.

469 Lawson DL, et al. Omega-3 polyunsaturated fatty acids augment endothelium-dependent vasorelaxation by enhanced release of EDRF and vasodilator prostaglandins. Eicosanoid 1991; 4: 217.

470 The Omega Diet. 1999. HarperCollins Publishers Inc., 10 East Third St, New York, NY.

471 Harris WS, et al. The Omega-3 Index: A new risk factor for deaths from coronary heart disease? Preventive Med 2004; 39: 212–220.

472 Estruch R, et al. Effects of a Mediterranean-style diet on cardiovascular risk factors: A randomized trial. Ann Intern Med 2006; 145: 1–11.

473 Smith SC, et al. CDC/AHA workshop on markers of inflammation and cardiovascular disease. Circulation 2004; 110: e550–e553.

474 Libby P, et al. Inflammation and Atherosclerosis. Circulation 2002; 105: 1135–1143.

475 Rifai N, et al. Inflammatory markers and coronary heart disease. Curr Opin Lipidol 2002; 13: 383–389.

476 Tzoulaki I, et al. C-reactive protein, interleukin-6, and soluble adhesion molecules as predictors of progressive peripheral atherosclerosis in the general population. Circulation 2005; 112: 976–983.

477 Cushman M, et al. C-reactive protein and the 10-year incidence of coronary heart disease in older men and women. Circulation 2005; 112: 25–31.

478 Ridker PM, et al. Rosuvastatin to prevent vascular events in men and women with elevated C-reactive protein. N Engl J Med 2008 Nov 9;359:2195-2207.

479 Anderson TJ, et al. Effect of chelation therapy on endothelial function in patients with coronary artery disease: PATCH substudy. J Am Coll Cardiol Feb 5, 2003; 41(3): 420–425.

480 Villarruz MV, et al. Chelation therapy for atherosclerotic cardiovascular disease. Cochrane Database Syst Rev 2002; (4): CD002785.

481 Atwood KC, et al. Why the NIH trial to assess chelation therapy (TACT) should be abandoned. Medscape J Med May 13, 2008; 10(5): 115.

482 Ford D, et al. Genetic heterogeneity and penetrance analysis of the BRCA1 and BRCA2 genes in breast-cancer families. Am J Hum Genet 1998; 62(3): 676–689.

483 www.cdc.gov/tobacco/sgr/sgr_2004/Factsheets/2.htm. Accessed March 27, 2005.

484 Godtfredsen NS, et al. Effect of smoking reduction on lung cancer risk. JAMA 2005; 294:

1505–1510.

485 http://progressreport.cancer.gov/doc. Accessed March 27, 2005.

486 Bernstein L, et al. Lifetime recreational exercise activity and breast cancer risk among black women and white women. J Natl Cancer Inst. November 2005; 97(22): 1671–1679.

487 McTiernan A. Breast cancer: Can anything help prevent it? April 1, 2006. www.consultantlive.com.

488 Callee EE, et al. Overweight, obesity and mortality from cancer in a prospectively studied cohort of US adults. N Eng J Med Apr 24, 2003; 348(17): 1625–1638.

489 Huang Z, et al. Nurses health study. JAMA; 278: 1407–1411.

490 Eliassen AH, et al. Adult weight change and risk of postmenopausal breast cancer. JAMA 2006; 296: 193–201.

491 McCann J. Obesity, cancer links prompt new recommendations. J of the Natl Cancer Inst 2001; 93(12): 901–902.

492 *Family Practice News*, Aug 1, 2000; 8.

493 Reiche EM, et al. Stress, depression, the immune system, and cancer. Lancet Oncol. 2004; 5(10): 617–625.

494 Kruk J, et al. Psychological stress and the risk of breast cancer: A case-control study. Cancer Detect Prev 2004; 28(6): 399–408.

495 Giovannuci E, et al. The role of fats, fatty acids, and total energy intake in the etiology of human colon cancer. Am J Clin Nutr 1997; 66: 1564S–1571S.

496 Campos FG, et al. Diet and colorectal cancer: Current evidence for etiology and prevention. Nutr Hosp 2005; 20(1): 18–25.

497 Gonzalez CA, et al. Meat intake and risk of stomach and esophageal adenocarcinoma within the European Prospective Investigation into Cancer and Nutrition (EPIC). J Natl Cancer Inst. March 1, 2006; 98(5): 345–354.

498 Cho E, et al. Red meat intake and risk of breast cancer among premenopausal women. Arch Int Med 2006 Nov; 166: 2253–2259.

499 Nothlings U, et al. Meat and fat intake as risk factors for pancreatic cancer: The Multiethnic Cohort Study. J Natl Cancer Inst. Oct 5, 2005; 97(19): 1458–1465.

500 Norat T, et al. Meat, fish, and colorectal cancer risk: The European Perspective into Cancer and Nutrition (EPIC). J Natl Cancer Inst. June 15, 2005; 97(12): 906–916.

501 http://progressreport.cancer.gov/doc. Accessed March 27, 2005.

502 www.hsph.harvard.edu/nutritionsource/fats.html. Accessed March 27, 2005.

503 Prentice RL, et al. Low-fat dietary pattern and risk of invasive breast cancer. (WHI) JAMA 2006; 295: 629–642.

504 Beresford SA, et al. Low-fat dietary pattern and risk of colorectal cancer. JAMA 2006; 295: 643–654.

505 Kim MK, et al. Dietary patterns and subsequent colorectal cancer risk by subsite: A prospective cohort study. Int J Cancer Jul 10,2005; 115(5): 790–798.

506 Dansinger ML, et al. Comparison of the Atkins, Ornish, Weight Watchers, and Zone diets for weight loss and heart disease risk reduction. JAMA 2005; 293: 43–53.

507 Lock K, et al. The global burden of disease attributable to low consumption of fruit and vegetables: Implications for the global strategy on diet. Bull World health Organ 2005; 83(2): 100–108.

508 http://progressreport.cancer.gov/doc. Accessed March 27, 2005.

509 Ludwig D. Dietary glycemic index and obesity. J Nutr 2000; 130: 280S–283S.

510 Franceschi S, et al. Dietary glycemic load and colorectal cancer risk. Ann Oncol 2001; 12: 173–178.

511 Augustin LS. Dietary glycemic index and glycemic load in breast cancer risk: A case control study. Ann Oncol Nov 2001; 12(11): 1533–1538.

512 Augustin LS, et al. Dietary glycemic index, glycemic load and ovarian cancer risk: A case-con-

trol study in Italy. Ann Oncol Jan 2003; 14(1): 78–84.

513 Augustin LS, et al. Glycemic index, glycemic load and risk of gastric cancer. Ann Oncol Apr 2004; 15(4): 581–584.

514 Schabath MB, et al. Dietary phytoestrogens and lung cancer risk. JAMA 2005; 294: 1493–1504.

515 Tucker KL, et al. The combination of high fruit and vegetable and low as saturated fat intakes is more protective against mortality in aging men than is either alone: The Baltimore Longitudinal Study of Aging. J Nutr 2005; 135(3): 556–561.

516 Rissanen TH, et al. Low intake of fruits, berries and vegetables is associated with excess mortality in men: The Kuopio Ischemic Heart Disease Risk Factor (KIHD) study. J Nutr 2003; 133(1): 199–204.

517 Pelicchi C, et al. Dietary intake of selected micronutrients and gastric cancer risk: An Italian case-control study. Ann Oncol Jul 31, 2008 [Epub ahead of print].

518 http://progressreport.cancer.gov/doc.

519 Van Den Brandt PA, et al. Salt intake, cured meat consumption, refrigerator use and stomach cancer incidence: A prospective cohort study (Netherlands). Cancer Causes Control 2003; 14(5): 427–438.

520 Kim MK, et al. Dietary patterns and subsequent colorectal cancer risk by subsite: A prospective cohort study. Int J Cancer Jul 10, 2005; 115(5): 790–798.

521 *Tufts University Health and Nutrition Letter*. Sept 2005; 23(7): 2.

522 Boffetta P. Epidemiology of environmental and occupational cancer. Oncogene 2004; 23(38): 6392–6403.

523 Darby S, et al. Radon in homes and risk of lung cancer: Collaborative analysis of individual data from 13 European case-control studies. BMJ 2005; 330(7485): 223.

524 Navarro A, et al. Meat cooking habits and risk of colorectal cancer in Córdoba, Argentina. Nutrition 2004; 20(10): 873–877.

525 Stolzenberg-Solomon RZ, et al. Meat and meat mutagen intake and pancreatic cancer risk in the NIH-AARP cohort. Cancer Epidemiol Biomarkers Prev Dec 2007; 16(12): 2264.

526 Martinez ME, et al. Meat intake, preparation methods, mutagens, and colorectal adenomas recurrence. Carcinogenesis Sep 2007; 28(9): 2019–2027.

527 Harris RE. Cyclooxygenase-2 (COX-2) and inflammogenesis of cancer. Subcell Biochem 2007; 42: 93–126.

528 http://progressreport.cancer.gov/doc. Accessed March 27, 2005.

529 Gallagher RP, et al. Tanning beds, sunlamps, and the risk of cutaneous melanoma. Cancer Epidemiol Biomarkers Prev. Mar 2005; 14(3): 562–566.

530 Saladi RN, et al. The causes of skin cancer: a comprehensive review. Drugs Today 2005; 41(1): 37–53.

531 Yu T, et al. The role of viral integration in the development of cervical cancer. Cancer Genet Cytogenet 2005; 158(1): 27–34.

532 Davila JA, et al. Hepatitis C infection and the increasing incidence of hepatocellular carcinoma: A population base study. Gastroenterology 2004; 127(5): 1372–1380.

533 Garland CF, et al. Serum 25-hydroxyvitamin D and colon cancer: Eight-year prospective study. Lancet 1989; 18: 1176–1178.

534 Hanchette CL, et al. Geographic patterns of prostate cancer mortality: Evidence for a protective effect of ultraviolet radiation. Cancer 1992; 70: 2861–2869.

535 Krishnan AV, et al. Calcitrol as a chemopreventive and therapeutic agent in prostate cancer: Role of anti-inflammatory activity. J Bone Miner Res Dec 2007; 22 Suppl 2: v74–80.

536 Grant WB. An ecologic study of the role of solar UVB radiation in reducing the risk of cancer using cancer mortality data, dietary supply data and latitude for European countries. In: MF Holick, ed. *Biologic Effects of Light*. 2001. Boston: Kluwer Academic Publishing, 2002: 267–276.

537 Garland CF, et al. Evidence of need for increased Vitamin D fortification of food based on pooled analysis of studies of serum 25-hydroxyvitamin D and breast cancer. Proc Amer Assoc Cancer Res 2006; 47.

538 Ingraham BA, et al. Molecular basis of the potential of vitamin D to prevent cancer. Curr Med Res Opin Jan 2008; 24(1): 139–149.

539 Grant WB. An estimate of premature cancer mortality in the US due to inadequate doses of solar ultraviolet-B radiation. Cancer. 2002; 94: 1867–1875.

540 Giovannucci E, et al. Prospective study of predictors of Vitamin D status and cancer incidence and mortality in men. J Natl Cancer Inst. April 5, 2006; 98(7): 451–459.

541 Erlinger TP, et al. C-reactive protein and the risk of incident colorectal cancer. JAMA 2004; 291(5): 585–590.

542 Khuder SA, et al. Nonsteroidal anti-inflammatory drug use and lung cancer: A meta-analysis. Chest 2005; 127(3): 748–754.

543 Nelson WG, et al. The role of inflammation in the pathogenesis of prostate cancer. J Urol 2004; 172(5 Pt 2): S6-11; discussion S11-2.

544 Pitt HA. Hepato-pancreato-biliary fat: The good, the bad and the ugly. HPB (Oxford) 2007; 9(2): 92–97.

545 Itxkowitz SH, et al. Inflammation and cancer IV. Colorectal cancer in inflammatory bowel disease: The role of inflammation. Am J Physiol Gastrointest Liver Physiol 2004; 287: G7–17.

546 Catassi C, et al. Association of celiac disease and intestinal lymphomas and other cancers. Gastroenterology 2005; 128 (Suppl): 79–86.

547 Nardone G, et al. Review article: Heliobacter pylori and molecular events in precancerous gastric lesions. Aliment Pharmacol Ther 2004; 20: 261–270.

548 Ernst PB, et al. The translation of Heliobacter pylori basic research to patient care. Gastroenterology 2006; 130: 188–206: quiz 212–183.

549 Sinicrope FA. Targeting cyclooxygenase-2 for prevention and therapy of colorectal cancer. Mol Carcinog 2006; 45: 447–454.

550 Hall MN, et al. A 22-year prospective study of fish, n-3 fatty acid intake, and colorectal cancer risk in men. Cancer Epidemiol Biomarkers Prev May 2008; 17(5): 1136–1143.

551 Edwards IJ, et al. Omega-3 fatty acids and PPAR gamma in cancer. PPAR Res 2008; 2008: 358052.

552 Li Q, et al. Inflammation-associated cancer NFkappaB is the lynchpin. Trends Immunol 2005; 26(6): 318.

553 Bugianesi E. Review article: Steatosis, the metabolic syndrome and cancer. Ailment Pharmacol Ther Nov 2005; 22 Suppl 2: 40–43.

554 Wei EK, et al. Low plasma adiponectin levels and risk of colorectal cancer in men: A prospective study. J Natl Cancer Inst Nov 16, 2005; 97(22): 1688–1694.

555 Elwing JE, et al. Type 2 diabetes mellitus: The impact on colorectal cancer adenoma risk in women. Am J Gastroenterol Jun 22, 2006.

556 Bugianesi E. Review article: Steatosis, the metabolic syndrome and cancer. Aliment Pharmacol Ther Nov 2005; 22 Suppl 2: 40–3.

557 World Health Organization. The Asian Pacific Perspective: Redefining Obesity and Its Treatment. Health Communications Australia Pty Ltd. February 2000.

558 WHO Expert Committee on Physical Status: The Uses and Interpretation of Anthropometry. Physical Status: The use and interpretation of anthropometry: Report of a WHO Expert Committee. Geneva, Switzerland: World Health Organization; 1995. World Health Organization Technical Health Status 854.

559 Bray GA, et al. Definitions and proposed current classification of obesity. In Bray GA, Blanchard C, James WPT, eds. Handbook of Obesity. New York, NY: Marcel Dekker Inc; 1997: 31–40.

560 National Heart, Lung, and Blood Institute. Clinical Guidelines on the Identification,

Evaluation, and Treatment of Overweight and Obesity in Adults: The Evidence Report. Bethesda, MD: National Institute of Health; 1998. NIH Publication 98-408. Available at www.nhlbi.nih.gov/guidelines/obesity/ob-gdlns.pdf. Accessed November 2001.

561 Calle EE, et al. Body-mass index and mortality and a prospective cohort of US adults. N Engl J of Med 1999; 341: 1097–1105.

562 Deitz WH, et al. Introduction: The use of body mass index to assess obesity in children. Am J Clin Nutr 1999; 70: 123S–125S.

563 Barlow SE, et al. Obesity evaluation and treatment: Expert Committee Recommendations. Pediatrics 1998; 102: e29.

564 Ruderman N, et al. The metabolically obese, normal weight individual revisited. Am J Clin Nutr 1998; 34: 1617–1621.

565 Caro JF. Insulin resistance in obese and nonobese man. J Clin Endocrinol Metab 1991; 73: 690–695.

566 Lapidis L, et al. Distribution of adipose tissue and risk of cardiovascular disease and death: A 12-year follow-up of participants in the population study of women of Gothenberg, Sweden. BMJ 1984; 289: 1257–1261.

567 Selvin E, et al. The effect of weight loss on C-reactive protein: A systemic review. Arch Intern Med 2007; 167: 31–39.

568 Pradham A. Obesity, metabolic syndrome, and type 2 diabetes: Inflammatory basis of glucose metabolic disorders. Nutr Rev Dec 2007 (11); 65(12): S152–S156.

569 Winer JC, et al. Adiponectin in childhood and adolescent obesity and its association with inflammatory markers and components of the metabolic syndrome. J Clin Endocrinol Metab Nov 2006; 91(11): 4415–4423.

570 Hung J, et al. Circulating adiponectin levels associate with inflammatory markers, insulin resistance and metabolic syndrome independent of obesity. Int J Obes (Lond) 2008 May; 32(5): 772–779.

571 Saltevo J, et al. Levels of adiponectin, C-reactive protein and interleukin-1 receptor antagonist are associated with insulin sensitivity: A population-based study. Diab Metab Rev Jul–Aug 2008; 24(5): 378–383.

572 Bahceci M, et al. The correlation between adiposity and adiponectin, tumor necrosis factor alpha, interleukin-6 and high sensitive C-reactive protein levels. Is adipocyte size associated with inflammation in adults? J Endocrinol Invest Mar 2007; 30(3): 210–214.

573 NHLBI Obesity Education Initiative Expert Panel on the Identification, Evaluation and Treatment of Overweight and Obesity in Adults. Clinical guidelines on the identification, evaluation and treatment of overweight and obesity in adults—the evidence report. Obes Res 1998; 6 (Suppl 2): 51S–209S.

574 World Health Organization. Obesity: Preventing and Managing the Global Epidemic, Report of a WHO Consultation. Geneva: World Health Organization. WHO Technical Report Series 894; 2000.

575 USA Today, Oct 30, 2000.

576 National Center for Health Statistics. Prevalence of overweight and obesity among adults: United States, 1999 (initial results from the 1999 National Health and Nutrition Survey). Hyattsville, MD: Center for Disease Control; 2000. Available at www.cdc.gov/nchs/products/pubs/pubd/hestats/obese/obse99.htm.

577 www.cpc.unc.edu/projects/china

578 Science, February 7, 2003.

579 Freedman DS, et al. Trends and correlates of class 3 obesity in the United States from 1990 through 2000. JAMA 2002; 288: 1758–1761.

580 Mokdad AH, et al. The continuing epidemic of obesity and diabetes in the United States. JAMA 2001; 286: 1195–1200.

581 McTigue KM, et al. The natural history of the development of obesity in a cohort of young

U.S. adults between 1981 and 1998. Ann Intern Med 2002; 136(12): 857–864.

582 Ogden CL, et al. Prevalence of overweight and obesity in the United States, 1999–2004. JAMA 2006; 295: 1549–1555.

583 WHO Expert Committee. Physical Status: The use and interpretation of anthropometry. World health organization Tech Rep Series. 1995; 854.

584 World Health Organization. Obesity epidemic puts millions at risk from related diseases. [Press release WHO/46, June 12, 1997]. Available at www.who.int/archives/inf-pr-1997/en/pr97-46.html.

585 US Department of Health and Human Services, Centers for Disease Control and Prevention, Office of Communications. Obesity epidemic increases dramatically in the United States: CDC director calls for national prevention effort. October 26, 1999. Available at: www.cdc.gov/ad/ac/media/pressrel/r991026.htm.

586 www.worldwatch.org/press/news/2000/03/04.

587 Rowland ML. Self-reported weight and height. Am J Clin Nutr 1990; 52: 1125–1133.

588 Palta M, et al. Comparison of self-reported and measured height and weight. Am J Epidemiol 1982; 115: 223–230.

589 Aday LA. Designing and Conducting Health Surveys: A Comprehensive Guide. San Francisco, CA. Jossey-Bass Publishers; 1989: 79–80.

590 *Tufts University Health and Nutrition Letter*. Sept 8; 26(1): 3.

591 Guo SS, et al. BMI during childhood, adolescence and young adulthood in relation to adult overweight and adiposity: The Fels Longitudinal Study. Int J Obes Relat Mmetab Disord 2000; 24: 162835.

592 Must A, et al. Long-term morbidity and mortality of overweight adolescents. A follow-up of the Harvard Growth Study of 1922 to 1935. N Engl J Med 1992; 327: 1350–1355.

593 Guo SS, et al. Predicting overweight and obesity in adulthood from body mass index values in childhood and adolescence. Am J Clin Nutr 2002; 76: 653–658.

594 Magarey AM, et al. Predicting obesity in early adulthood from childhood and parental obesity. Int J Obesity 2003; 27: 505–513.

595 National Center for Health Statistics. Prevalence of overweight among children and adolescents: United States, 1999. www.cdc.gov/nchs/products/pubs/pubd/hestats/overweight99.htm.

596 Wang Y, et al. Trends of obesity and underweight in older children and adolescents in the United States, Brazil, China and Russia. Am J Clin Nutr 2002; 75: 971–977.

597 Chinn S, et al. Prevalence and trends in overweight and obesity in three cross-sectional studies of British children, 1974 to 1994. BMJ 2001; 322: 24–26.

598 Ibid.

599 Wang Y, et al. Trends of obesity and underweight in older children and adolescents in the United States, Brazil, China and Russia. Am J Clin Nutr 2002; 75: 971–977.

600 Marata M. Secular trends in growth and changes in eating patterns of Japanese children. Am J Clin Nutr 2000; 72 (Suppl): 1379S–1383S.

601 DeOnis M, et al. Prevalence and trends of overweight among preschool children in developing countries. A J Clin Nutr 2000; 72: 1032–1039.

602 Magarey AM, et al. Prevalence of overweight and obesity in Australian children and adolescents: Reassessment of 1985 and 1995 data against new standard international definitions. Med J Aust 2001; 174: 561–564.

603 DeOnis M, et al. Prevalence and trends of overweight among preschool children in developing countries. A J Clin Nutr 2000; 72: 1032–1039.

604 Wang Y, et al. Trends of obesity and underweight in older children and adolescents in the United States, Brazil, China and Russia. Am J Clin Nutr 2002; 75: 971–977.

605 DeOnis M, et al. Prevalence and trends of overweight among preschool children in developing countries. A J Clin Nutr 2000; 72: 1032–1039.

606 Bundred P, et al. Prevalence of overweight and obese children between 1989 and 1998:

Population based series of cross-sectional studies. BMJ 2001; 322: 1–4.

607 Strauss RS, et al. Epidemic increase in childhood overweight, 1986–1998. JAMA 2001; 286: 2845–2848.

608 James WPT, et al. Socioeconomic determinants of health: The contribution of nutrition to inequalities of health. BMJ 1997; 314: 1545–1549.

609 Ogden CL, et al. High body mass index for age among US children and adolescents, 2003–2006. JAMA 2008; 299(20): 2401–2405.

610 Daniels SR, et al. Lipid screening and cardiovascular health in childhood. Pediatrics July 2008; 122(1): 198–208.

611 Gordon-Larsen P, et al. Determines of adolescent physical activity and inactivity patterns. Pediatrics 2000; 105: e83.

612 Doak C, et al. The underweight/overweight household: An exploration of household sociode-mographic and dietary factors in China. Public Health Nutr 2002; 5: 215–221.

613 Popkin BM. An overview on the nutrition transition and its health implications: The Bellagio meeting. Public Health Nutr 2002; 5 (Suppl): 93–103.

614 Eckel RH, et al. American Heart Association call to action: Obesity as a major risk factor for coronary heart disease. Circulation 1998; 97: 99–100.

615 Donahue M, et al. Obesity and cardiovascular disease. Am Heart Journal 2001; 142(6): 1088–1090.

616 www.ConsumerFreedom.com

617 Allison D, et al. Annual deaths attributable to obesity in United States. JAMA 1999; 282: 1530–1538.

618 Surgeon General's Call to Action to Prevent and Decrease Overweight and Obesity, 2001.

619 World Health Organization. Obesity epidemic puts millions at risk from related diseases. Press release. WHO/46; June 12, 1997.

620 Institute of Medicine. Weighing the options: Criteria for evaluating the weight management programs. Washington DC: National Academy Press, 1995.

621 American Heart Association. Press Release: 10 AM ET, June 1, 1998. Available at www.ameri-canheartorg/Whats_News/AHA_News_Releases/obesity.html.

622 Van Italle T. Obesity and Therapy, 2nd ed. Stunkard AJ and Wadden TA, eds. New York, NY: Raven Press, 1993.

623 Calle EE, et al. Body mass index and mortality in a prospective cohort of US adults. N Engl J Med 1999; 341: 1097–1105.

624 Folsom AK, et al. Associations of general and abdominal obesity with multiple health out-comes in older women: The Iowa Women's Health Study Arch Int Med 2000; 160: 2117–2128.

625 Calle EE, et al. Body mass index and mortality in a prospective cohort of US adults. N Engl J Med 1999; 341: 1097–1105.

626 Gu D, et al. Body weight and mortality among men and women in China. JAMA 2006; 295: 776–783.

627 Manson JE, et al. Body weight and mortality among women. N Engl J Med 1995; 333: 677–685.

628 Rimm EB, et al. Body size and fat distribution as predictors of coronary heart disease among middle-aged and older US men. Am J Epidemiol 1995; 141: 1117–1127.

629 Al Suwaidi J, et al. Association between obesity and coronary atherosclerosis and vascular remodeling. Am J of Cardiol 2001; 88: 1300–1303.

630 Wei M, et al. Relationship between low cardiorespiratory fitness and mortality in normal-weight, overweight and obese men. JAMA 1999; 282(16): 1547–1553.

631 Al Suwaida J, et al. Obesity is an independent predictor of coronary endothelial function in patients with normal or mildly diseased coronary arteries. J Am Coll Cardiol 2001; 37: 1523–1528.

632 Kenchaiah S, et al. Obesity and the risk of heart failure. N Engl J Med 2002; 347: 305–313.

633 Lauer MS, et al. The impact of obesity on left ventricular mass and geometry: The Framingham heart study. JAMA 1991; 266: 231–236.

634 Iacobellis G, et al. Influence of excess fat on cardiac morphology and function: Study in uncomplicated obesity. Obes Res 2002; 10: 767–773.

635 Wang TJ, et al. Obesity and the risk of new-onset atrial fibrillation. JAMA 2004; 292(20): 2471–2477.

636 Stamler R, et al. Weight and blood pressure. Findings in hypertension screening of one million Americans. JAMA 1978; 240: 1607–1610.

637 Thompson D, et al. Lifetime health and economic consequences of obesity. Arch Int Med 1999; 159: 2177–2183.

638 Resnick H, et al. Relation of weight gain and weight loss on subsequent diabetes risk in overweight adults. J Epidemiol Community health 2000; 54: 596–602.

639 Ford ES, et al. Weight change and diabetes incidence: Findings from a national cohort. Am J Epidemiol. 1997; 146: 214–222.

640 Jung RT. Obesity is a disease. Br Med Bull 1997; 53: 307–321.

641 National Institute of Health. Clinical guidelines on the identification, evaluation and treatment of overweight and obesity and adults: The evidence report. Bethesda, MD: National Heart, Lung and Blood Institute and National Institute of Diabetes and Digestive and Kidney Diseases; 1998.

642 Henegar JR, et al. functional and structural changes in the kidney in the early stages of obesity. J Am Soc Nephrol 2001; 12: 1211–1217.

643 Kambham N, et al. Obesity-related glomerulopathy: An emerging epidemic. Kidney Int. 2001; 59: 1498–1509.

644 Davi G, et al. Platelet activation in obese women. JAMA 2002; 288: 2008–2014.

645 Ibid.

646 Yudkin JS, et al. C-reactive protein in healthy subjects: Associations with obesity, insulin resistance and endothelial dysfunction. Arterioscler Thromb Vasc Biol 1999; 19: 972–978.

647 Visser M, et al. Elevated C-reactive protein levels in overweight and obese adults. JAMA 1999; 282: 2131–2135.

648 Strong JP, et al. Prevalence and extent of atherosclerosis in adolescents and young adults: Implications for prevention from the Pathobiological Determinants of Atherosclerosis in Youth Study. Circ 2000; 102: 374–379.

649 Sorof M, et al. Isolated systolic hypertension, obesity and hyperkinetic hemodynamic states in children. J Pediatr 2002; 140: 660–666.

650 Chu NF, et al. Clustering of cardiovascular disease risk factors among obese schoolchildren: The Taipei Children's Heart Study. Am J Clin Nutr 1998; 67: 1141–1146.

651 Uwaifo GI, et al. Impaired glucose tolerance in obese children and adolescents. N Eng J Med 2002; 347: 290–292.

652 USA Today, June 18, 2001.

653 Schwimmer JB, et al. Health-related quality of life of severely obese children and adolescents. JAMA 2003; 289(14): 1813–1819.

654 Kaplowitz PB, et al. Earlier onset of puberty in girls: Relation to increased body mass index and race. Pediatrics 2001; 108: 347–353.

655 De la Eva RC, et al. Metabolic correlates with obstructive sleep apnea in obese subjects. J Pediatr 2002; 140: 654–659.

656 Russel DL, et al. The relation between skeletal maturation and adiposity in African American and Caucasian children. J Pediatr 2001; 139: 844–848.

657 Callee EE, et al. Overweight, obesity and mortality from cancer in a prospectively studied cohort of US adults. N Engl J Med Apr 24, 2003; 348(17): 1625–1638.

658 Huang Z, et al. Nurse's Health Study JAMA 1997; 278: 1407–1411.

659 Pan SY, et all. Association of obesity and cancer risk in Canada. Am J Epidemiol. 2004; 159(3): 259–268.

660 McCann J. Obesity, cancer links new recommendations. J of the Natl Cancer Inst 2001; 93(12): 901.

661 *Family Practice News*, Aug. 1, 2000: 8.

662 Must A, et al. The disease burden associated with overweight and obesity. JAMA 1999; 282: 1523–1529.

663 Ibid.

664 *Family Practice News*, Aug. 15, 2001: 13.

665 Bacon CG, et al. Sexual function in men older than 50 years of age: Results from the health professionals follow-up study. Ann Intern Med 2003; 139(3): 161–168.

666 Oster G, et al. The clinical and economic burden of obesity in a managed-care setting. Am J Manag Care 2000; 6: 681–689.

667 Thompson D, et al. Lifetime health and economic consequences of obesity. Arch Int Med 1999; 159: 2177–2183.

668 Thompson D, et al. Lifetime health and economic consequences of obesity. Arch Intern Med 1999; 159: 2177–2183.

669 Zhao W, et al. Economic burden of obesity-related chronic diseases in Mainland China. Obes Rev Mar 2008; 9 Suppl 1: 62–67.

670 Kennedy ET, et al. Popular diets: Correlation to health, nutrition and obesity. J Am Diet Assoc 2001; 101: 411–420.

671 www.mypyramid.gov/professionals/index.html.

672 Kennedy ET, et al. Popular diets: Correlation to health, nutrition and obesity. J Am Diet Assoc 2001; 101: 411–420.

673 Dansinger ML, et al. Comparison of the Adkins, Ornish, Weight Watchers, and Zone diets for weight loss and heart disease risk reduction. 2005; 293: 43–53.

674 Kaplan JP, et al. Caloric imbalance and public health policy. JAMA 1999; 282: 1579–1581.

675 United States Department of Health and Human services. Physical activity and health: A report of the Surgeon General. Document No. S/N 017-023-00196-5. Atlanta, Georgia: US Department of Health and Human Services. Center for Disease Control and Prevention, National Center for Chronic Disease Prevention and health promotion, 1996.

676 Klem M, et al. A descriptive study of individuals successful at long-term maintenance of substantial weight-loss. Am J Clin Nutr 1997; 66: 239–246.

677 Kennedy, ET, et al. Popular diets: Correlation to health, nutrition and obesity. J Am Diet Assoc. 2001; 101: 411–420.

678 Nielsen Report on Television. New York, NY: Nielsen Media Research; 1998.

679 Hu, FB, et al. Television watching and other sedentary behaviors in relation to the risk of obesity and type 2 diabetes mellitus in women. JAMA 2003; 289(14): 1785–1791.

680 Tucker LA, et al. Television viewing and obesity in adult males. Am J Public Health 1989; 79: 516–518.

681 Tucker LA, et al. Television viewing and obesity in adult females. Am J Public Health 1991; 81: 908–911.

682 Ching PLYH, et al. Activity level and risk of overweight in male health professionals. Am J Public Health 1996; 86: 25–30.

683 Gortmaker S, et al. Television viewing as a cause of increasing obesity among children in the United States, 1986–1990. Arch Pediatr Adolesc Med 1996; 150: 356–362.

684 Anderson RE, et al. Relationship of physical activity and television watching with body weight and level of fitness among children. JAMA 1998; 279: 938–942.

685 Hernandez B, et al. Association of obesity with physical activity, television programs and other forms of video viewing among children in Mexico City. Int J Obesity 1999; 23: 845–854.

686 Ainsworth BE, et al. Compendium of physical activities. Med Sci Sports Exerc 1993; 25:

71–80.

687 Hu, FB, et al. Television watching and other sedentary behaviors in relation to the risk of obesity and type 2 diabetes mellitus in women. JAMA 2003; 289(14): 1785–1791.

688 Ching PLYH, et al. Activity level and risk of overweight in male health professionals. Am J Public Health 1996; 86: 25–30.

689 Hu, FB, et al. Television watching and other sedentary behaviors in relation to the risk of obesity and type 2 diabetes mellitus in women. JAMA 2003; 289(14): 1785–1791.

690 Falciglia GA, et al. Television commercials and eating behavior of obese and normal-weight women. J Nutr Educ 1980; 12: 196–199.

691 Wiecha JL, et al. The hidden and potent effects of television advertising. Arch Pediatr Adolesc Med 2006; 160: 436–442.

692 Kotz K et al. Food advertisements during children's Saturday morning television programming: Are they consistent with dietary recommendations? J Am Diet Assoc 1994; 94: 1296–1300.

693 Lewis MK, et al. Food advertising on British children's television: A content analysis and experimental study with nine-year-olds. Int J Obesity 1998; 22: 206–214.

694 Coon KA, et al. Relationships between use of television during meals and children's food consumption patterns. Pediatrics 2001; 107: e7.

695 Eremis S, et al. Is obesity a risk factor for psychpathology among adolescents? Pediatr Int. 2004; 46(3): 296–301.

696 Hu FB, et al. Dietary fat intake and the risk of coronary heart disease in women. N Eng J Med 1997; 337: 1491–1499.

697 Salmeron J, et al. Dietary fat intake and risk of type 2 diabetes in women. Am J Clin Nutr 2001; 73: 1019–1026.

698 Ludwig DS. The glycemic index: Physiological mechanisms relating to obesity, diabetes, and cardiovascular disease. JAMA 202; 287: 2414–2423.

699 Ludwig DS, et al. High glycemic index foods, overeating and obesity. Pediatrics 1999; 103: e26.

700 Liu S, et al. A prospective study of dietary glycemic load, carbohydrate intake and risk of coronary heart disease in women. Am J Clin Nutr 2000; 71: 1455–1461.

701 Salmeron J, et al. Dietary fiber, glycemic load, and risk of the non-insulin dependent diabetes mellitus in women. JAMA 1997; 277: 472–477.

702 Barclay AW, et al. Glycemic index, glycemic load and chronic disease risk – A meta-analysis of observational studies. Am J Clin Nutr 2008 Mar; 87(3): 627–637.

703 Dickinson S, et al. High glycemic index carbohydrates increase nuclear factor-kappa B activation in mononuclear cells of lean, healthy subjects. Am J Clin Nutr May 2008; 87(5): 1188–1193.

704 Bray GA, Bray CA. *An Atlas of Obesity and Weight Control.* Boca Raton, FL: Parthenon Publishing, 2003.

705 *UC Berkeley Wellness Letter*, Aug 2008; 24(1): 1.

706 Rayssinguier Y, et al. High fructose consumption combined with low dietary magnesium intake may increase the incidence of the metabolic syndrome by inducing inflammation. Magnes Res Dec 2006; 19(4): 237–243.

707 New findings bitter, sweet for fructose fans. *Tufts University Health and Nutrition Letter* Sept 2007; 25(7): 1.

708 Putnam JJ, Allshouse JE. Food consumption, prices, and expenditures, 1970–1997. Washington, D.C.: Food and Consumers Economics Division, Economic Research Service, US Department of Agriculture, 1999.

709 Borrud L, et al. What we eat: USDA surveys food consumption changes. Commun Nutr Inst 1997; 27: 4–5.

710 Harnack L, et al. Soft drink consumption among US children and adolescents: Nutritional

consequences. J Am Diet Assoc 1999; 99: 436–441.

711 Guthrie JF, et al. Food sources of added sweeteners in the diets of Americans. J Am Diet Assoc 2000; 100: 43–51.

712 Bowman SA. Diets of individuals based on energy intakes from added sugars. Fam Econ Nutr Rev 1999; 12: 31–38.

713 Lutsey PL, et al. Dietary intake and the development of the metabolic syndrome: The Atherosclerosis Risk in Communities Study. Circulation Feb 12, 2008; 117(6): 754–761.

714 Dhingra R, et al. Soft drink consumption and risk of developing cardiometabolic risk factors and the metabolic syndrome in middle-aged adults in the community. Circulation 2007; 116: 480–488.

715 Lawton CL, et al. A medium-term intervention study on the impact of high- and low-fat snacks varying in sweeteners and fat content: Large shifts in daily fat intake, but good compensation for daily energy intake. Br J Nutr 1998; 80: 149–161.

716 Birch LL, et al. Children's food intake following drinks sweetened with sucrose or aspartame: Time course of effect. Physiol Behav 1989; 45: 387–395.

717 Anderson GH, et al. Aspartame: Effect on lunch-time food intake, appetite and hedonistic response in children. Appetite 1989; 13: 93–103.

718 Raben A, et al. Sucrose compared with artificial sweeteners: Different effects on ad libitum food intake and body weight after 10 weeks of supplementation in overweight subjects. Am J Clin Nutr 2002; 76: 721–729.

719 Blundell JE, et al. Paradoxical effects of an intense sweetener (aspartame) on appetite. Lancet 1986; 1: 1092–1093.

720 Rogers PJ, et al. Separating the actions of sweeteners and calories: Effects of saccharin and carbohydrates on hunger and food intake on human subjects. Physiol Behav 1989; 45: 1093–1099.

721 Tordoff MG, et al. Oral stimulation with aspartame increases hunger. Physiol Behav 1990; 47: 555–559.

722 Beridot-Therond ME, et al. Short-term effects of the flavor of drinks on ingestive behaviors in man. Appetite 1998; 31: 67–81.

723 Lavin JH, et al. The effects of sucrose- and aspartame-sweetened drinks on energy intake, hunger, and food choice of female, slightly restrained eaters. Int J Obes Relat Metab Disord 1997; 21: 37–42.

724 Teschemacher H. Opioid receptor ligands derived from food proteins. Curr Pharm Des 2003; 9(16): 1331–1344.

725 Kitts DD, et al. Bioactive proteins and peptides from food sources. Applications of bioprocesses used in isolation and recovery. Curr Pharm Des 2003; 9(16): 1309–1323.

726 Lin L, et al. Beta-casomorphins stimulate and enterostatin inhibits the intake of dietary fats in rats. Peptides 1998; 19(2): 325–331.

727 Schusdziarra V, et al. Effect of beta-casomorphins and analogs on insulin release in dogs. Endocrinology 1983; 112: 885–889.

728 Block G. Foods contributing to energy intake in the US: Data from NHANES III and NHANES 1999–2000. J of Food Comp and Anal 2004; 17: 439–447.

729 National Center for Health Statistics, 1994. Plan and Operation of the Third National Health and Nutrition Examination Survey, 1998–94. Vital Health Stat I (32). Hyattsville, MD: U.S. Department of Health and Human Services. DHHS Publication No. (PHS) 94–1308.

730 National Center for Health Statistics, 2002. NHANES 1999–2000 Public Data Release File Documentation. Available at: www.cdc.gov/nchs/data/nhanes/gendoc.pdf.

731 J Pediatr 2001; 138(4): 493–498.

732 USA Today, July 24, 2000. Reporting a study released that day by the Archives of Diseases in Childhood.

733 Marmonier C, et al. Snacks consumed in a non-hungry state have poor satiating efficiency:

Influence of snack composition on substrate utilization and hunger. Am J Clin Nutr 2002; 76: 518–528.

734 Goris AHC, et al. Under-eating and under-recording of habitual food intake in obese men: Selective underreporting of fat intake. Am J Clin Nutr 2000; 71: 130–134.

735 *Family Practice News*, Feb 11, 2006.

736 McNutt SW, et al. A longitudinal study of the dietary practices of black and white girls nine and 10 years old at enrollment: The NHLBI Growth and Health Study. J Adolesc Health 1997; 20: 27–37.

737 Zoumas-Morse C, et al. Children's pattern of macronutrient intake and associations with restaurant and home eating. J Am Diet Assoc 2001; 101: 923–925.

738 Franklin BA. The downside of our technological revolution? An obesity conducive environment. Am J of Card 2001; 87: 1093–1095.

739 Mozaffarian D, et al. Trans fatty acids and cardiovascular disease. NEJM April 13, 2006; 354(15): 1601–1613.

740 Master-Harte LD, et al. Sucrose analgesia for minor procedures in newborn infants. Ann Pharmacother 2001; 35: 947–52.

741 Max M, et al. Tas1r3, encoding a new candidate taste receptor, is allelic to the sweet responsiveness locus, Sac. Nat Genet 2001; 28: 58–63.

742 Gangwisch JE, et al. Inadequate sleep as a risk factor for obesity: Analysis of NHANES 1. Sleep 2005; 28: 1289–1296.

743 Williamson DF, et al. Am J Epidemiol 1995; 141: 1128–1141.

744 Allison DB, et al. Weight loss increases and fat loss decreases all-cause mortality rate: Results from two independent cohort studies. Int J Obes Relat Metab Disord 1999; 23: 603–611.

745 Williamson DF, et al. Intentional weight loss and mortality among overweight individuals with diabetes. Diabetes Care 2000; 23: 1499–1504.

746 Oster G, et al. Lifetime health and economic benefits of weight-loss among obese persons. Am J Public Health 1999; 89: 1536–1542.

747 Diabetes prevention Program Research Group. Reduction in the incidence of type 2 diabetes with lifestyle intervention or metformin. N Engl J Med 2002; 346: 393–403.

748 Esposito K, et al. Effects of weight-loss and lifestyle changes on vascular inflammatory markers in obese women. JAMA 2003; 289: 1799–1804.

749 Davi G, et al. Platelet activation in obese women. JAMA 2002; 288: 208–2014.

750 Lean MEJ, et al. Obesity, weight loss and prognosis in type II diabetes. Diabetes Med 1990; 7(3): 228–233.

751 American Gastroenterology Association medical position statement on obesity. Gastroenterology 2002; 123: 879–881.

752 Mikhail N, et al. Obesity and hypertension, Progress in Cardiovascular Diseases. 1999; 42(1): 39–58.

753 www.who.int/topics/diabetes_mellitus/en. Accessed Jan 22, 2008.

754 www.who.int/mediacentre/factsheets/fs312/en/index.html. Accessed Jan 19, 2008.

755 www.who.int/diabetes/actionnow/en/mapdiabprev.pdf. Accessed Jan 19, 2008.

756 www.who.int/diabetes/facts/world_figures/en/index5.html.

757 Saydah SH, et al. Poor control of risk factors for vascular disease among adults with previously undiagnosed diabetes. JAMA 2004; 291: 335–342.

758 Rosenbloom AL, et al. Emerging epidemic of type 2 diabetes in youth. Diabetes Care Feb 1999; 22(2): 345–354.

759 Diabetes and Obesity: Time to Act, International Diabetes Federation-International Association for the Study of Obesity 2004.

760 ADA Economic costs of diabetes in the US in 2002. Diabetes Care 2003; 26: 917–932.

761 Tuomilehto J, et al. Prevention of type 2 diabetes mellitus by changes in lifestyle among subjects with impaired glucose tolerance. NEJM 2001; 344(18): 1343–1350.

762 Reaven G. Banting Lecture 1988. Role of insulin resistance in human disease. Diabetes 1988; 37: 1595–1607.

763 Avogaro P, et al. Acta Diabetol Lat 1967; 4: 36–41; Haller H. Epidemiology and associated risk factors of hyperlipoproteinemia. Z Gesante Inn Med 1977; 32: 124–128.

764 DOC News. New ADA initiative moves beyond metabolic syndrome. www.diabetes.org/doc-news. Accessed July 2006.

765 Ibid.

766 Meigs JB, et al. Risk variable clustering in the insulin resistance syndrome. The Framingham Offspring Study Diabetes 1997; 46: 1594–1600.

767 Hanley AJ, et al. Factor analysis of metabolic syndrome using directly measured insulin sensitivity: The Insulin Resistance Atherosclerosis Study Diabetes 2002; 51: 2642–2647.

768 Laukkanen JA, et al. Metabolic syndrome and the risk of prostate cancer in Finnish men: A population-based study. Cancer Epidemiol Biomarkers Prev Oct 2004; 13(10): 1646–1650.

769 Gooktas S, et al. Prostate cancer and adiponectin. Urology Jun 2005; 65(6): 1168–1172.

770 Bugianesi E. Review article: Steatosis, the metabolic syndrome and cancer. Aliment Pharmacol Ther Nov 2005; 22 Suppl 2: 40–43.

771 Soliman PT, et al. Association between adiponectin, insulin resistance and endometrial cancer. Cancer Jun 1, 2006; 106(11): 2376–2381.

772 Morita T, et al. The metabolic syndrome is associated with increased risk of colorectal adenoma development: The Self-Defense Forces health study. Asian Pac J Cancer Prev Oct–Dec 2005; 6(4): 485–459.

773 Lipscombe LL, et al. Diabetes mellitus and breast cancer: A retrospective population-based cohort study. Breast Cancer Res Treat Aug 2006; 98(3): 349–356.

774 Stolzenberg-Solomon RZ, et al. Insulin, glucose insulin resistance and pancreatic cancer in male smokers. JAMA 2005; 294: 2872–2878.

775 Expert Panel on Detection, Evaluation, and Treatment of High Blood Cholesterol in Adults JAMA 2001; 285: 2486–2497.

776 Definition, Diagnosis and Classification of Diabetes Mellitus and Its Complications, Report of a WHO Consultation. Geneva, Switzerland: Department of Noncommunicable Disease Surveillance, World Health Organization; 1999.

777 Grundy SM, et al. Diagnosis and management of the metabolic syndrome: An American Heart Association/National Heart, Lung and Blood Institute Scientific statement. Circulation. 2005; 112: 2735–2752.

778 Alberti KG, et al. The metabolic syndrome – A new worldwide definition. Lancet 2005; 366: 1059–1062.

779 Festa A, et al. Chronic subclinical inflammation as part of the insulin resistance syndrome: The Insulin Resistance Atherosclerosis Study. (IRAS) Circulation 2000; 102: 42–47.

780 Howard G, et al. Ability of alternative indices of insulin sensitivity to predict cardiovascular risk: Comparison with the "minimal model" Insulin Resistance Atherosclerosis Study (IRAS) Investigators Ann Epidemiol 1998; 8: 358–369.

781 Hanley AJ, et al. Homeostasis model assessment of insulin resistance in relation to the incidence of cardiovascular disease: The San Antonio Heart Studies. Diabetes Care 2002; 25: 1177–1184.

782 Hanley AJ, et al. Factor analysis of metabolic syndrome using directly measured insulin sensitivity: The Insulin Resistance Atherosclerosis Study. Diabetes 2002; 51: 2642–2647.

783 Chu JW, et al. Glycoprotein abnormalities associated with insulin resistance in healthy volunteers identified by the Vertical Auto Profile-II Methodology. Clin Chem 2003; 49(6): 1014–1017.

784 Ford ES, et al. Prevalence of the metabolic syndrome among US adults: Findings from the third National Health and Nutrition Examination Survey. JAMA 2002; 287: 356–359.

785 Dresner A, et al. Effects of free fatty acids on glucose transport and IRS-1-associated phos-

phatidylinositol 3-kinase activity. J Clin Invest 1999; 103: 253–259.

786 Song Y, et al. a prospective study of red meat consumption and type 2 diabetes in middle-aged and elderly women: The women's health study. Diabetes Care 2004 Sep; 27(9): 2108–2115.

787 Van Dam RM, et al. Dietary fat and meat intake in relation to risk of type 2 diabetes in men. Diabetes Care Mar 2002; 25(3): 417–424.

788 Tuomilehto J, et al. Prevention of type II diabetes mellitus by changes in lifestyle among subjects with impaired glucose tolerance. NEJM 2001; 344(18): 1343–1350.

789 Hamman RF Genetic and environmental determinants of non-insulin dependant diabetes mellitus. (NIDDM) Diabetes Metab Rev 1992; 8: 287–338.

790 Ishizaka N, et al. Association between cigarette smoking, metabolic syndrome, and carotid atherosclerosis in Japanese individuals. Atherosclerosis Aug 2005; 181(2): 381–388.

791 Yoo S, et al. Comparison of dietary intakes associated with metabolic syndrome risk factors in young adults: The Bogalusa Heart Study. Am J Clin Nutr Oct 2004; 80(4): 841–848.

792 Kang ES, et al. Relationship of serum high sensitivity C-reactive protein to metabolic syndrome and microvascular complications in type 2 diabetes. Diab Res Clin Pract Aug 2005; 69(2): 151–159.

793 Choi HK, et al. Gout and the risk of type 2 diabetes among men with high cardiovascular profile. Rheumatology (Oxford) Aug 18, 2008 [Epub ahead of print].

794 Shoelson SE, et al. Inflammation and insulin resistance. J Clin Invest 2006; 116: 1793–1801.

795 Pradham AD, et al. C-reactive protein is independently associated with fasting insulin in non-diabetic women. Arterioscler Thromb Vasc Biol 2003; 23: 650–655.

796 Festa A, et al. Chronic subclinical inflammation as part of the insulin resistance syndrome: The Insulin Resistance Atherosclerosis Study. (IRAS) Circulation 2000; 102: 42–47.

797 Festa A, et al. Elevated levels of acute-phase proteins and plasminogen activator inhibitor-1 predict the development of type 2 diabetes: The insulin resistance atherosclerosis study. Diabetes 2002; 51: 1131–1137.

798 Lutsey PL, et al. Dietary intake and the development of the metabolic syndrome: The Atherosclerosis Risk in Community Study. Circulation Feb 12, 2008; 117(6): 754–761.

799 Diamant M, et al. The association between abdominal visceral fat and carotid stiffness in mediated by circulating inflammatory markers in uncomplicated type 2 diabetes. J Clin Edocrinol Metab 2005; 90: 1495–1501.

800 Van Dam RM, et al. Dietary fat and meat intake in relation to risk of type 2 diabetes in men. Diabetes Care 2002; 25(3): 417–424.

801 Schulze MB, et al. Processed meat intake and incidence of Type 2 diabetes in younger and middle-aged women. Diabetologia 2003; 46(11): 1465–1473.

802 Song Y, et al. A prospective study of red meat consumption and type 2 diabetes in middle-aged and elderly women: The women's health study. Diabetes Care Sep 2004; 27(9): 2108–2115.

803 Van Dam RM, et al. Dietary fat and meat intake in relation to risk of type 2 diabetes in men. Diabetes Care Mar 2002; 25(3): 417–424.

804 Elliott SS, et al. Fructose, weight gain, and the insulin resistance syndrome. Am J Clin Nutr 2002; 76(5): 911–922.

805 Miller A, et al. Dietary fructose and the metabolic syndrome. Curr Opin Gastroenterol Mar 2008; 24(2): 204–209.

806 Rayssiguier Y, et al. High fructose consumption combined with low dietary magnesium intake may increase the incidence of metabolic syndrome by inducing inflammation. Magnès Res Dec 2006; 19(4): 237–343.

807 Wolever TM, et al. Long-term effect of varying the source or amount of dietary carbohydrate on postprandial plasma glucose, insulin, triacylglycerol, and free fatty acid concentrations in subjects with impaired glucose tolerance. Am J Clin Nutr 2003; 77(3): 612–621.

808 Kondo N, et al. Association of inflammatory marker and highly sensitive C-reactive protein with aerobic exercise capacity, maximum oxygen uptake and insulin resistance in healthy

middle-aged volunteers. Circ J. Apr 2005; 69(4): 452–457.

809 LaMonte MJ, et al. Cardiorespiratory fitness is inversely associated with the incidence of metabolic syndrome. Circulation 2005; 112: 505–512.

810 Reaven GM. The insulin resistance syndrome: Definition and dietary approaches to treatment. Annu Rev Nutr 2005; 25: 391–406.

811 Diabetes 2005; 54: 603–608.

812 Tsiara S, et al. Influence of smoking on predictors of vascular disease. Angiology 2003; 54(5): 507–530.

813 Storlien LH, et al. Fatty acids, triglycerides and syndromes of insulin resistance. Prostaglandins Leukot Essen Fatty Acids Oct 1997; 57(4–5): 379–385.

814 Waite N, et al. The impact of fish-oil supplements on insulin sensitivity. J Hum Nutr Diet Jul 2008; 21(4): 402–403.

815 Anderson RA. Chromium in the prevention and control of diabetes. Diabetes Metab Feb 2000; 26(1): 22–27.

816 Liese AD, et al. Whole-grain intake and insulin sensitivity: The Insulin Resistance Atherosclerosis Study. Am J Clin Nutr Nov 2003; 78(5): 965–971.

817 Kang ES, et al. Relationship of serum high sensitivity C-reactive protein to metabolic syndrome and microvascular complications in type 2 diabetes. Diab Res Clin Pract Aug 2005; 69(2): 151–159.

818 Ludwig DS, et al. Dietary fiber, weight gain, and cardiovascular disease risk in young adults. JAMA Oct 27, 1999; 282(16): 1539–1546.

819 Diabetes Care 2006; 29: 775–780.

820 Ludwig DS. Diet and development of the insulin resistance syndrome. Asia Pac J Clin Nutr 2003; 12 Suppl: S4.

821 Kuo CS, et al. Insulin sensitivity in Chinese ovo-lacto vegetarians compared with omnivores. Eur J Clin Nutr Feb 2004; 58(2): 312–316.

822 Teegarden D. Calcium intake and reduction in weight or fat mass. J Nutr Jan 2003; 133(1): 249S–251S.

823 Pereira MA, et al. Dairy consumption, obesity, and the insulin resistance syndrome in young adults: The CARDIA Study. JAMA Apr 2002; 287(16): 2081–2089.

824 Liu S, et al. A prospective study of dairy intake and the risk of type 2 diabetes in women. Diabetes Care Jul 2006; 29(7): 1579–1584.

825 Colli JL, et al. International comparisons of prostate cancer mortality rates with dietary practices and sunlight levels. Urol Oncol. May–Jun 2006; 24(3): 184–194.

826 Colli JL, et al. Comparisons of prostate cancer mortality rates with dietary practices in the United States. Urol Oncol. Nov–Dec 2005; 23(6): 390–398.

827 Gallus S, et al. Milk, dairy products and cancer risk (Italy). Cancer Causes Control. May 2006; 17(4): 429–437.

828 Cho E, et al. Dairy foods, calcium, and colorectal cancer: A pooled analysis of 10 cohort studies. J Natl Cancer Inst Jul 7, 2004; 96(13): 1015–1022.

829 Shin MH, et al. Intake of dairy products, calcium, and vitamin D and risk of breast cancer. J Natl Cancer Inst Sep 4, 2002; 94(17): 1301–1311.

830 Tsuda H, et al. Milk components as cancer chemoprotective agents. Asian Pac J Cancer Prev 2000; 1(4): 277–282.

831 Lopez-Ridaura R, et al. Magnesium intake and risk of type 2 diabetes in men and women. Diabetes Care Jan 2004 ; 27(1): 134–140.

832 He K, et al. Magnesium intake and incidence of metabolic syndrome among young adults. Circulation 2006; 113: 1675–1682.

833 Van Dam RM, et al. Coffee consumption and risk of type II diabetes: A systematic review. JAMA Jul 6, 2005; 294(1): 97–104.

834 Wu T, et al. Caffeinated coffee, decaffeinated coffee, and caffeine in relation to plasma C-pep-

tide levels, a marker of insulin secretion, in US women. Diabetes Care. Jun 2005; 28(6): 1390–1396.

835 Farnsworth E, et al. Effect of a high-protein, energy-restricted diet on body composition, glycemic control, and lipid concentrations in overweight and obese hyperinsulinemic men and women. Am J Clin Nutr Jul 2003; 78(1): 31–39.

836 Khan A, et al. Cinnamon improves glucose and lipids of people with type 2 diabetes. Diabetes Care Dec 2003; 26(12): 3215–3218.

837 Mattila C, et al. Serum 25-hydroxyvitamin D concentration and subsequent risk of type 2 diabetes. Diabetes Care 2007; 30: 2569–2570.

838 Pittas A, et al. Vitamin D and calcium intake in relation to type 2 diabetes risk in women. Diabetes Care 2006; 29: 650–656.

839 Pittas AG, et al. The effects of calcium and vitamin D supplementation on blood glucose and markers of inflammation in non-diabetic adults. Diabetes Care Jul 2007; 30(7): e81.

840 Van Cauter E, et al. Roles of circadian rhythmicity and sleep in human glucose regulation. Endocrinology Review 1997; 18: 716–738.

841 Lutsey PL, et al. Dietary intake and the development of the metabolic syndrome: The Atherosclerosis Risk in Community Study. Circulation Feb 12, 2008; 117(6): 754–761.

842 Dhingra R, et al. Soft drink consumption and risk of developing cardiometabolic risk factors and the metabolic syndrome in middle-aged adults in the community. Circulation 2007; 116: 480–488.

843 Tsimikas S, et al. Oxidized phospholipids, Lp(a) lipoprotein, and coronary artery disease. NEJM July 7, 2005; 353(1): 46–57.

844 Von Eckardstein A, et al. Lipoprotein (a) further increases the risk of coronary events in men with high global cardiovascular risk. J Am Coll Card 2001; 37(2): 434–439.

845 Griffen BA, et al. Role of plasma triglycerides in the regulation of plasma low density lipoprotein (LDL) subfractions: Relative contribution of small, dense LDL to coronary heart disease risk. Atherosclerosis 1994; 106(2): 241–253.

846 Hodis HN. Triglyceride rich lipoprotein remnant particles and risk of atherosclerosis. Circulation 1999; 99: 2852–2854.

847 Camppos H, et al. Predominance of large LDL and reduced HDL-2 cholesterol in normolipemic men with cholesterol artery disease. Arterioscler Thromb Vasc Biol 1995; 15(8): 1043–1048.

848 American Diabetes Association. Economic consequences of diabetes mellitus in the US in 1997. Diabetes Care 1998; 21: 296–309.

849 American Medical News, March 16, 1998.

850 USA Today, May 1, 2002: 5D.

851 USA Today, October 24 2002: 2D.

852 USA Today, May 14 2003.

853 www.mdnetguide.com. Accessed March 2002.

854 Anderson JW, et al. Health advantages and disadvantages of weight reducing diets: A computer analysis and critical review. J Am Coll Nutr 2000; 19: 578–590.

855 Klem ML, et al. A descriptive study of individuals successful at long-term maintenance of substantial weight loss. Am J Clin Nutr 1997; 66: 239–246.(Taken from the American College of Sports Medicine Position Stand. Appropriate strategies for weight loss and prevention of weight regain for adults. Med Sci Sprts Exerc 2001; 33: 2145–2156.)

856 Dansinger ML. Comparison of the Adkins, Ornish, Weight Watchers and Zone diets for weight loss and heart disease risk reduction. JAMA 2005; 293: 43–53.

857 Dietary references intakes for energy, carbohydrate, fiber, fat, fatty acids, cholesterol, protein, and amino acids. Institute of Medicine of the National Academies. The National Academy Press. Washington, D.C.

858 Gaby AR. Adverse effects of dietary fructose. Alt Med Rev 2005 Dec; 10(4): 294–306.

859 Rayssiguier Y, et al. High fructose consumption combined with low dietary magnesium intake may increase the incidence of metabolic syndrome by inducing inflammation. Magnes Res 2006 Dec; 19(4): 237–43.

860 *UC Berkeley Wellness Letter* 2008 Aug; 24(11): 1.

861 New findings bitter sweet for fructose fans. Tufts Univ Health and Nutrition Letter 2007 Sept; 25(7): 1.

862 Nunes AP, et al. Analysis of genotypic potentiality of stevoside by comet assay. Food Chem Toxicol 2007 Apr; 45(4): 662–6.

863 *USA Today*, April 22, 2008.

864 www.MyPyramid.gov.

865 Jenkins D, et al. Glycemic index of foods: A physiologic basis for carbohydrate exchange. Am J Clin Nutr 1981; 34: 362–366.

866 FAO/WHO Expert consultation. Carbohydrates in human nutrition: Report of a joint FAO/WHO expert consultation, Rome, April 14–18, 1997. Rome: Food and Agriculture Organization, 1998. (FAO Food and Nutrition paper 66).

867 Liu S, et al. A prospective study of dietary glycemic load, carbohydrate intake and the risk of coronary heart disease in women. Am J Clin Nutr 2000; 71: 1455–1461.

868 Salmeron J, et al. Dietary fiber, glycemic load, and the risk of NIDDM in men. Diabetes Care 1997; 20: 545–550.

869 Ludwig D. Dietary glycemic index and obesity. J Nutr 2000; 130: 280S–283S.

870 Franceschi S, et al. Dietary glycemic load and colorectal cancer risk. Ann Oncol 2001; 12: 173–178.

871 Augustin LS. Dietary glycemic index and glycemic load in breast cancer risk: A case control study. Ann Oncol Nov 2001; 12(11): 1533–1538.

872 Augustin LS, et al. Dietary glycemic index, glycemic load and ovarian cancer risk: A case-control study in Italy. Ann Oncol Jan 2003; 14(1): 78–84.

873 Augustin LS, et al. Glycemic index, glycemic load and risk of gastric cancer. Ann Oncol Apr 2004; 15(4): 581–584.

874 Dickson S, et al. High glycemic index carbohydrates increase nuclear factor-kappaB activation in mononuclear cells of young, lean healthy subjects. Am J Clin Nutr May 2008; 87(5): 1188–1193.

875 Foster-Powell K, et al. International table of glycemic index and glycemic load values: 2002. Am J Clin Nutr 2002; 76: 5–56.

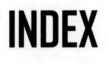

INDEX

About the Author

D r. Duke Johnson has dedicated more than twenty years of his life to stopping the epidemic spread of chronic diseases around the world. He is an expert on the different medical traditions practiced globally and on the state of world health, with patients living in more than thirty different countries. His preventive health teaching regularly reaches more than 3 million people in fifty-five countries.

Dr. Johnson is Medical Director of the 30,000-square-foot, $14 million Nutrilite Health Institute Center for Optimal Health in Southern California and is a highly requested lecturer, having spoken to more than one hundred thousand people in thirty different countries on five continents. He has significant media experience with articles in many well-respected magazines and many large international newspapers.